Review of Hemodialysis fc Nurses and Dialysis Personnel

D0878211

Sixth Edition

C.F. Gutch, MD, FACP

Professor Emeritus, Department of Internal Medicine
University of South Dakota School of Medicine
Sioux Falls, South Dakota

Martha H. Stoner, RN, PhD

Associate Professor, School of Nursing
University of Colorado Health Sciences Center
Denver, Colorado

Anna L. Corea, RN, MN, CNAA

Quality Management Projects Specialist
Total Renal Care, Inc.
Torrance, California
and
Assistant Clinical Professor
School of Nursing
University of California–Los Angeles
Los Angeles, California

Ⅶ Mosby

St. Louis Baltimore Boston Carlsbad
Chicago Minneapolis New York Philadelphia Portland
London Milan Sydney Tokyo Toronto

Mosby
Dedicated to Publishing Excellence

Editor-in-Chief, Nursing: Sally Schrefer
Editor-in-Chief, Nursing Databases: Darlene Como
Developmental Editor: Barbara Watts
Project Manager: Gayle Morris

Printed in the United States of America
Composition by Wordbench
Printing by Plus Communications

Mosby, Inc.
11830 Westline Industrial Drive
St. Louis, Missouri 63146

International Standard Book Number 0-8151-2099-0

99 00 01 02 / 9 8 7 6 5 4 3 2 1

Contributors

Kathy Bender, RN, BSN, CNN
Clinical Support Specialist
Amgen
Thousand Oaks, California

Lowanna S. Binkley, RN, MA, CNN
Manager, Professional Services
Amgen
Thousand Oaks, California

Christopher R. Blagg, MD, FRCP
Executive Director
Northwest Kidney Centers
Professor of Medicine
University of Washington
Seattle, Washington

Eileen D. Brewer, MD
Chief, Renal Section
Department of Pediatrics
Baylor College of Medicine
Medical Director, Renal Dialysis
Texas Children's Hospital
Houston, Texas

Linda S. Christensen, RN, CNN
Staff Nurse, Acute Dialysis Program
University of California–Los Angeles
Los Angeles, California

Kenneth E. Cotton, MA, MBA, MPA
Assistant Professor of Health Care Management
Metropolitan State College of Denver
Denver, Colorado

Helen Currier, RN, CNN
Assistant Director, Renal Dialysis
Texas Children's Hospital
Houston, Texas

Jim Curtis, CHT, CNCT
Area Administrator
FMC Dialysis Services West – NW Area
Portland, Oregon

Lesley C. Dinwiddie, RN, MSN, FNP, CNN
Clinical Instructor
Nephrology Division, Dept. Of Medicine
University of North Carolina
Chapel Hill, North Carolina

Ronald Emerson, AD, CHT
Dialysis Technician
Total Renal Care, Inc.
University of California–Los Angeles
Los Angeles, California

Nancy Gallagher, RN, BS, CNN
St. Joseph Medical Center, FHS-W
Director, Regional Nephrology Services
Tacoma, Washington
President, Nephrology Nurses Certification Board, 1997-1998
Pitman, New Jersey

Peter W. Gardner
Former Research Technician
VA Medical Center, West Los Angeles
Los Angeles, California

Susan K. Hansen, RN, MBA, CNN
Clinical Marketing Manager, Hemodialysis Business
Renal Division
Baxter Healthcare
Lake Forest, California

Mara Hersh-Rifkin, MSW, LCSW
University of California–Los Angeles
Health Network
Los Angeles, California

Margaret S. Holloway, RN, MN
Administrator, Pediatric and Home Dialysis
Total Renal Care, Inc.
University of California–Los Angeles
Los Angeles, California

Martin V. Hudson, CNBT
Chairperson
National Nephrology Certification Organization
New York, New York

Kathy Laws, RN, BS, CNN
Area Administrator
Total Renal Care, Inc.
San Diego, California

Mary M. Macaluso, RN, BSN, CPDN, CNN
Nephrology Nurse Specialist
Spectra Renal Management Division of Fresenius Medical Care
Conyers, Georgia

Gwen Elise McNatt, RN, MS, CNN, CFNP
Transplant Nurse Practitioner
Organ Transplant Center
Northwestern Memorial Hospital
Adjunct Clinical Instructor
College of Nursing
University of Illinois at Chicago
Chicago, Illinois

Allen R. Nissenson, MD, FACP
Professor of Medicine
Director, Dialysis Program
University of California–Los Angeles
Los Angeles, California

Patt Peterson, RN
Manager, Professional Services
Medisystems Corporation
Seattle, Washington

Eileen Peacock, RN, MSN, CNN, CIC, CPHQ
Director of Integrated Quality Development
Total Renal Care, Inc.
Berwyn, Pennsylvania

Ginnette Pepper, RN, PhD
Assistant Professor
School of Nursing
University of Colorado Health Science Center
Denver, Colorado

Christy A. Price, RN, MSN
Nephrology Clinical Specialist
Independent Nurse Consultant
Salt Lake City, Utah

Georgina Randolph, RN, MSN, MBA, CNN
Divisional Vice President
Total Renal Care, Inc.
San Diego, California

Karen Robbins, RN, MS, CNN
Educator/Manager Hartford Dialysis Unit
Hartford Hospital
Hartford, Connecticut

Mark Rolston, CHT
Renal Care Group
Nashville, Tennessee

Karen Schardin, RN, BSN, CNN
Administrator
Dialysis Clinic, Inc.
Carson City, Nevada

Sandra Smolka-Hill, RN, MSN, CNN
Administration, Acute Unit
Total Renal Care, Inc.
University of California–Los Angeles
Los Angeles, California

Julia Walsh Starr, RN, MSN
Staff Nurse, Acute Unit
Total Renal Care, Inc.
University of California–Los Angeles
Los Angeles, California

Beverly Wells Storck, RN, BSN
Nurse Manager
University of North Carolina
Chapel Hill, North Carolina

Jo Anne E. Strutz, RN
Former Assistant Nurse Manager
Dialysis Program
University of California–Los Angeles Medical Center
Los Angeles, California

Cedric Tuck-Sherman, MBA
Vice President, Business Development
Velos Medical Informatics
New York, New York

Philip M. Varughese, BS, CHT
Dialysis Technical Manager
Mt. Sinai Hospital Medical Center
New York, New York
President
National Association of Nephrology Technicians/Technologists, 1997-1998
Dayton, Ohio

Susan C. Vogel, RN, MHA, CNN
Administrator
South Valley Regional Dialysis Center
Encino, California

Susan E. Weil, RD, CS
Renal Dietitian Specialist
Dialysis and Kidney Transplant Programs
University of California–Los Angeles
Health Network
Los Angeles, California

Mary Ann Wierszbiczki, RN, MN
Nephrology Clinical Nurse Specialist
Irvine Renal Dialysis
University of California–Irvine
Orange, California

Gail S. Wick, BNS, RN, CNN
Vice President
Clinical Quality Programs
Fresenius Medical Care North America
Lexington, Massachusetts

Reviewers

Lowana S. Binkley, RN, MA, CNN
Manager, Professional Services
Amgen
Thousand Oaks, California

Annie W. Tu, RN, MSN, CNN
Renal Clinical Nurse Specialist
University of Washington Medical Center
Seattle, Washington

Curtis A. Johnson, Pharm D
Professor, Pharmacy and Medicine
University of Wisconsin-Madison
Center for Health Science
Madison, Wisconsin

Foreword

The opportunity to write this foreword for the sixth edition has provided a time for reflection on my involvement with the end stage renal disease population. I entered the field of dialysis in 1972, just prior to the passage of the Medicare funding for dialytic therapy. Passage of HR 1 was a time of joy and overwhelming relief. It was no longer necessary for committees to choose who would receive treatment while others were destined to succumb to renal failure. The days of the "GOD Squads" were over. At this time the focus of our care was technical and the gold standard for staff orientation and clinical reference material was *Review of Hemodialysis for Nurses and Dialysis Personnel* by Gutch and Stoner. It was the dialysis bible.

Beginning in 1973, the number and acuity of people receiving dialysis increased markedly and required an increased number and classification of personnel to care for the ESRD population. This was a busy and exciting time to be involved in nephrology nursing.

Throughout these 25 years the technological advances have been remarkable and have increased our ability to provide efficient dialytic therapy. We have seen the advent of volumetric machines, high-efficiency and high-flux dialyzers, and computerization. We have changed our focus from technical excellence to quality care, adequacy of treatment and patient outcomes. Our language has changed to reflect the technological advances. We now speak of adequacy of treatment reflected in Kt/V or URR. We have protocols to manage anemia with erythropoietin and intravenous iron and calcium/phosporous balance with calcijex.

We have grown from a "mom and pop" operation to a corporate giant. We have lost some of our homespun family milieu and have become more business-like in our approach. We provide a better product to serve the masses, but have sacrificed some of the gentler, more comfortable milieu.

We have changed with the times, and the care we provide patients has changed accordingly. Multidisciplinary teams provide holistic care and care across a continuum of modality changes and the lifespan. The population served spans the age continuum from pediatrics to geriatrics. The cumulative research and best practice models have come to fruition in the DOQI guidelines that will guide our practice in the future.

Advances in peritoneal dialysis and the advent of newer, more effective immunosuppressive agents for transplantation have increased the success of those treatment modalities. Patients now have three successful treatment options.

As the numbers of people with ESRD who are receiving dialysis continue to grow, so does the need for qualified dialysis personnel to provide high-quality and cost-effective care. This latest edition of *Review of Hemodialysis for Nurses and Dialysis Personnel* will no doubt continue to be a resource for orienting new employees and for ongoing learning for all dialysis personnel.

In keeping with our changing times and fast-paced information highway, this newest edition of *Review of Hemodialysis for Nurses and Dialysis Personnel* has several new chapters. Reflections of our expanding population are seen in the chapters on pediatrics, geriatrics, diabetes, and transplantation. In addition, the chapter on computers and new technology will help project the "baby boomers" into cyberspace.

I would like to congratulate Dr. Gutch, Dr. Stoner and Ms. Corea on providing the nephrology community with another classic reference to aid our efforts in providing care along the continuum for patients with ESRD. Thank you for this unique and important contribution to our never-ending quest for knowledge.

Pat Weiskittel RN, MSN, CNN, CS
President-elect
American Nephrology Nurses Association
1998

Foreword to the First Edition

This book is written in a different way from most books. It poses questions and then answers those questions with the aim of giving a good understanding of the basic principles, basic diseases, and basic problems in the treatment of kidney patients by dialysis. I found it a great pleasure to read. I believe the book will be very useful, since we all tend to forget such basic information. We take for granted words that are used each day; yet if we study their derivation, their origin, and their deeper meaning, we cannot fail to obtain a better understanding of the processes with which we are involved.

It is an honor and a pleasure to wish this book by Dr. C. F. Gutch and nurse M. H. Stoner much success. May it become the dictionary for both the dialyzer and the dialyzed.

W. J. Kolff, MD, PhD

Professor of Surgery and Research
Professor of Engineering
Head, Division of Artificial Organs
and Director, Institute for
Biomedical Engineering
University of Utah,
Salt Lake City, Utah
1971

To our patients
each of whom in his or her own way has
contributed to the further development of dialysis
and the treatment of kidney failure

Preface

The first edition of this *Review* stated as its objective, "to bring to nurses, technicians, and patients—either already involved in or first entering dialysis—a general background, some basic principles, and a broad overview of dialysis and its application." The objective is continued in Edition 6.

The number of contributors has increased, bringing new expertise and a broad background of experience to the text. Several new chapters and much new material have been added. The original question and answer format is retained.

Our gratitude is expressed to the contributors, who tolerated delays, confusion and change with patience. Many friends, colleagues, patients, manufacturers, vendors and others provided help and encouragement; our sincere thanks go to each of them. Particular thanks to Lo Binkley and Anna Tu for their critical global reviews and Curtis Johnson for his expert review of Chapter 12. Appreciation is expressed to several Mosby developmental editors who, during times of turmoil, worked to bring the manuscript forward. Special thanks to Barbara Watts, who successfully brought it to fruition.

Contents

14 COMPLICATIONS OF CHRONIC DIALYSIS THERAPY, 192

15 TRANSPLANTATION, 213

16 PERITONEAL DIALYSIS AND HOME DIALYSIS THERAPIES, 230

17 DIABETES AND HEMODIALYSIS, 254

18 INFECTION CONTROL AND UNIVERSAL PRECAUTIONS, 264

19 PSYCHOSOCIAL ASPECTS OF DIALYSIS THERAPY, 279

20 PEDIATRIC HEMODIALYSIS, 288

21 ESRD IN THE ELDERLY, 300

22 MANAGEMENT OF QUALITY IN DIALYSIS CARE, 307

23 RENAL CARE AND INFORMATION TECHNOLOGY, 312

REFERENCES AND RECOMMENDED READINGS, 321

NEPHROLOGY ORGANIZATIONS AND RESOURCES, 329

GLOSSARY, 345

INDEX, 359

The Hemodialysis Team

Martha H. Stoner

Dialysis, the process of cleansing the blood of accumulated waste products, is a complex treatment requiring a team of highly trained individuals with a variety of skills. For this chronic treatment to be successful, the interdisciplinary team must work with the patient and family, supporting them in the areas of clinical need, psychosocial needs, and religious beliefs. Team members will include, but not be limited to, the physician, nurse, technician, dietitian, social worker, and administrator. Other team members might include a biomedical technician, psychologist, dentist, child development specialist, pharmacist, physician's assistant, vocational rehabilitation counselor, member of the clergy, coach, school teacher, or others who have special skills needed to help the patient reach maximum potential. Finally, the patient and family members are integral components of the dialysis team; without them, all the efforts of the other team members would be fruitless.

ROLE OF THE PHYSICIAN

To begin with, the nephrologist assesses the patient and determines when end-stage renal disease (ESRD) has been reached and requires the initiation of dialysis treatment. A nephrologist is an internist with further specialty training of 2 to 3 years in the field of nephrology. Evidence points increasingly to the importance of having patients seen and followed by a nephrologist early in the course of chronic renal failure (CRF), and long before progression to ESRD. With early nephrological intervention, appropriate medical therapy can be instituted, perhaps improving or at least maintaining renal function and slowing the need for dialysis.

Once the need for dialysis is determined, the nephrologist is responsible for writing the orders for the dialysis prescription—those components of the procedure that make it therapeutic. These include the specific dialyzer, flow rate, the anticoagulation during dialysis, the duration or length of time of dialysis, the frequency, and whatever unique instructions may be required for the specific vascular access.

How is a dialysis facility structured?

Every dialysis facility has a medical director who is ultimately responsible for medical care in the facility. Each dialysis facility has written policies and procedures that guide staff members in the clinical practice and patient care, and that monitor established standards of care, quality assurance, equipment and maintenance standards, reuse, and any pertinent medication or treatment protocols. These policies are written by the team and approved by the facility and nursing administrator, as required by the Joint Commission for Accreditation of Healthcare Organizations (JCAHO) for a special care unit. Whenever a patient in acute renal failure or a severely uremic patient is dialyzed in the hospital setting, a physician should be readily available to handle crises or complications of the dialysis.

ROLE OF THE NURSE

What are the functions of the dialysis nurse?

While nurses are responsible for the direct care of patients undergoing dialysis, much of this care is performed by technical staff under the supervision of the nurse. Patient and family education, and ongoing reinforcement and support for self-care are more critical services provided by the nurse. In addition, the nurse is responsible for ongoing assessment of the patient and is generally the one who initiates multidisciplinary case conferences when the patient's physical, emotional, or social condition indicates the need.

Nursing administration or nursing services organizations may differ among dialysis units. In those facilities using a *primary nursing* model, each patient has a specifically designated primary nurse who is responsible for overall patient care. On the other hand, *case management* is also appropriate for the care of dialysis patients. This model expands the nursing care/responsibility beyond the dialysis unit to the hospital, ambulatory care or outpatient facilities, and home. Case management ensures continuity of care from both a quality of care and an economic perspective. Whichever model is utilized, the goal of nursing is to serve as an advocate for those patients who require assistance and to empower them to become their own advocates.

With an increasing emphasis being placed on Continuous Quality Improvement (CQI) as one means to ensure delivery of quality care to patients, nurses are taking the lead in this activity. Nurses are also seen in the roles of business manager, research coordinator, fiscal administrator, and chief technician in some settings.

What kinds of experience and background are essential for a nurse to be successful in dialysis?

While some facilities may have different requirements for the nurses filling various positions within a dialysis facility, there are minimal qualifications required by all. A dialysis nurse should be a professional nurse with a minimum of 1 year experience in medical-surgical nursing. A license to practice nursing in the state is required, and certification within a specialty, such as nephrology, critical care, etc., is preferred. A background in critical care nursing or emergency department nursing is particularly useful, and for the nurse who functions in a managerial role, experience with personnel development, leadership roles, and other supervisory positions can be helpful in ensuring success in the position in a dialysis unit.

Less experienced nurses who assume a role as a beginning practitioner need an environment that offers extensive orientation, education, close supervision, and support.

What other qualities should the dialysis nurse possess?

Other important qualifications include the ability to interact effectively with patients and personnel, as well as a demonstrated interest and skill in patient teaching and problem-solving. Self-confidence and patience also are important in a dialysis nurse. Caring for dialysis patients and their families can be highly stressful because of the intensity of care required, the chronicity of ESRD, and the patient's struggles with independence versus dependence. Dialysis nurses should be exemplars of the blend between the art and science of nursing. A significant scientific knowledge base and technical skill must be complemented by a caring, compassionate sensitivity, personal resiliency, and an ability to cope with stress; all are useful characteristics in a dialysis nurse.

Furthermore, some interest in teaching and an ability to teach are essential attributes. The dialysis nurse is frequently called upon to provide learning experiences for patients, family members, other dialysis personnel, diverse health care professionals, and the public. The dialysis nurse must have supervisory skills to make appropriate assignments to technicians and other personnel and to evaluate accurately the care provided by them.

Are there established standards of practice for dialysis nurses?

Regulations governing the administration of the ESRD Program under Medicare describe a number of standards and criteria related to qualifications of professional staff, acceptable patient care policies and procedures, and unit administration. However, Medicare does not issue standards of practice for dialysis nurses.

Professional nursing organizations promote high standards of nephrology nursing practice. In 1987, the Nephrology Nursing Certification Board (NNCB) was established for the purpose of developing, implementing, and coordinating all aspects of certification for nephrology nurses in the United States, and in 1988, the American Nephrology Nurses Association published its first Standards of Care. A nephrology nurse who meets the qualifications and passes the NNCB's written examination is entitled to use the initials CNN (Certified Nephrology Nurse) as a professional credential.

More recently, the Dialysis Outcomes Quality Initiative (DOQI), put forth by the National Kidney Foundation in October 1997, offered some clinical practice guidelines in the areas of anemia management, hemodialysis adequacy, peritoneal dialysis adequacy, and vascular access. These are practice guidelines only and are not intended to be requirements or to be specific to nursing practice, but rather they are guidelines for the general care of the ESRD patient undergoing dialysis. (See page 333 for additional information on NKF-DOQI.)

What education is available for nurses interested in dialysis?

Most dialysis units provide specialized learning opportunities for nurses as supervised on-the-job instruction during the period of orientation. Some units offer formal educational programs for dialysis personnel other than their own employees. These more formal programs include both theory and clinical practice. The curriculum should include instruction in the following areas: renal anatomy and physiology, including pathophysiology; fluid, electrolyte, and acid-base balance; dialysis theory; vascular access; dialysis procedures and techniques; recognition of complications and emergency conditions, and appropriate prevention and intervention; psychosocial problems; dietary regimens; medications; and interpersonal relations, including effective intervention in patients with chronic illness.

Some community colleges offer dialysis training programs that teach the theoretical basics of dialysis, with clinical practicums provided by the dialysis facility supporting the student. With the approaching millennium and the push for professional nurses to have a minimum of a baccalaureate degree in nursing at the entry level, interest is growing in formalizing a nephrology nursing curriculum at the graduate level. Vanderbilt University (Nashville) has offered a nephrology nursing specialty arm in its nurse practitioner program. Other schools of nursing are also addressing nephrology nursing as a specialty area in the graduate program.

Continuing education programs for dialysis nurses are available through a variety of educational and professional organizations. These include the Council on Nephrology Nursing and Technology of the National Kidney Foundation, American Nephrology Nurses Association, as well as local chapters of these organizations. In addition, the Association of Critical Care Nurses, Infection

Control Nurses, and other such organizations offer some programs of interest to nephrology nurses.

What is the role of the dialysis nurse administrator?

A nursing leader responsible for patient care coordination may assume several titles, depending on the facility's structure. Whether as the nursing administrator, the Director of Nurses (DoN), charge nurse or nursing coordinator, this nurse will have the primary responsibility for direct patient care. Supporting a professional practice model will ensure that patients receive optimal care.

Modeling knowledgeable, skillful care of patients is a vital aspect of the role of the nurse administrator, along with recruitment and retention of an adequate number of well-prepared patient caregivers—both nurses and technicians. It is also the responsibility of the nurse administrator to equip personnel with knowledge through learning opportunities and, finally, provide resources in the form of supplies and time, enabling staff to give the desired quality of patient care.

ROLE OF THE DIALYSIS UNIT ADMINISTRATOR

A dialysis unit administrator is responsible for ensuring the fiscal soundness of the dialysis facility. The administrator may make purchasing decisions, and it is desirable that these be made with an understanding of the clinical implications of such decisions. A unit administrator usually comes prepared with either a clinical or a fiscal background. Occasionally, an administrator with a clinical background will also acquire an MBA or other fiscal or business educational preparation. This individual is thus prepared with both the clinical expertise to make decisions in the best interest of patients, as well as decisions based on what is best for the facility as a business.

ROLE OF THE TECHNICIAN

What are the roles of the dialysis technician?

Technicians have been members of the dialysis team since dialysis programs began. Two major roles have existed for technicians; one is directed at assembly and maintenance of the equipment while the other role focuses on patient care. In some settings, technicians combine patient and equipment care responsibilities. The timely and accurate assembly of dialysis equipment is vital to any dialysis program. Ongoing maintenance of costly equipment is a highly valued element of a dialysis program. Technicians work with all members of the dialysis team; in most settings they are most closely aligned with nurses. Patient care activities are delegated and supervised by professional nurses.

What abilities are required of the dialysis technicians?

Knowledge of mechanics and technological skill are essential for technicians who assume responsibility for equipment setup and maintenance. An understanding of the principles of physics and computer technology are desirable qualifications for technicians. Interpersonal skills are necessary for good relations with patients and their families. Patient care technicians must have some understanding of human anatomy and physiology and the pathophysiology of ESRD. For patient safety, a technician also possesses patient monitoring skills and clinical judgment.

Are there established standards of practice for technicians?

Dialysis technicians are bound by the standards of practice issued by the state in which they practice, if the state has practice guidelines. Technicians are also bound by the DOQI guidelines, as well as by unit-specific policies and procedures. Currently, two organizations offer technician certification exams.

What educational opportunities are available for dialysis technicians?

Dialysis programs offer on-the-job training for newly hired and inexperienced technicians. Certificate programs for dialysis technicians are available through some community colleges, and continuing education programs are conducted by health care agencies, specialty organizations, and technical colleges. The National Association of Nephrology Technologists (NANT) offers many educational programs both locally and nationally. In addition, large nephrology meetings may provide advanced learning opportunities for the technician who is seeking an expansion of responsibilities or who is functioning in an expanded role. These include, but are not limited to, the Peritoneal Dialysis Symposium, National Kidney Foundation Clinical Meetings, the American Society of Nephrology meeting, and the meetings sponsored by the Association for Advancement of Medical Instrumentation (AAMI).

ROLE OF THE RENAL DIETITIAN

What is the role of the renal dietitian?

A renal dietitian serves in a consultative role to patients and their families as well as to other members of the dialysis team. Dietitians provide an indispensable function in supporting the patient through all phases of ESRD. Dietary management is instrumental in delaying the need for dialysis. Furthermore, even once dialysis is initiated, ongoing assessment of the nutritional status of the patient and education of the patient and family are contributions made by the renal dietitian. See Chapter 12 for a more detailed description of the role of nutrition and the renal dietitian in the care of the person with ESRD.

ROLE OF THE SOCIAL WORKER

Two major activities have been described by the Council of Nephrology Social Workers:

- to develop awareness of the psychosocial aspects of chronic renal disease and
- to develop and carry out methods for dealing with these problems and needs as key to the role of the renal social worker.

How do these two goals relate to the social worker in a treatment center?

The social worker assists the patient and family in their adjustment to the illness. This involves a psychosocial assessment, provision of emotional support, and educational reinforcement. A thorough working knowledge of all available resources is essential. The social worker participates with other treatment team members in short- and long-term planning with the patient and his or her family. Evaluation of the patient's social background is important in successful development of the treatment plan. The social worker apprises other team members of special facets of patient or family behavior, history, and functioning that may influence the individual patient's care and course of treatment.

What are the qualifications necessary for the nephrology social worker?

A qualified social worker is defined by ESRD regulations as a person who is licensed, if applicable, by the state in which practicing and:

- has completed a course of study with specialization in clinical practice and holds a master's degree from a graduate school of social work accredited by the Council on Social Work Education; or
- has served for at least two years as social worker, one year of which was in a dialysis unit or transplant program before September 1, 1976, and has established a consultative relationship with a social worker who qualified under item 1.

Continuing education programs are available through the Council of Nephrology Social Workers.

Should psychiatric resources be available?

An awareness of one's own mortality and a life restricted by dependence on a machine are some of the issues that confront the dialysis patient. The social worker assists patients and families in adapting to illness-imposed lifestyle changes, such as alterations in family and societal roles. Psychiatric consultation or team conferences with psychiatric staff are important resources for the social worker and dialysis team for several reasons.

First, most dialysis patients are subjected to situational stress. Despite this fact, psychiatric intervention may be perceived by the patient as an unnecessary and unwelcome intrusion. The social worker assists patients in resolving problems and in dealing with crises but should have psychiatric resources available for consultation or referral when needed.

Second, some patients become increasingly dependent or noncompliant during periods of their illness. During such times, the social worker should work with the patient, family and other team members to help understand the behavior. Ultimately, the patient is responsible for much of his or her own management, and this should be emphasized by the social worker.

Finally, because sexual dysfunction can be a problem for patients undergoing maintenance dialysis, the social worker may be the team member whom the patient and/or family approaches for counseling.

ETHICS, RIGHTS AND RESPONSIBILITIES

For the ESRD patient and family, life with maintenance dialysis requires major changes in activity and lifestyle. These disruptions are sometimes unpleasant as well as unanticipated. Frequently the dialysis unit and involved personnel are perceived by the patient as a cause of his or her unsatisfactory situation. Frustration and conflict are prone to develop and must be resolved.

Is written consent necessary before starting dialysis?

Informed written consent for any invasive procedure, including dialysis, is always required. For emergency dialysis, if the patient is too ill, the next of kin or another person who has durable power of attorney may sign the consent for treatment.

It is important that staff members, as well as patients and families, understand the importance of informed consent, since patients and families often have misconceptions or unrealistic ideas about dialysis and what procedures may be involved. The exact format of the consent form is determined by the unit or institution's legal advisor. It should clearly document that an adequate discussion and explanation of benefits, complications, risks, and alternatives are provided to and understood by the patient. Separate consent is necessary for access procedures or modification. Update of the dialysis consent form is necessary if there is a significant change in procedure that might affect the patient, such as dialyzer reuse.

What are some of the rights of the patient?

- To be fully informed about his or her illness.
- To be informed as to the nature of the treatment and the usual risks.
- To be fully informed about alternative methods of treatment.
- To know that personal privacy will be respected and professional confidentiality maintained.
- To have input into the treatment regimen.

May a patient voluntarily decide to discontinue dialysis?

Many professionals, but not all, believe that a rational adult who, for reasons that are valid to him or her, elects to stop treatment with full understanding of the consequences should have that right. The ethical and legal issues are complex; not all ESRD workers agree, and in some instances courts have ordered dialysis to be continued.

What are some responsibilities of personnel to patients?

- To make the patient as fully informed as possible, as long as it is consistent with high-quality care.
- To ensure that all safeguards are met fully and to provide high-quality dialysis service.
- To be supportive of patient and family in their adjustment to the illness, its treatment, and the accompanying changes in their lives. This involves teaching them about the disease and its treatment so that they can make informed decisions and set realistic goals.

What are some responsibilities of the patient?

- To understand and to follow the instructions of the physicians, nurses, and other personnel providing care.
- To strive for a high degree of independence through learning and to assume responsibility for self-care as far as possible.
- To respect the rights and privacy of other patients.

Finally, what are some interpersonnel responsibilities?

- One person, usually a nurse, must be in charge. Problems should be taken to this individual to prevent misconceptions or ambiguity.
- All personnel must carry out assigned responsibilities to the best of individual ability, provide the best possible patient care, and contribute to the overall smooth operation of the unit.
- All personnel should strive for a pleasant environment that allows for interaction among patients, personnel, and visitors while maintaining an appropriate level of efficiency and professionalism.

Basic Chemistry of Body Fluids and Electrolytes

K. E. Cotton and C. F. Gutch

Normal kidneys maintain the balance between body water and the substances dissolved in it within the narrow limits necessary for life. Kidneys also excrete the waste products of protein metabolism. Dialysis partially substitutes for these two important functions when the normal kidneys fail. Fundamental to understanding the processes used by the kidney—natural or artificial—is a basic knowledge of the chemistry involved and the measurements used.

METRIC SYSTEM

To begin with, a solid review of the basic system of measurement is necessary. The metric system is used in chemical and physical measurements that relate to body physiology. Length is expressed by the basic unit of the *meter*. The basic unit of mass is the *gram*, and the *liter* is the basic unit of volume. Table 2-1 lists common metric terms and their interrelationship.

The metric system is entirely decimal. Prefixes indicate smaller or larger units (Table 2-2).

To relate the metric system to more familiar uses, the following approximations may be helpful:
- A man who is 6 feet 4 inches tall is about 1.95 m in height.
- A dime is about 1 mm thick.
- A 154-pound person weighs 70 kg.

The following are *commonly used conversion factors* to change metric units to the English system of pounds, inches, and quarts.
- 1 meter (m) = 39.37 inches (in)
- 1 inch (in) = 2.54 centimeters (cm)
- 1 liter (L) = 1.057 quarts (U.S.) (qt)
- 1 gallon (gal) = 3.785 liters (L)
- 1 kilogram (kg) = 2.2 pounds (lb)
- 1 ounce (oz) = 28.35 grams (g)
- 1 fluid ounce (fl oz) = 29.57 milliliters (ml)

Table 2-1 Commonly Used Metric Units

Quantity	Unit	Symbol	Relationship of Units
Length	Millimeter	mm	1 mm = 0.001 m
	Centimeter	cm	1 cm = 0.01 m
	Meter	m	1 m
	Kilometer	km	1 km = 1000 m
Area	Square centimeter	cm^2	$1\ cm^2 = 0.0001\ m^2$
	Square meter	m^2	$1\ m^2$
	Square kilometer	km^2	$1\ km^2 = 1\ 000\ 000\ m^2$
Volume	Milliliter	ml	1 ml = 0.001 L
	Deciliter	dl	1 dl = 0.01 L
	Liter	L	1 L
	Cubic meter	m^3	$1\ m^3 = 1000\ L$
Mass	Milligram	mg	1 mg = 0.001 g
	Gram	g	1 g
	Kilogram	kg	1 kg = 1000 g

Adapted from White WL, Erickson ME, Stevens SC: *Chemistry for the clinical laboratory,* ed 4, St. Louis, 1976, Mosby.

Temperature is expressed in degrees centigrade. Zero degrees centigrade is the freezing point of water and 100°C is its boiling point. The following is a comparison of some centigrade temperatures with the Fahrenheit scale:

	°F	°C
Boiling point of water	212	100
Normal body temperature	98.6	37
Freezing point of water	32	0
	0	–18

For conversion of Fahrenheit values to centigrade and vice versa, use the formula:

Fahrenheit temperature = 9/5(centigrade temperature) + 32
Centigrade temperature = 5/9(Fahrenheit temperature) – 32

CHEMISTRY

All physical things are composed of a finite number of kinds of matter. Matter is anything that possesses weight and occupies space. The basic kinds of matter are called elements. An element cannot be further divided without changing its chemical properties. There are 108 known elements. They may exist alone, in mixtures, or in chemical combinations (compounds). Some elements exist alone in their natural form as a solid, liquid, or gas. For instance, gold nuggets are pure, crystalline gold (Au). Metallic mercury (Hg) is a liquid under ordinary conditions. Helium (He) is a monatomic gas. The physical state depends upon the melting or boiling point. Many elements do not exist in an uncombined state, but only as compounds. Oxygen as it exists in air is not monatomic oxygen (O) but a compound of two oxygen atoms, O_2. Almost all hydrogen (H) exists in compounds, such as water (H_2O).

Table 2-2   Metric Decimal Prefixes

Multiplication Factors	Prefix	Symbol
1		
$0.1 = 10^{-1}$	deci	d
$0.01 = 10^{-2}$	centi	c
$0.001 = 10^{-3}$	milli	m
$0.000\ 001 = 10^{-6}$	micro	μ
$0.000\ 000\ 001 = 10^{-9}$	nano	n
$0.000\ 000\ 000\ 01 = 10^{-12}$	pica	p

Adapted from Young DS: Implementation of SI units for clinical laboratory data, *Ann Intern Med* 106:114, 1987.

What is an atom?

An atom is the smallest particle of an element that retains the properties of that element. Atoms are composed of (1) a central nucleus containing protons and neutrons and (2) electrons that move in an orbital fashion around the nucleus. An atom resembles a miniature solar system. The sun represents the nucleus; the paths of the planets represent the orbiting electrons. Several electrons may occupy the same orbital path.

Protons are a part of all nuclei and have a positive charge equivalent to that of an electron. An electron is a particle of infinitesimal small mass with a negative charge. A neutron is equal to a proton in mass, but is electrically neutral.

What is a compound?

A compound is a chemical combination of elements. The proportion of elements is fixed for each compound. For example, water, H_2O, always exists in a 2:1 ratio of hydrogen and oxygen.

What is a molecule?

A molecule is the smallest unit of a substance that retains its chemical properties. A molecule of oxygen, O_2, has different chemical properties than an atom of oxygen, O.

What is atomic weight?

Atomic weights relate to one another based on an arbitrary scale that assigns a weight of 12 atomic mass units (amu) to the carbon isotope 12 (^{12}C). On this scale, protons and neutrons each weigh 1 amu; electrons have negligible mass. The hydrogen atom (^1H) is 1 amu, and the oxygen atom (^{16}O) is 16 amu. One atomic mass unit is sometimes called a dalton (d), after John Dalton, an early developer of the atomic concept.

What does atomic number indicate?

The atomic number is the number of protons in the nucleus of an atom. This is a unique number that characterizes each element. This number of protons in a nucleus determines the chemical nature of the atom; by contrast, the number of neutrons affects only the weight of an atom. When two atoms with the same number of protons have different numbers of neutrons, and hence have different weights, they are called isotopes.

How does atomic weight relate to molecular weight?

To calculate molecular weight, add the weights of each atom that make up that molecule. For instance, water, H_2O, consists of two hydrogen atoms and one oxygen atom. From this, we can calcualate that the molecular weight of water is 18 d (1 + 1 + 16). If the amu weight of an element is expressed in grams, it is called a gram atomic weight; for compounds, the term is gram molecular weight. This does not make calculating more complex, however. For instance, sixteen grams of oxygen contain the same number of particles as does 1 g of hydrogen, since oxygen weighs 16 times as much as hydrogen.

The number of particles in any gram atomic weight is very large. It is, however, a precise number: 6.023×10^{23}. This is known as Avogadro's number.

What is the practical use of Avogadro's number?

Avogadro's number defines the relationship between the atomic or molecular weight in amu units and in grams. One gram molecular weight of a nonionized solute dissolved to make 1 L of solution has a solute concentration of 6.023×10^{23} particles per liter. For urea (nonionizable), with a molecular weight of 60, this is 60 g of solute in 1 L of solution.

For substances that dissociate into ions, this principle applies to each ion type. Thus sodium chloride, NaCl, forms almost twice Avogadro's number of particles per gram molecular weight because the Na^+ and Cl^- ions separate (dissociate) upon dissolving.

What determines the physical state of a molecule?

Every molecule possesses kinetic energy, the energy of movement. The speed of a molecule depends on the temperature. An increase in temperature increases molecular speed; cooling reduces molecular speed. The rapid movement of each molecule acts to keep all particles separate from one another.

There are also powerful attractive forces between particles. These attractive forces tend to aggregate molecules. In a crystal of ice the attractive forces are greater than the separating forces, and the molecules remain trapped in the crystal structure. When heat is added, kinetic energy increases until the separative forces are greater than the attractive forces. This is the process of melting. Further addition of heat increases the kinetic energy until some molecules acquire sufficient energy to escape the liquid state entirely by boiling and producing steam.

Conversely, as cooling occurs, steam condenses into water, then crystallizes into ice. These steps occur as kinetic energy and molecular speed are reduced, and the attractive forces become more important.

What is an ion?

An ion is a particle that has an electric charge. It may be a charged atom, such as a sodium ion, or a charged compound, such as a lactate ion. The formation of an ion, called ionization, is illustrated by the formation of sodium and chloride ions.

The sodium atom has a solitary electron in its outermost orbit. The adjacent orbit is filled with eight electrons, a stable number for this ion. Atoms increase their stability when their outermost orbits are filled with a stable number of electrons. The stability of sodium can be increased by giving up its solitary outer electron and leaving a filled orbit. This loss of an electron results in an excess of positive charge. In this case, there is a +1 charge remaining on the sodium ion after it has given up this outer electron.

Chlorine has an outer shell that is one electron short of being filled. If it accepts an electron, it gains stability. It also gains a net negative charge, −1.

All substances must stay very close to electrical neutrality; one type of ion does not exist separate from the other. Where there are positive ions, there are an equal number of negative ions nearby.

A crystal of NaCl has no free ions. As the crystal dissolves, Na^+ and Cl^- ions are liberated from the bond structure. This is also called ionization.

What is ionic bonding?

There is an attraction between positive and negative ions. In a crystal of table salt (NaCl) there are enough attractive forces to maintain a precisely ordered structure in the crystal. The ions need not be permanently attached to each other, just close to each other.

What is a covalent bond?

Some atoms cannot easily fill the outermost orbital ring because they have several electrons to gain or lose. Oxygen (O) has six electrons in its outermost ring and must gain two; carbon has only four and must either gain or lose four electrons. These atoms gain stability by *sharing* electrons with another atom.

The bonds in a water molecule (H_2O) are covalent bonds. The oxygen atom fills its outermost orbital by sharing the electron of two hydrogen atoms. Each hydrogen atom gains stability by sharing one electron from the oxygen to fill its shell with two electrons. This bond between hydrogen and oxygen exists only when there is a precise relationship between the three participants in the bond. Covalent bonds are generally quite stable and stronger than ionic bonds.

What is an equivalent (combining) weight?

An equivalent weight is the gram atomic weight of a substance divided by the charge. Ions with more than one charge per ion can react with more than one singly charged ion of opposite charge. The equivalent weight notation equalizes the weight of all ions according to their *weight per charge*.
The calcium ion has an atomic weight of 40 and a charge of +2. One [atom] of calcium can react with [two ions] of chloride to form calcium chloride ($CaCl_2$). In the equivalent notation, one equivalent of calcium (20 g) reacts with one equivalent of chloride (35.5 g) to form 55.5 g of $CaCl_2$.

What is a polar molecule?

In a polar molecule the charge is not quite equally distributed. For example, in water, the two electrons shared between the hydrogen and the oxygen are attracted closer to the oxygen atom. This gives a slight negative charge to the oxygen atom and a slight positive charge to the hydrogen atoms.

The effect of this slight charge distribution is also determined by the geometry of the molecule. For instance, in carbon dioxide the atoms are lined up in a row, O=C=O. Any effect of the charge separation is masked since the positive and negative areas overlap. On the other hand, in the water molecule the atoms are not lined up in a row but form an angle of 105 degrees (Fig. 2-1). This results in a slight positive charge on the hydrogen side of the atom and a slight negative charge on the oxygen side. The combination of charge separation and geometry makes the molecule electrically unbalanced and thereby polar.

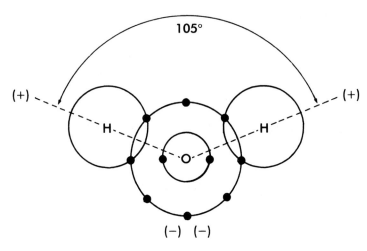

Fig. 2-1 Polar effect; covalent bond in water molecule.

Of what importance is this polar nature?

Look at the water molecule example once again. The polarity of water allows negative ions to be attracted toward the positive end of the water molecule and positive ions toward the negative end. This is an important force in dissolving substances into ions. The effect of polar solvents is that of another separating force that allows ionization to occur at lower temperatures. The importance of this effect can be seen by attempting to dissolve sodium chloride (NaCl) in a nonpolar solvent such as alcohol.

Define a solution.

A solution is a homogeneous mixture of dissolved particles (solute) and a liquid (solvent). In physiologic solutions, the solvent is usually water. Physiologic saline contains 0.85 g of NaCl in 100 ml of water.

How is the concentration of a solution measured?

Nonionized particles have been measured in terms of weight of solute per volume of solvent. Blood glucose and urea commonly have been measured as milligrams per 100 ml (mg/dl). For ionized particles it is important to know the relative number of particles present and the contribution of their charge. These are measured more precisely by the use of molarity and normality, and are usually expressed as mEq/L (milliequivalents per liter). See page 15, "What is an equivalent (combining) weight?"

What are S.I. units?

"S.I. units" is the abbreviation for le Systeme Internationale d'Unites. This is an extension of the metric system to provide uniformity of units of measurement and their easy interconversion. Since 1987 S.I. has been used to report data by most clinical laboratories in the United States. In this system the amount of a substance is written as moles per liter rather than mass, such as g/L or mg/dl. See Appendix A for some common chemistry conversion factors.

What is molarity?

A solution is 1 molar (1M) if 1 g atomic weight of a solute is dissolved to make a solution of 1 L. A 1M solution of any nonionized solute has the same number of particles in the solution, specifically Avogadro's number.

What is normality?

A solution containing one equivalent of ions in a 1 L solution is 1 normal (1N). For a singly charged ion, such as chloride, a 1N solution is also 1M. For a doubly charged ion, such as calcium (valance of 2), a 1N solution is 0.5M.

A substance that dissolves in water to form ionized particles is an electrolyte. Sodium chloride (NaCl) dissolves in water to yield Na^+ and Cl^- ions. Positive ions are called cations, negative ions are called anions. Body fluids contain various cations such as Na^+, K^+, Ca^{++}, and such anions as Cl^- and HCO_3^-.

Are urea and creatinine electrolytes?

No. Both urea and creatinine are soluble in water, but they do not form charged particles.

What is conductivity?

Conductivity is the property of a solution to conduct an electric current. It is illustrated by an electrolytic cell. Fig. 2-2 shows such a cell—a container of solution with two electrodes. The electrodes are connected by wires through a battery and an ammeter; the ammeter measures flow of current through the circuit. If the only communication between electrodes is through very pure water, little or no current flows; there is no way for electrons to pass through the water.

If sodium chloride is added to the water, current will flow. Sodium ions are attracted to the negative electrode (cathode), where each ion accepts an electron. At the same time, chloride ions are attracted to the positive electrode (anode), where each gives up an electron.

Fig. 2-2 Electrolytic cell. (Adapted from Cotton KE, Gutch CF: Topics in hemodialysis: milliequivalents, conductivity and osmolality, *J Extracorp Tech* 3:148, 1974.)

The ease with which electrons flow in a solution depends upon the kinds of electrolytes present and their concentration. Conductivity monitors are vital components of dialysis fluid delivery systems that must produce solutions of constant, precise solute content.

What is osmolality?

Diffusion (spreading out) of particles occurs from an area of higher concentration to an area of lower concentration. A strong electrolyte solution has a reduced water concentration, since some of the water has been replaced by solute. If two solutions of different concentrations are separated by a membrane permeable only to water, water flows from the area of greatest water concentration to the area of *least* water concentration. This is the same as saying that water flows from the area of least solute concentration to the area of greatest solute concentration.

Osmolality is a measure of the ability of a solution to "attract" water. It depends upon the *number of particles* present. A molal solution is made by dissolving 1 g molecular weight (1 mole) in 1 kg of solvent. (NOTE: There is a technical difference between a *molal* solution, 1 mole solute/1 kg *solvent*, and the *molar* solution mentioned in a previous paragraph, represented by 1 mole solute/1 L *solution*.) A molal solution of nonionizable substance (such as urea or glucose) has an osmotic effect of 1 osmole/kg. If the solute is ionizable, there will be more particles, and the osmotic effect will be increased. A molal solution of NaCl will have an effect of nearly 2 Osm/L because almost all the NaCl dissociates into sodium ions and chloride ions as it goes into solution.

Most physiologic solutions have an osmolality far under 1 Osm/kg. Normal blood plasma has an osmolality of approximately 290 mOsm/kg (290 mmol/kg in S.I. units).

How is the osmolality of a solution determined?

As solute is added to water, the freezing point decreases in linear fashion, proportionate to osmolality. A "freezing point osmometer" actually measures the minute changes in the freezing point as solute concentration is changed. The readout is given in mOsm/kg, or mmol/kg. Osmolality may be used to cross-check the concentration of dialysis fluid.

Does water dissociate into ions?

To a very slight degree, yes. Pure water has a hydrogen ion (H^+) concentration of 1.0×10^{-7} moles per liter (mol/L). There is a similar concentration of hydroxide ion (OH^-) since each is derived from one water molecule: H_2O (H^+ + OH^-.

If the H^+ concentration exceeds that of pure water, the solution is acidic. If the concentration is less, it is *basic*, or alkaline.

Of what importance is the hydrogen ion concentration?

Normal H^+ concentration in human extracellular fluid is 36 to 45 *nanomol/L* (pH 7.35 to 7.45). All metabolic processes of the body require this precise range of H^+ concentration. If the concentration becomes too great or too small, massive derangements of metabolism occur. The extremes of [H^+] compatible with life lie between 16 and 160 nanomol/L (pH 7.80 to 6.80).

Two body organs are involved in H+ regulation: the lungs and the kidneys. The lungs eliminate carbon dioxide (the major end product of metabolism) as rapidly as it is produced, and in so doing regulate the partial pressure of carbon dioxide in blood. The pCO_2 determines the concentration of carbonic acid (H_2CO_3) in body water. The kidneys regulate the concentration of bicarbonate (HCO_3^-) in body fluid, and eliminate the nonvolatile (fixed) acid and the basic products of metabolism. Kidney failure causes retention of hydrogen ions; this is called metabolic acidosis.

What is an acid?

An acid is a substance that can donate a hydrogen ion, and a base is a substance that can accept a hydrogen ion. An acid may be called a proton donor and a base, a proton receptor. Remember that the hydrogen atom consists of a positively charged nucleus, or proton, and a single, negatively charged orbiting electron. The hydrogen ion (H^+) is the proton without the orbiting electron.

Define pH.

pH is the term used by chemists for expressing very small H^+ concentration and is defined as *the negative logarithm to the base 10 of the H^+ concentration* (pH = –Log H$^+$). Pure water has H$^+$ concentration of 10^{-7} mol/L, or 10 nm/L; its pH is 7.00.

At pH less than 7.00 (H$^+$ greater than 100 nmol/L), a solution becomes acidic (meaning, of course, that protons are available for donation). If the hydrogen ion concentration is reduced (pH greater than 7.00), protons can be accepted, and the solution is basic (see Fig. 2-3).

pH measures only the free H$^+$ in solution. If some H$^+$ is bound and not ionized, it does not affect the pH. The pH of normal blood is 7.4, with a range of 7.35 to 7.45.

How is the pH value used clinically?

If the pH is less than 7.35, the solution is clearly acidic and H$^+$ is increased. Conversely, if pH is greater than 7.45, the solution is basic (alkaline) and H$^+$ is decreased; see Fig. 2-3. In calculating replacement therapy for either a metabolic alkalosis or acidosis, it is important to quickly quantitate the H$^+$ excess or deficit. This is done by simple calculations.

Normal pH of 7.40 represents 40 nmol/L of H$^+$. As pH goes down, H$^+$ increases. For each 0.10 decrement in pH, multiply 40 by 1.25 to get the increment in H$^+$. Thus, for pH = 7.30: 40 x 1.25 = 50 nmol H$^+$. For pH = 7.20: 50 x 1.25 = 63 nmol H$^+$. For each 0.10 pH change, the multiplication is done stepwise.

With decreasing H$^+$ (increasing pH), the factor becomes 0.8. Thus, for pH = 7.50: 40 x 0.8 = 32 nmol H$^+$. This is continued in the same stepwise fashion for pH 7.60, 7.70, and so forth. For values between 0.10 pH units, calculate the upper and lower values and extrapolate—for pH 7.25, H$^+$ is halfway between 50 and 63, or 56 nmol/L.

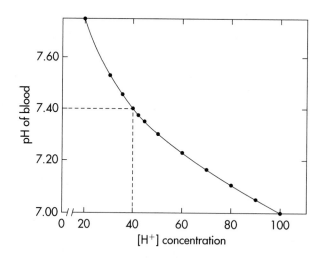

Fig. 2-3   Hydrogen ion concentration (nEq/L) vs. pH. (Redrawn from White WL, Erickson ME, Stevens SC: *Chemistry for the clinical laboratory*, ed 4, St. Louis, 1976, Mosby.)

What is a buffer?

Buffers are substances that, in solution, maintain a constant hydrogen ion concentration despite addition of either acid or base.

How does a buffer maintain the pH?

Some substances dissolved in water are nearly completely ionized, such as sodium chloride. Other substances are readily dissolved but are poorly ionized (lactic acid—about 1% ionized in solution). Buffers in the physiologic range include a mixture of monohydrogen phosphate ($HOP_4^=$) and dihydrogen phosphate ($H_2PO_4^-$). An equilibrium exists between these two forms: $HOP_4^= + H^+ = H_2PO_4^-$.

If acid is added to the solution, the equilibrium shifts to the right. Some H^+ is bound to $HOP_4^=$ and no longer affects the pH. This keeps the pH near its original value. If some H^+ is removed from the solution, the equilibrium is shifted to the left, H^+ is liberated, and the pH change is minimal.

BODY WATER

How much water does the body contain?

Water is the major constituent of the body. It comprises 45 to 75% of the weight of an adult. The proportion varies inversely with the amount of body fat. A 70-kg man (154 lb) has about 42 L of total body water (60% of weight). Women have less. Infants and very young children have the highest proportion of body water.

What purpose does this fluid serve?

Body tissue is made up of living cells. Complex chemical processes within these cells produce energy in the form of heat, motion, and regeneration. Oxygen and nutrients are metabolized; carbon dioxide and other wastes are produced. Water within the cell is the medium for these chemical processes.

Water also surrounds and bathes all cells, protecting them from the hazards of the external world. It is the vehicle for transportation of nutrients from—and wastes to—the outside environment.

How is water distributed in the body?

About 55% of total body water (TBW) is intracellular and 45% is extracellular. Some 17% of the extracellular fluid (ECF) exists as fluid in bone and connective tissue and as transcellular fluid (pleural, peritoneal, pericardial), which do not interchange readily. For clinical purposes, the ECF represents approximately one third of TBW, or 20% of body weight. Intracellular fluid is about two thirds of TBW or 40% of body weight.

How is body water measured?

The techniques involve tracer dilution methodology. A suitable marker, a dye or radioisotope, is injected in known concentration. The extent to which it is diluted in a specific body compartment over time is used to calculate the approximate fluid volume of that compartment.

$$\text{Volume of compartment} = \frac{\text{Mass of "x" given} - \text{Mass of "x" lost (urine, etc.)}}{\text{Concentration of "x" in compartment}}$$

Plasma volume can be measured with tagged albumin. TBW may be measured with about 1 percent precision. Good markers for ECF and for intracellular fluid (ICF) are not available; these volumes are estimated using the distribution proportions given in the previous paragraph.

What is the composition of extracellular fluid?

Plasma water and interstitial fluid are nearly the same. Sodium is the major cation (145 mEq/L). Chloride and bicarbonate are the major anions. About 7 percent of plasma volume is protein and lipid material that does not cross the capillary wall. The protein molecules are anionic; to maintain electrical neutrality, there are slightly fewer sodium and chloride ions in plasma than in interstitial fluid. Clinical calculations of electrolytes usually ignore these small differences and assume that plasma electrolytes are representative of the total ECF.

What determines the distribution of water between plasma and the interstitial compartment?

This depends on the balance between (1) colloid (protein and lipid) osmotic pressure, (2) intracapillary blood pressure, and (3) tissue turgor pressure. This is known as the Starling effect.

What are the constituents of intracellular fluid?

The composition of ICF varies with the specific tissue. Muscle values are commonly used in calculations. Potassium, the major intracellular cation, is 155 mEq/L; magnesium is 40 mEq/L, and sodium is only 10 mEq/L. Organic phosphates and protein are the important anions; chloride and bicarbonate total only 10 mEq/L.

How are the electrolyte concentrations kept different inside and outside the cell?

The cell membrane is impermeable to protein and the organic phosphate complexes, confining them inside the cell. There are metabolically active (energy-consuming) "pumps" in the cell wall that transport sodium ions from within the cell to the outside, while moving potassium ions from the exterior to the cell's interior.

Does water pass across the cell membrane?

Yes, water moves quickly in either direction to maintain total osmolal equality on both sides of the membrane (Fig. 2-4).

Are there nonelectrolytes in body fluids?

Yes, these include glucose, amino acids, and other nutrients and metabolic wastes such as urea. Their concentration is relatively low compared with the electrolytes.

What is meant by fluid balance?

A normal diet contains 500 to 1000 ml of water in the food itself. Some 300 to 500 ml of water is produced each day by metabolism of food and from tissue breakdown. Other fluid taken in, such as coffee, tea, juice, or other drink, obviously represents water intake and averages 1500 to 2000 ml/day.

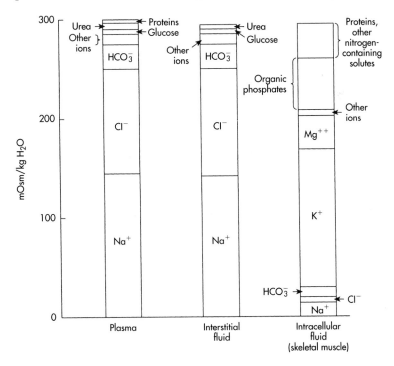

Fig. 2-4 Osmotic composition of major body fluids. (Redrawn from Laiken ND, Fanestil DF: *Best and Taylor's physiological basis of medical practice*, ed 12, Baltimore, 1991, Williams & Wilkins.)

Between 700 and 1000 ml of water is lost each day through evaporation from the lungs and by insensible perspiration. Vigorous activity or a rise in temperature causes additional loss (measurable in liters if the environmental temperature increase is severe). A minimum of 400 ml of fluid or more must be excreted as urine each day to prevent the accumulation of metabolic wastes.

The electrolyte composition, pH, osmolality, etc., are precisely maintained in the body's internal fluid environment. The kidneys keep this balance, called *homeostasis*. The kidney conserves fluid or excretes excess as needed. When kidney failure occurs, meticulous attention to the balance of fluid intake and losses becomes a necessity.

Renal Physiology and the Pathology of Renal Failure

C. F. Gutch

"What is man, when we come to think upon him,
but an ingenious machine for turning with infinite
artfulness the red wine of Shirez into urine."

From "Dreamers" in *Seven Gothic Tales* by Izak Dineson.

Before any discussion of the pathology of renal failure, it is important to review the functions that normal kidneys perform. There are two prime functions: (1) elimination of metabolic wastes and other toxic materials and (2) maintenance of a stable composition of the body's internal fluid environment (Fig. 3-1).

In addition, kidneys also have several endocrine functions including: (1) production of *renin*, which affects sodium, fluid volume, and blood pressure; (2) *erythropoietin* formation, which controls red cell production in the bone marrow; (3) production of *prostaglandins*; and (4) involvement in the *kallikrein-kinin system*.

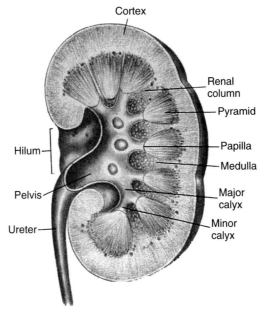

Fig. 3-1 Longitudinal section of normal kidney.

Also, the normal kidney is a receptor site for several hormones: (1) antidiuretic hormone (ADH), produced by the pituitary, reduces the excretion of water; (2) aldosterone, produced by the adrenal cortex, promotes sodium retention and enhances secretion of potassium and hydrogen ion; (3) parathyroid hormone increases phosphorus and bicarbonate excretion and stimulates conversion of vitamin D to the active 1, 25 vitamin D_3 form.

What is a nephron?

The nephron is the functional unit of the kidney. There are over a million such units in each of the two kidneys. Each nephron has two main parts, the glomerulus and the tubule. The glomerulus consists of a network of thin-walled capillaries closely surrounded by a pear-shaped epithelial membrane called Bowman's capsule. The space between the two layers of Bowman's capsule opens into the proximal tubule, which makes a series of convolutions in the cortex of the kidney. It straightens out, then makes a U turn, known as Henle's loop, in the kidney medulla. It becomes convoluted again adjacent to its own glomerulus and finally joins other distal tubules to form a collecting duct to carry the freshly formed urine to the kidney pelvis (Fig. 3-2). Each kidney pelvis funnels the urine into its ureter, which connects with the urinary bladder. The urethra conveys the urine from the bladder to the exterior.

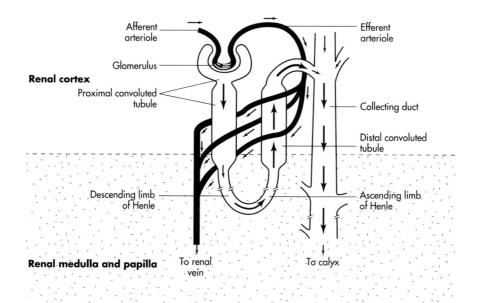

Fig. 3-2 Diagram of nephron with afferent arteriole, glomerulus, efferent arteriole, and collecting duct.

What does the glomerulus do?

Blood enters the capillary tuft through an afferent arteriole. Because of the blood pressure in the capillaries and because of their thin walls, ultrafiltration occurs. Water and solutes of molecular weight less than 68,000 d (albumin) pass freely into Bowman's space. This fluid is the *glomerular filtrate*, and its rate of production is the glomerular filtration rate (GFR). A man of average size has about 180 L of filtrate per day, or 125 ml/min. Ninety-nine percent of this filtrate is reabsorbed in the tubules.

What is the function of the tubules?

Their main functions are reabsorption and secretion. Of the 180 L of glomerular filtrate produced each day, about 2 L remain as the final urine. The rest of the water is reabsorbed along with glucose, amino acids, small proteins, and most electrolytes. The remaining filtrate becomes concentrated and begins to resemble the ultimate urine as it progresses down the tubule. Final adjustments of water-to-solute load occur in the distal tubule under the influence of ADH. The tubules conserve water and electrolytes by returning them to the blood. Hydrogen ion and metabolic wastes are excreted along with a volume of water appropriate to the total body need.

What happens in kidney failure?

Renal failure may be **acute** or **chronic**. In both there is enough loss of nephron function to upset the normal steady state of the body's internal environment. Waste products of protein metabolism accumulate.

This is termed *azotemia*, indicating retention of nitrogenous products (azote = nitrogen). Azotemia is a major component of the uremic syndrome.

What is uremia?

Uremia, or the uremic syndrome, encompasses a complex of symptoms and findings resulting from disordered biochemical processes when kidney function fails.

Is retention of urea the cause of uremia?

Severity of the uremic symptoms roughly parallels the rise in blood urea. Urea clearly contributes to some of the symptoms—malaise, lethargy, anorexia, insomnia—but it is not the primary toxin of uremia. Numerous other substances are retained in the body when kidney function fails. More than 200 potential uremic toxins have been identified.

How is acute renal failure defined?

It is *any sudden, severe impairment of kidney function*. Onset is rapid, over hours or a few days. Classically there is oliguria (less than 400 ml of urine per 24 hours). However, nearly half the cases are a nonoliguric variety. Nonoliguric renal failure is less fulminant and less difficult to manage than the oliguric form; dialysis is often not necessary.

What causes acute renal failure?

There are three categories of causes: (1) prerenal, (2) intrarenal (intrinsic), and (3) postrenal.

Prerenal causes reduced blood flow to the kidney sufficiently to impair function. The most common causes include low extracellular fluid volume (as in severe dehydration), heart failure, and blockage of the renal arteries.

Postrenal causes blocked flow of urine leaving the kidney. Obstruction may be at the ureter, bladder, or urethral level.

Identification of prerenal and postrenal causes is important because often they may be corrected quickly, without residual damage to the kidneys.

Intrinsic acute renal failure (ARF) is caused by direct damage to kidney tissue. This might occur with an acute inflammation (rapidly progressive glomerulonephritis). Much more often, it is the result of severely compromised blood flow (hemorrhagic shock) or direct toxicity to kidney parenchymal cells; this can come from some antibiotics, myoglobin, or ethylene glycol. The result is *acute tubular necrosis*, which causes 75 percent of all acute renal failure. Commonly called ATN, this condition is caused by injury to cells of the kidney tubules. The cell damage may be toxic (from chemicals or drugs) or ischemic (from severely reduced blood flow). Actual necrosis of cells does not always occur, but functional impairment is severe.

What brings on acute tubular necrosis?

The most frequent causes include surgery, trauma, sepsis, cardiovascular collapse, and nephrotoxic injury. Multisystem failure with sepsis is a frequent cause of ATN and a high mortality.

Nephrotoxins include hemoglobin (from hemolysis of red cells) and myoglobin from muscle breakdown (rhabdomyolysis) as a result of crush injury, heat stroke, seizure, etc. Many diagnostic and therapeutic agents, antibiotics (aminoglycosides especially), anesthetics, contrast media, cancer chemotherapy agents—as well as street drugs—are toxic to the kidney in varying degrees.

How is acute renal failure recognized?

Most cases are found in hospital Intensive Care Units. Monitoring of fluid intake/output, urine electrolytes, and serum solutes can furnish early clues.

Serum creatinine may increase 50 to 100 μmol/L, and urea may increase by 3.7 to 10.7 mmol/L each day. When tissue breakdown is extensive, serum potassium, phosphate, sulfate, and hydrogen ion rise rapidly.

What is the course of acute renal failure?

Acute renal failure from pre-renal or post-renal causes reverses quickly when the precipitating factor is corrected. Most intrinsic renal failure, or ATN, is recoverable. However, other effects of the injury or the medical or surgical catastrophe that precipitated the renal failure may continue. These — with the complications of infection, sepsis, and hemorrhage — often have a very high mortality rate.

How does chronic renal failure differ from ARF?

Progressive and irreversible loss of function occurs over many months or years. As the number of functioning nephrons decreases, each remaining unit must clear an increasing solute load. Eventually the limit to the amount of solute that can be cleared is reached, and the concentration in body fluids must rise. Azotemia and clinical uremia result. Fortunately, the slow rate of progression allows the body to adapt somewhat. Symptoms may be relatively mild proportionate to the chemical abnormalities.

What is end-stage renal disease (ESRD)?

In the course of chronic kidney disease the renal insufficiency often may be managed by diet, sodium restriction, phosphate control, and medication for a considerable time. As function falls to 10 to 15 percent of normal, the end is reached; dialysis or transplantation is necessary if the patient is to survive.

What are some causes of end-stage renal disease?

In the United States, diabetic nephropathy causes about 42 percent of the end stage renal disease bringing people to maintenance dialysis. Hypertension contributes about 26 percent, and various forms of glomerulonephritis, about 11 percent (Fig. 3-3).

What are the clinical manifestations of ESRD?

These are the features of a gradually developing uremic syndrome. Fatigue, slowed thinking, and pruritus occur early. All organ systems become involved. A wide complex of symptoms and findings evolves (Table 3-1).

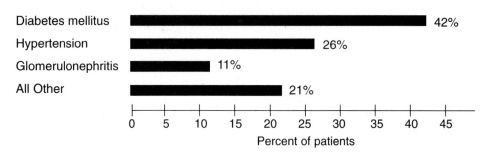

Fig. 3-3 Primary causes of end-stage renal disease in the United States for 1996. (Data from US Renal Data System, *USRDS 1998 Annual Data Report*, Bethesda, MD, 1998, National Institute of Health, National Institute of Diabetes and Digestive and Kidney Diseases.)

What abnormalities of water and electrolytes occur?

- Decreased weight occurs from loss of tissue mass.
- TBW is increased with a higher proportion of extracellular fluid.
- Total body potassium is reduced; serum value may be elevated.
- Hydrogen ion is retained. Serum [H+] is usually about 56 nmol/L (pH 7.25) because some of it becomes intracellular in an exchange for potassium and from buffering by bone salts.
- Serum calcium is low, partly because of decreased intestinal absorption. Phosphorus excretion is sharply curtailed. The resulting high phosphate level contributes to parathyroid stimulation, bone disease and soft tissue calcification.
- Serum magnesium is slightly elevated.

What cardiovascular abnormalities occur with uremia?

Hypertension affects a majority of patients. Expanded extracellular fluid volume associated with sodium retention is a factor. Many patients have increased plasma renin activity. Nephrectomy is occasionally necessary to control resistant hypertension.

Atherosclerosis is a major factor in morbidity and mortality. A defect in liver lipoprotein lipase is a likely cause of increased serum triglycerides. Coronary artery disease, stroke, and peripheral arterial disease are increased.

Myocardial dysfunction presents as left ventricular hypertrophy, resulting from hypertension, anemia, and atherosclerosis. Progression to cardiac failure is usual.

Pericardial effusion of small degree is detected by ultrasound in many patients. Clinical pericarditis presents with sudden left chest pain and an audible rub. The fluid is usually bloody; if volume is large, tamponade may result.

Table 3-1   Some Clinical Manifestations of the Chronic Uremic Syndrome

Cardiovascular System	Gastrointestinal System
Shortness of breath	Poor appetite
Cough	Nausea, vomiting
Edema	Sore mouth
High blood pressure	Peptic ulcer
Chest pain	Pancreatitis
Arrhythmias	

Neurologic System	Endocrine System
Numbness, tingling	Amenorrhea, impotence
Burning feet	Insulin resistance
Restless legs	Growth retardation
Twitching, tremors	Bone disorders
Weakness	
Memory defects	
Confusion	
Seizures	

Immune System	Hematologic System
Infection resistance decreased	Easy bruising
Burnout of immune disorders	Anemia
Neoplasms increased	Bleeding tendency

What metabolic disturbances are features of uremia?

There are three primary types.

Carbohydrate abnormalities. Nondiabetics with ESRD have abnormal glucose metabolism. Cellular sensitivity to insulin is reduced. After a glucose load, peak blood sugar is near normal, but the rate of decline is slow.

When ESRD is the result of insulin-dependent diabetes mellitus (onset before age 35), peripheral cellular resistance to insulin is especially severe. Violent swings between hypo- and hyperglycemia are frequent. Total insulin needs decrease somewhat after the patient begins dialysis, but wide swings of blood glucose and problems with insulin dosage continue because of the decreased ability of the kidney to metabolize insulin and consequent increase in the half-life of insulin.

Most diabetic ESRD in the United States is of noninsulin-dependent type. Such patients are usually obese and have a resistance to insulin. Most are improved by weight reduction and increased activity. Many patients respond to oral hypoglycemic agents.

Lipid metabolism. Type 4 hyperlipoproteinemia is common. The elevated very low density lipoproteins (VLDLs) are somewhat different from the usual VLDLs, which may be a result of reduced hepatic lipoprotein lipase activity, possibly related to insulin resistance. Carnitine deficiency has also been suggested to have a role.

Protein metabolism. Protein calorie malnutrition is common. Loss of lean tissue mass is masked by an increase in body water with occult edema. Serum albumin tends to be low because of poor protein intake, although impaired hepatic synthesis may play a part. Several nonessential amino acids are elevated, while certain essential polypeptides are decreased.

What are the hematologic abnormalities in uremia?

Anemia is the most common and severe hematologic defect. Production of erythropoietin is decreased in the failed kidney, causing reduced red blood cell (RBC) formation in bone marrow. Red blood cell life span is also reduced from the normal 120 days to half that number. In turn, aluminum excess causes microcytosis of red blood cells (RBCs) and resistance to administered recombinant erythropoietin.

Finally, bleeding problems are the result of platelet defects in release or adhesion. The defect corrects quickly with dialysis.

Why are infections a problem?

Leukocyte abnormalities include reduced white blood cell (WBC) count in some patients. Granulocytes have reduced response to infection and low bactericidal activity. In fact, infection is the second most common cause of death in ESRD patients. Susceptibility is enhanced by malnutrition and by immune system defects.

What are the immunologic defects?

There are both humoral and cellular defects. In addition to increased susceptibility to infection, there is burnout in some immune disorders, such as lupus, and failure to respond to the hepatitis vaccine. Risk of cancer is increased. White blood cell function is decreased in uremia, but improves after dialysis with biocompatible membranes.

What are some gastrointestinal manifestations of uremia?

Uremic individuals have poor appetite and are often nauseated. Altered taste and dry mouth are common. Gastrointestinal bleeding, often occult, is aggravated by medications (aspirin, heparin) and by the platelet defects. Functional constipation is frequent in patients on dialysis.

What neurologic changes occur with uremia?

Fatigue, slow mentation, sleep disturbances, anxiety, depression, and agitation are common. Seizures occur if azotemia increases rapidly. Electroencephalographic changes (increased slow wave activity) occur and are related to increased parathyroid hormone (PTH) level. Calcium content of brain tissue is increased, and brain aluminum is elevated.

Peripheral neuropathy may present as burning feet, twitching, restless legs, reduced vibratory sensation, and decreased reflexes. The latter relate to slowed nerve conduction velocity, present in most ESRD patients. A motor neuropathy or myopathy may present as weakness of proximal muscles of arms and legs.

What skeletal changes are seen with uremia?

All ESRD patients have bone changes of some degree. These are part of the broad entity, renal osteodystrophy. Kidney failure causes retention of phosphate. There is also failure of conversion of vitamin D_3 to 1,25 dihydroxycholecalciferol, the metabolically active form of vitamin D. This causes reduced calcium uptake at the intestine. Even very slight reduction in plasma ionized calcium results in increased secretion of PTH by the parathyroids. PTH stimulates osteoclast cells in bone to mobilize calcium, leaving a fibrotic marrow space. This is *osteitis fibrosa*.

Osteomalacia results from the defect in the formation of $1,25(OH)_2 D_3$, causing impaired mineralization of new bone tissue (osteoid). Osteomalacia is also induced by aluminum accumulation.

Bone pain, fractures, and vertebral compressions are frequent in severe renal osteodystrophy. After some time on dialysis, some patients develop carpal tunnel syndrome, or shoulder or hip girdle pain. This relates to β-2 microglobulin accumulation with amyloid deposits in bone, joints, and periarticular tissues. Small bone cysts and an erosive arthropathy visualize on imaging.

What endocrine abnormalities occur in uremia?

Changes in insulin production and effect, and parathyroid hormone perturbations have been mentioned. Most other endocrine systems are also affected by uremia. These include:

- Plasma norepinephrine levels are increased; epinephrine values are inconsistent.
- Cortisol levels are near normal, with a normal response to adrenocorticotropic hormone (ACTH). Aldosterone is increased.
- Both glucagon and gastrin values are elevated. This results from loss of renal metabolic clearance.
- Hypothyroidism is more frequent in ESRD patients than in the general population. Euthyroid individuals on dialysis have low total thyroxine

(T_4) and T_3 values and reduced free T_3, while free T_4 is normal. Conversion of T_4 to T_3 in peripheral tissue is reduced. Thyroid-binding globulin is low. Thyroid-stimulating hormone (TSH) is mostly normal, but the response to thyroid-releasing hormone (TRH) is reduced.

- Besides ACTH and TSH, the anterior pituitary produces four other hormones that are affected by uremia. Growth hormone and prolactin are increased. There is both increased production and decreased elimination. No systemic effect has been attributed to the elevation of either hormone.

Follicle-stimulating hormone (FSH) and luteinizing hormone (LH) each have critical roles in the pituitary-gonadal axis in both sexes. Production of abnormal estrogen and progesterone, or testosterone, by the gonads in uremia adversely influences the feedback mechanisms to the pituitary gland. LH levels are elevated in both men and women. FSH values are normal or minimally increased in both. End effects include testicular atrophy, low sperm count, and impotence in men, and dysmenorrhea or amenorrhea in women. Infertility is usual for both men and women. There is accumulating evidence that patients receiving recombinant human erthyropoietin have fewer sexual problems of this sort. Much of the data is subjective. A number of objective studies support reductions of prolactin and growth hormone after administration of erythropoietin, but the mechanism is not clear. It is also unclear whether the effects that have been noted are the result of correction of anemia or are due to some specific effect of erythropoietin.

Principles of
Hemodialysis

C. F. Gutch

REVIEW OF HEMODIALYSIS

Thomas Graham, a London chemist, reported the principles of the semipermeable membrane in 1861 and gave the process of selective diffusion the name
dialysis. Then, in 1913, Abel, Rowntree, and Turner devised an apparatus for the
dialysis of blood, using a number of collodion tubes, through which blood was
flowed while a saline solution bathed the outside of the tubes. (See Fig. 4-1.)
This device was used successfully to treat animals with uremia. Later, Kolff and
Berk developed the first clinically successful artificial kidney, after the development of heparin for anticoagulation and the ready availability of cellulose in the
form of cellophane tubing. They employed a rotating drum of wood slats around
which a spiral of cellophane tubing was wrapped. The lower portion of the drum
was immersed in a bath of dialysis fluid, while the blood was propelled along
the tubing by rotating of the drum. In 1948, Skeggs and Leonards first developed a parallel plate dialyzer; the first disposable dialyzer was the Travenol
twin-coil unit, marketed in 1956. About 1965, Gambro began production of disposable parallel plate devices, while at the same time hollow-fiber artificial kidneys were developed in the United States.

Fig. 4-1 Vividiffusion apparatus of Abel, Rowntree, and Turner. (Adapted from Nosé Y:
Manual on artificial organs, vol 1: The artificial kidney, St. Louis, 1969, Mosby.)

SOLUTE TRANSFER

What does hemodialysis mean?

Hemo, of course, means blood. *Dialysis* connotes a separation or filtration process. Metabolic wastes or toxins are filtered from the blood by a semipermeable membrane and carried away by the dialysis fluid.

What waste products are removed by dialysis?

A large number of substances accumulate in uremia (see Chapter 3). The molecular size of many of these is less than 500 daltons. They diffuse readily across cellulosic membranes. Particles in the range of 500 to 2000 d, sometimes called middle molecules, diffuse poorly across such membranes. Polypeptides in this size range have been suspected of causing some uremic symptoms, although this has never been proven. Molecules larger than 3000 daltons are not generally regarded as toxic, with the exception of beta$_2$-microglobulin (11,800 daltons) and its relation to amyloid, bone disease and anemia.

What is a semipermeable membrane?

The semipermeable membrane acts as a sieve. It may be thought of as having submicroscopic openings or pores. Solute particles larger than these openings cannot pass through and are retained. Those particles small enough to pass do so at a rate inverse to their size: very small particles traverse more rapidly than those somewhat larger.

How does the semipermeable membrane function in hemodialysis?

The patient's blood is passed through a compartment formed by the membrane. Dialyzing fluid surrounds this compartment. Red cells, white cells, platelets, and most plasma proteins are too large to pass through the pores of the membrane. Water and small particles such as electrolytes cross by diffusion (see Fig. 4-2), as do urea (60 d), creatinine (113 d), and glucose (184 d).

What is diffusion?

Molecules in solution are in constant motion and seek to spread uniformly throughout the solution. The rate of spread depends on the concentration, size, and electric charge of the particles. Diffusion of particles across a semipermeable membrane is the basis of dialysis.

Why are all the solutes and water in blood not removed by the dialyzer?

The dialysis fluid is an electrolyte solution similar in composition to normal plasma water. Water molecules cross the membrane in both directions, as do

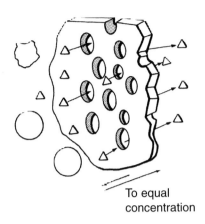

To equal
concentration

Fig. 4-2 Semipermeable membrane.

electrolytes and other small particles. Only if the concentration of a particular kind of particle is greater on one side than on the other will there be a net flow from the side of high concentration to the side of lower concentration. This is the concentration gradient.

Are there membranes permeable to middle and large molecules?

There are several synthetic materials that are used for high flux dialysis. These include polyacrylonitrile (PAN), polycarbonate, polysulfone, polyamide, polymethylmethacrylate (PMMA), and other membrane materials.

What is mass transfer rate or solute flux?

Artificial kidneys are designed to remove metabolic wastes from the body, restore water and electrolyte balance, and correct acid/base disturbances. The dialysis process involves transport of unwanted or excess solute and excess water from the blood across a semipermeable membrane. The engineering term for such transport is *mass transfer*, and the rate of movement is the mass transfer rate, or solute flux.

What factors affect mass transfer rate?

Flux, at a constant temperature, is governed by the solute concentration gradient and the physical characteristics of the dialyzer. The latter include effective membrane surface area, membrane permeability, blood and fluid flow rates, and flow geometry. The mass transfer rate varies continually throughout the course of a clinical dialysis procedure.

TRANSPORT

What is meant by diffusive transport?

As noted above, solute particles diffuse through the dialysis membrane from the side of higher concentration to the lower. This movement is termed diffusive transport or, less commonly, conductive transport.

What determines the rate of diffusive transport?

The rate of transfer depends on:
- The concentration gradient across the membrane for each solute.
- The surface area of the membrane; the greater the area, the more solute moved per unit time.
- The mass transfer coefficient for the solute of interest for the particular membrane. The mass transfer coefficient increases for thinner or more porous membranes. It also is affected by the flow rates of both blood and dialysis fluid.

What is convective transport?

When water moves across a membrane because of a pressure gradient (ultrafiltration), there is a friction effect on solute molecules, called *solvent drag*. This associated solute movement is termed *convective transport* (Latin *convectus*, "carried together").

What is the sieving coefficient?

The amount of solute convected across a membrane in proportion to the quantity of fluid ultrafiltrated depends on particle size relative to pore size. If the pore/particle ratio is high, there is no restriction of solute transfer and the sieving coefficient is said to be 1.0. If none of the particles can be squeezed through, the sieving coefficient is zero.

What is the importance of convective transport?

Solute particles larger than 500 daltons may have a low sieving coefficient, but because of their low diffusive transport, the convective component becomes a major fraction of their total transfer. Convective transport is of prime importance in high-flux hemodialysis and in the techniques of continuous arteriovenous hemofiltration, CAV hemodialysis, and diafiltration.

What is meant by clearance?

Clearance is an empirical measure indicating a calculated volume of blood completely cleared of a substance (x) in 1 minute. It is a *theoretical* volume, not a real volume.

How is the clearance concept applied to a hemodialyzer?

The clearance of x, referred to as Kx, is expressed as:

$$Kx = \frac{Q_b \cdot (C_i - C_o)}{C_i}$$

where Q_b = blood flow rate (ml/min)
C_i = concentration of x at blood inflow (mg/dL)
C_o = concentration of x at outflow blood line (mg/dL)

This expression does not allow for convective transport and is not applicable for high-flux devices.

How is clearance determined for high-flux dialyzers?

The equation is modified to take account of ultrafiltration, thus:

$$Kx = \frac{(Q_{bi} \cdot C_{bi}) - (Q_{bo} \cdot C_{bo})}{C_{bi}}$$

where Q_{bi} = blood flow rate in inlet
C_{bi} = concentration of x in blood at inlet
Q_{bo} = blood flow rate at outlet
C_{bo} = concentration of x in outflow blood

This is termed the *whole blood clearance*. However, solutes diffuse from or are convected by only the water component of blood. Red cells are 72% water; plasma is 93% water. Therefore, for 100 ml (1 dL) of blood of hematocrit 30%:

$$0.72 \times 30 = 21.6$$
$$+ \ 0.93 \times 70 = 65.1$$

volume of blood water cleared = 86.7 ml

It is much more accurate, when evaluating high-flux equipment, to calculate Kx, from the dialysis fluid side:

$$Kx = \frac{Q_{do} \cdot C_{do}}{C_{bi}}$$

where Q_{do} = dialysate outflow rate
C_{do} = concentration of x in dialysate outflow
C_{bi} = concentration of x in inflow blood

ULTRAFILTRATION

Controlled fluid removal at dialysis is essential. Coil dialyzers had high internal resistance; the pressure necessary to maintain blood flow established a positive hydrostatic gradient, causing water to cross the membrane. This was called *ultrafiltration*. Kiil dialyzers had low internal resistance, and negative pressure on the fluid side provided the hydrostatic gradient. Most current dialyzers utilize elements of both positive blood compartment pressure and negative fluid compartment pressure (Fig. 4-3).

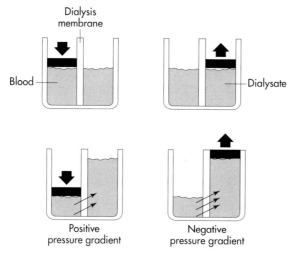

Fig. 4-3 Ultrafiltration. (Adapted from Nosé Y: *Manual on artificial organs, vol 1: The artificial kidney,* St. Louis, 1969, Mosby.)

How does the hydrostatic gradient operate?

The difference in hydrostatic pressure, blood to fluid, represents the *transmembrane pressure* (TMP). The rate of ultrafiltration is a function of: (1) mean transmembrane pressure, (2) a coefficient peculiar to the particular membrane, (3) membrane area, and (4) the geometry of the dialyzer.

$$TMP = \left(\frac{P_{bi} + P_{bo}}{2} \right) - \left(\frac{P_{di} + P_{do}}{2} \right)$$

where P_{bi} = pressure at the blood inlet
P_{bo} = pressure at the blood outlet
P_{di} = pressure at the fluid inlet
P_{do} = pressure at the fluid outlet

What is the relationship between the hydrostatic pressure and the ultrafiltration rate?

For a particular dialyzer, at any given TMP, a certain amount of fluid will be removed per unit time at specific blood and fluid flow rates. During the investigational phase of a new dialyzer, an average ultrafiltration rate per mm Hg TMP is calculated. This is the ultrafiltration coefficient (k_{UF}) and is unique to each dialyzer. The relationship is expressed:

$$UFR = k_{UF} \cdot TMP$$

where   UFR = ultrafiltration rate (ml/hr)
$\qquad$ k_{UF} = ultrafiltration coefficient (ml/mm Hg TMP)
$\qquad$ TMP = transmembrane pressure (mm Hg)

This relation is depicted in Fig. 4-4. The curves start at about 25 mm Hg rather than at zero TMP because of the osmotic effect of plasma proteins attracting fluid into the blood compartment. For Cuprophan and similar membranes, the ultrafiltration coefficient is 2 to 8 ml/hour/mm Hg, and the slope is a straight line. The k_{UF} of cellulose acetate is about double that amount. High-flux dialyzers have a k_{UF} of 20 to 70 ml/hour/mm Hg; the slope is much steeper, but reaches a plateau at very high TMP. At such levels the solvent drag effect causes caking of plasma protein on the membrane, reducing permeability.

How does the blood flow rate relate to hydrostatic pressure?

The Hagen-Poiseuille equation expresses this:

$$Q = \frac{\pi(\Delta p)R^4}{8\,\mu L} \qquad \text{or} \qquad \Delta p = \frac{Q \cdot 8\,\mu L}{\pi R^4}$$

where   Q = volumetric flow rate
$\qquad$ Δp = fluid pressure drop
$\qquad$ R = internal radius of tube
$\qquad$ μ = fluid viscosity
$\qquad$ L = length of channel

In clinical use of dialyzers this may be applied:

$$\text{Flowrate } (Q_B) = \frac{\text{Pressure (P)}}{\text{Resistance (R)}}$$

Most hemodialysis systems use a blood pump. The blood pump is occlusive; each revolution of the pump moves an approximate volume of blood. The

Fig. 4-4   Ultrafiltration vs. TMP cellulosic and high-flux membranes. UF starts at about 25 mm Hg because of plasma oncotic pressure. (Redrawn from Jacobson JR, Striker GE, Klahr S, editors: *The principles and practice of nephrology,* St. Louis, 1995, Mosby.)

left side of the equation is determined by the speed of the blood pump. The pressure generated (P) will be that necessary to overcome the resistance (R) in the blood circuit.

What affects the resistance in the blood circuit?

The two major components are: (1) the viscosity of the blood and (2) the geometry of the blood pathway.

1. Viscosity is largely a matter of hematocrit. The viscosity of blood of 30% hematocrit is approximately 2.3–2.5 centipose, about 2 to 2 1/2 times that of water.
2. Several aspects are important to the geometry of the blood pathway:
   - Length of the pathway. Hollow-fiber dialyzers have low resistance because of the short (15 to 50 cm) pathway.
   - Number of pathways. With a large number of pathways, the divided resistance is lower. Hollow-fiber dialyzers have several thousand pathways and have low resistance.
   - Cross-sectional area of the pathway. A large cross-sectional pathway has low resistance; a small one has high resistance. For hollow-fiber dialyzers, the control factor is the internal radius of the fiber.

How is the amount of ultrafiltration controlled during hemodialysis?

In the past, control of ultrafiltration was sought by manipulating the transmembrane pressure (TMP). Blood outlet and fluid inlet pressures, critical variables in the calculation, are often inexact. The k_{UF} information provided by manufacturers is most often based on in vitro studies and may differ from actual patient experience by as much as plus or minus 30 percent. Even with conventional cellulosic membranes and blood flow rates of 200 to 300 ml/min, wide discrepancies between planned and actual fluid removal may occur. With use of high-efficiency or high-flux dialysis, precision in ultrafiltration management became crucial, leading to development of equipment to directly control ultrafiltration on a minute-to-minute basis.

How do ultrafiltration controls function?

There are two basic systems: (1) volumetric or balancing type and (2) servo-feedback or flow sensor type (see Chapter 5).

In the volumetric system, inflow and outflow through the fluid compartment are exactly balanced by special pumps. A separate pump removes fluid from this closed loop at a rate set by the operator. This creates negative pressure in the fluid loop, causing ultrafiltration across the membrane to match the rate of fluid removal.

The servo-feedback system uses very sensitive flowmeters to constantly monitor dialysis fluid inflow and outflow. This information feeds into a microprocessor that subtracts dialysate inflow (Q_{di}) from dialysate outflow (Q_{do}) to determine rate of ultrafiltration (Q_{uf}) continuously. The desired ultrafiltration rate is programmed by the operator; the microprocessor adjusts TMP so that measured Q_{uf} matches desired Q_{uf}.

Direct ultrafiltration control systems, when operating correctly, achieve a plus or minus 10 percent accuracy in volume of fluid removal.

What shifts occur between intracellular/extracellular fluid compartments during hemodialysis?

Ultrafiltration can rapidly remove fluid from the vascular compartment. If the rate of removal exceeds the repletion rate from interstitial space, hypovolemia and hypotension occur. Infusion of hypertonic saline will increase osmolality in both the vascular and extravascular spaces. This, in turn, will attract fluid from the much longer intracellular pool and avoid the hypovolemia that causes the low blood pressure.

What is sodium modeling?

This procedure involves the development of a computer model of sodium and water movement between compartments during dialysis. Sodium content of the dialysis fluid is varied during the procedure according to the preprogrammed plan. This may be done in either of two ways: (1) addition of a special NaCl concentrate to the dialysis fluid by an infusion pump, or (2) varying the proportion of the usual concentrate as the fluid is mixed, thus changing the final sodium concentration. For example, a commonly used proportioning yields a dialysis fluid sodium of 140 mEq/L; a 10 percent increase in the amount of concentrate as it is mixed increases the final fluid sodium to 154 mEq/L, with only minor quantitative changes in other electrolyte concentrations such as potassium and calcium.

How is acid-base balance achieved during hemodialysis?

When continuous fluid proportioning systems were introduced in 1963, bicarbonate could not be used in the concentrate because the calcium and magnesium precipitated. Sodium acetate, which the body metabolizes to bicarbonate, was substituted, avoiding the precipitation problem. Acetate-based concentrate became standard for many years. It had several disadvantages, particularly the production of cardiovascular instability.

Introduction of short, rapid dialysis and high-flux dialysis made the return to bicarbonate-based fluid mandatory for these procedures. Bicarbonate dialysate is now the standard of practice at most facilities.

How is bicarbonate used in dialysis fluid production?

The concentrate to be used is packaged in two parts. The "acid concentrate" contains chemicals other than sodium bicarbonate, plus a small amount of acid. The "bicarbonate concentrate" has the sodium bicarbonate and some sodium chloride (necessary to increase conductivity for monitoring purposes). Three streams of fluid are blended by the proportioning equipment: (1) water (34 parts); (2) acid concentrate (1 part); and (3) bicarbonate concentrate (1.8 parts).

Different types of equipment utilize concentrates of different composition and different mixing proportions. *Accidental use of mismatched concentrate is a potentially fatal error.*

What is reverse filtration?

During high-flux dialysis the ultrafiltration control system prevents excessive net fluid removal. The process generates a blood/dialysis fluid profile within the dialyzer that is positive (blood-to-fluid) near the blood inlet, but which may, under some circumstances, become negative (fluid-to-blood) toward the outlet. The movement of dialysis fluid into the blood is termed "reverse filtration."

What is the significance of reverse filtration?

The water used in preparation of dialysis fluid is not sterile. Addition of bicarbonate concentrate encourages and supports bacterial proliferation. Endotoxin and breakdown products form and may be carried across the high-flux membrane into the bloodstream when reverse filtration occurs. Pyrogen reactions as well as other adverse effects may occur.

How can the effects of reverse filtration be countered?

A molecular filter (ultrafilter) can be placed in the fluid delivery line just ahead of the dialyzer. These devices use ultrafiltration membranes to remove suspended particles of molecular size, but not dissolved solutes. Bacteria and pyrogen or pyrogen fragments are rejected by the ultrafilter (see Chapter 6).

QUANTIFICATION OF DIALYSIS

Since the 1970s there have been many efforts to define how much dialysis is needed to keep a given patient in an adequate state of health. Some of these included the "square meter hour hypothesis," the "middle molecule hypothesis," the Dialysis Index, and others. One of these is the urea Kt/V index.

What is the urea Kt/V index?

Urea is a good small molecule marker because its level correlates well with the nutritional state of the individual and with protein catabolism. The urea Kt/V index is the result of complex mathematical modeling of urea kinetics. K is the dialyzer clearance of urea (ml/min), t represents dialysis time (in minutes), and V indicates the volume of distribution of urea in body fluid. V is not a real volume that can be measured. It is derived from pharmacokinetic modeling and involves more than one fluid pool and rates of transfer between them. These cannot be directly measured.

Enthusiasm varies for the use of the Kt/V index to predict the amount of dialysis time necessary. An optimum value for maximum patient well-being over an extended period of time has not been established. Most target values proposed in the past have proven inadequate. The N.I.H. Conference Committee in 1996 recommended a minimum Kt/V of 1.2. For more information regarding Kt/V, see later discussions of nutrition management.

Dialyzers, Dialysate, and Delivery Systems

Mark Rolston, Peter W. Gardner, Patt Peterson, and C. F. Gutch

The dialyzer is a selective filter for removing toxic or unwanted solutes from the blood. The filtration process uses a semipermeable membrane between blood flowing on one side and dialysis fluid, called dialysate, flowing on the opposite side. The delivery system *prepares* dialysate of correct chemical composition, and then *delivers* it at proper temperature and other parameters to the dialyzer.

All dialyzers consist of a series of parallel flow paths designed to provide a large surface area between blood and membrane, and membrane and dialysate. There are two basic flow path geometries: (1) rectangular cross section, seen in parallel plate dialyzers, and (2) circular cross section, seen in hollow fiber dialyzers.

How does dialyzer surface area relate to flow path design?

For rectangular flow path design, the surface area is:

$$A = 2 \cdot L \cdot W \cdot N$$

where L = length of each flow path
W = width of flow path
N = number of flow paths

For circular cross section:

$$A = 2 \cdot \pi \cdot R \cdot L \cdot N$$

where R = radius of circular passage

How is dialyzer blood volume affected by blood passage design?

Blood volume (V_b) is determined by:

$$V_b = W \cdot H \cdot L \cdot N \text{ (rectangular passages)}$$

where   H = blood film thickness (height)

and

$$V_b = \pi \cdot R^2 \cdot L \cdot N \text{ (circular passages)}$$

Is flow resistance related to the flow path design?

From Poiseuille's law, the drop in pressure (P_b) for rectangular cross section is expressed:

$$\Delta P_b = Q_b \cdot \frac{12 \cdot \mu \cdot L}{N \cdot W \cdot H}$$

where μ = blood viscosity (poise)

Qb = blood flow rate (ml/min)

For circular cross section, the equation becomes:

$$\Delta P_b = Q_b \cdot \frac{8 \cdot \mu \cdot L}{N \cdot \pi \cdot R^4}$$

PARALLEL PLATE DIALYZERS

What are characteristics of plate dialyzers?

They are assembled in layers, like a sandwich. Sheets of membrane are placed between supporting plates, which have ridges, grooves, or cross hatches to support the membrane and allow the flow of dialysate along it. The contained volume of blood is small, and heparin requirements are also usually small. The main disadvantage of plate dialyzers is that they are not well suited for reuse.

HOLLOW-FIBER DIALYZERS

The hollow-fiber artificial kidney (HFAK) is by far the most commonly used dialyzer. HFAKs are available in a wide variety of sizes and membranes.

What serves as the semipermeable membrane in the HFAK?

Tiny hollow fibers of about 150 to 250 μm in diameter are used. They are formed from a variety of materials, cellulosic and synthetic. Wall thickness may be as little as 7 μm, although some synthetics have walls of 50 μm or more (Fig. 5-1).

Fig. 5-1   Hollow-fiber dialyzer.

What are advantages of hollow-fiber dialyzers?

The contained blood volume is very low in relation to their surface area because of their geometry. Resistance to blood flow is low because of the large number of blood passages. Ultrafiltration can be precisely controlled. They are well adapted to reuse.

What are disadvantages of the HFAK?

- Meticulous deaeration of the fiber bundle is required before beginning a dialysis procedure. Otherwise, fibers may air lock and not admit blood.
- There may be uneven distribution of blood at the inflow header space, with reduced perfusion of some of the center fibers.
- Residual toxic products of ethylene oxide sterilization retained in the potting material of the headers can cause adverse patient reactions.

Are there other ways to sterilize hollow fiber dialyzers?

Yes. Some producers use gamma irradiation. Other manufacturers employ steam sterilization. Both methods are effective.

MEMBRANES FOR HEMODIALYSIS

Membranes used in hemodialysis are of two basic types: (1) organic cellulose derivatives, and (2) synthetic membranes.

Willem Kolff used cellulose sausage casings for the first successful clinical dialysis. Cellulosic membranes continue to be basic for many dialyzers. Synthetic membranes were developed in the search for efficient, large-volume sea water desalinization by reverse osmosis. The development of volume-controlled ultrafiltration equipment for hemodialysis made the use of these high hydraulic permeability membranes practical. They, in turn, have made high-flux hemodialysis, hemofiltration and continuous renal replacement therapy (CRRT) viable options in renal treatment.

What is the nature of a cellulosic membrane?

Cellulose $(C_6H_{10}O_5)_n$ is a complex carbohydrate polymer that is the structural material of plants. Commercial cellulose is obtained from wood products and cotton. Treatment with heat and chemicals produces a liquid slurry, which is coagulated and formed into sheets, or extruded through dies as hollow fibers. Different kinds of processing result in membranes of various thicknesses, water absorptive qualities, and permeabilities.

What accounts for the permeability of cellulosic membranes?

Electron microscopy shows that the fibers of cellulose membranes swell when wet, forming a tortuous maze. The "pores" are actually twisting, irregular tunnels that force a water or a solute molecule to travel a distance several times the thickness of the membrane to get through it.

What are some cellulose membranes now used in hemodialysis?

Cuprophan has been widely used. The cellulose is treated with ammonia and copper oxide during manufacture; Cuprammonium rayon and Hemophan are modifications. Saponified cellulose ester, cellulose acetate and triacetate are other widely used cellulose materials.

What are the advantages and disadvantages of cellulose membranes?

One distinct advantage is the fact that they have been used for many years, and their transport characteristics are well known. They are also relatively inexpensive. However, all the cellulosic membranes have some degree of bioincompatibility with blood. This poses a number of problems, which will be discussed later in this chapter.

What are features of synthetic membranes?

These synthetics are thermoplastics. They have a thin, smooth luminal surface supported by a sponge-like wall structure. Those used for hemodialysis include polyacrylonitrile (AN, PAN), polysulfone, polyamide, polymethylmethacrylate (PMMA), and others. Convective transfer accounts for their overall mass transport. All have ultrafiltration coefficients of 20 to 70 ml/hr/mm Hg or more. They are well adapted to reuse. Synthetics have much fewer bioincompatibility problems than cellulose membranes.

What are negative aspects of synthetic membranes?

There are several negative aspects:
- They are expensive in comparison to cellulosics.
- Automated ultrafiltration control is required because of the very high water permeability.
- Adsorption of proteins to the membrane surface can be a problem.
- The high permeability creates a risk of backfiltration from dialysate to blood.

MEMBRANE BIOCOMPATIBILITY

Each time blood comes in contact with a foreign surface, an inflammatory response is elicited. This response is used to gauge the biocompatibility of a hemodialysis membrane. When there is an intense reaction and a high level of inflammation, the membrane is said to be bioincompatible. When the response and inflammation are mild, the membrane is classified as biocompatible. The level of membrane biocompatibility may be associated with both short- and long-term consequences.

How does one measure the level of inflammatory response resulting from blood/membrane interaction during hemodialysis?

The intensity of the reaction is measured by the level of complement generation following initiation of hemodialysis. Markers used to evaluate complement activation are C3a, C5a, and the "Membrane Attack Complex"—C5b through C9—in the patient's blood.

What is complement activation?

The complement system is a series of plasma proteins that react sequentially to cause a variety of biological events. This system works with the immune system to defend the body from substances that the body determines to be "non-self." When blood encounters a hemodialysis membrane, the response elicited is similar to that occurring when the body's immune system is challenged by bacteria.

What are some of the intra-dialytic manifestations of complement activation?

The first clinical manifestation to be associated with complement activation is leukopenia. Immediately after starting hemodialysis using cellulosic membrane, patients' white cell counts drop sharply. This begins to correct after about fifteen minutes. By the end of a four-hour dialysis, the white cell count will be back to the initial level or perhaps slightly higher, due to a compensatory response by the bone marrow.

This leukopenia is transient, but it may be important to patients with compromised cardiac or pulmonary systems. C5a, an end product of the complement cascade, activates white cells. When white cells are activated, they become "sticky." These cells aggregate, or clump, and are sequestered in the first capillary bed they encounter, usually the lungs. The clumps of white cells reduce pulmonary capillary perfusion, and reduce the patient's ability to efficiently exchange oxygen and CO_2 between blood and alveolar air. This may be manifested as an intra-dialytic hypoxemia.

Other intra-dialytic problems likely associated with complement activation include chest pain, back pain, coagulation abnormalities, and in severe cases, anaphylaxis. Activation of complement peaks at fifteen minutes and can last as long as 90 minutes. The amount of complement generated relates to the type and surface area of the membrane being used.

Which membranes induce the highest levels of complement activation?

Cellulose and cellulose-based membranes induce more complement activation than do synthetic membranes. The chemical composition of the cellulosic surface is similar to that of the cell wall of bacteria: both are chains of polysaccharide structures. The body responds to blood-cellulose contact much the same as it does to invasion by bacteria. Free hydroxyl groups on the membrane surface are likely the primary source of the intense complement activation. Chemical alterations to buffer the free hydroxyl groups are used to create "modified cellulosic membranes" like cellulose acetate and hemophan. Membranes of cellulose acetate have some of the surface hydroxyl linked with acetyl groups. Hemophan membranes have amino groups attached to the reactive sites to buffer them. Both of these modifications reduce the amount of complement generated; however, these membranes are still less effective than synthetics in minimizing complement production.

Why do synthetic membranes induce less complement than cellulosic membranes?

Being synthetic, they lack the reactive sites found on cellulose-based membranes; thus the amount of complement generated during hemodialysis is less than with cellulosic membrane.

What are some of the long-term considerations when selecting a membrane for hemodialysis?

Long-term use of bioincompatible membranes may be associated with an increased incidence of infection and malignancy, and impaired nutritional status. Patients dialyzed on cellulose membranes have a higher incidence of beta$_2$ amyloid disease than those on synthetics. The increased risk of infection and malignancy is thought to be due to repeated attacks on the patient's immune system.

When patient blood is repeatedly exposed to bioincompatible surfaces, the body responds as though under attack. The immune system kicks in, complement is generated, and the inflammatory response is triggered. There can be tissue damage, and future stimuli may elicit only a limited response, thus predisposing the individual to infection and potential malignancy.

Malnutrition is a major contributor to morbidity and mortality of persons on hemodialysis. Even with adequate protein intake, malnutrition is a problem and seems to relate to an accelerated catabolic process, most evident on dialysis days. A catabolic effect associated with bioincompatible membrane is well documented. Degradation of 15–20 grams of muscle protein during a 150-minute exposure to cellulose membrane has been described (Guiterrez A et al., 1990). Beta$_2$ amyloid disease is important in long-term morbidity. Clinical manifestations include arthropathies, bone lesions and pathological fractures, soft tissue swelling, and carpal tunnel syndrome. Incidence of B$_2$AD is 25 percent greater for persons dialyzed with cellulosic membranes than synthetics (Floege J et al., 1991). Possible reasons for the difference include:

- Cellulose membranes do not have the capability to remove molecules as large as β$_2$-microglobulin.
- Cellulose membranes induce high levels of complement generation, and some products of complement activation may be responsible for the release of β$_2$-microglobulin from monocytes.

How does membrane biocompatibility affect patients with some residual renal function?

In one study, patients dialyzed on cellulose acetate membranes appeared to lose residual renal function more rapidly than those dialyzed with polysulfone membrane.

Does biocompatibility of the membrane affect patients in acute renal failure?

This is not clear. There is a consensus that the more compatible membranes do contribute to better recovery and survival. Less complement activation, less white cell activation, and less inflammation associated with more biocompatible membranes are believed responsible.

DIALYZER REUSE

What are the advantages of reuse?

Fundamentally, the average cost per dialysis is substantially reduced. The "first-use syndrome," an infrequent phenomenon of chest or back pain, nausea, and malaise occurring in the first half hour of a run with a new cellulose dialyzer, is absent or rare with reused dialyzers.

What are disadvantages of reuse?

Processing, testing, identification, and storage of reused units requires space and personnel time. Consumption of high-quality water is greatly increased. Sterilizing agents, particularly formaldehyde, are a hazard to personnel and to patients. Quality control of manual processing is difficult to ensure. Automated systems minimize these problems, but at high initial cost.

Are there guidelines for reuse procedures?

Yes. Guidelines were defined by the Association for the Advancement of Medical Instrumentation (AAMI) and subsequently given the force of law by the Food and Drug Administration (FDA). See Chapter 7, "Dialyzer Preparation", for more on reuse of dialyzers.

DELIVERY SYSTEMS

The delivery system prepares and delivers dialysate to the dialyzer unit. Most systems provide dialysate for a single patient; others have the capacity to supply several dialyzer stations simultaneously.

What are the functions of dialysate?

Dialysate carries away the waste materials and fluid removed from the blood by the dialysis procedure, prevents the removal of essential electrolytes, and averts excess water removal during the procedure. These functions are achieved by making the chemical composition of the dialysate correspond as nearly as possible to that of normal plasma water.

What chemicals are used?

There are usually five compounds involved: sodium chloride, sodium bicarbonate or sodium acetate, calcium chloride, potassium chloride, and magnesium chloride. Glucose may be included in some formulations.

How are the chemicals made into dialysate?

Manufacturers provide dialysis concentrate in various sized containers. The sodium chloride content is near saturation, and the other constituents are in proportion to their final concentration in the dialysate. There is some equipment for making concentrate on site from dry chemicals, reducing transportation costs. The use of acetate rather than bicarbonate in concentrate avoids the problem of precipitation of calcium and magnesium due to the high pH of bicarbonate. The acetate is physiologically compatible with blood, and is metabolized to bicarbonate in the liver. However, acetate dialysate is not suited for rapid, high-efficiency dialysis or high-flux dialysis. The serum bicarbonate becomes depleted, and the acetate level's elevation may exceed the rate at which it can be metabolized by the liver. Only a small proportion of patients in the United States continue on acetate dialysate.

How is bicarbonate-based dialysate prepared?

Calcium and magnesium will not remain in a solution with bicarbonate because of the low hydrogen ion content. To solve this, two separate concentrates are used. The proportioning (delivery) system is more complex, since it must mix and monitor three liquids instead of only two.

What chemicals are in the bicarbonate concentrates?

The "A" (indicating acidified) concentrate contains most of the sodium, all of the calcium, magnesium and potassium, chloride, and a small amount of acetic acid to maintain pH low enough to keep the calcium and magnesium in solution when mixed into dialysate.

The "B" (bicarbonate) concentrate contains the sodium bicarbonate. Some systems include part of the sodium chloride as well as the "B" concentrate; this raises the total conductivity, making it easier to monitor the concentrate. Table 5-1 shows the tabular formula used with one volume-volume type dilution.

In the proportioning system, the "B" concentrate is usually diluted partially with water; the "A" concentrate is then proportioned into the mixture just before it goes to the dialyzer. In the closed system, CO_2 cannot bubble off, the reaction between sodium bicarbonate and acetic acid cannot proceed to completion, and the hydrogen ion content keeps the calcium in solution.

Table 5-1 Tabular Formula for One Volume-Volume Type Dilution

| Component | mEq/L in Final Dilution | | | | | | |
	Na^+	K^+	Ca^{++}	Mg^{++}	Cl^-	HCO_3^-	CH_3COO^-
Concentrate B	59				20	39.0	
Concentrate A	81	2.0	3.5	0.7	87.2		4.0
Final	140	2.0	3.5	0.7	107.2	35.0	

What are the potential problems with bicarbonate dialysate?

Liquid "B" concentrate is not stable; some manufacturers add a small amount of special polymer as a stabilizer. Others provide dry $NaHCO_4$ as the powder, to be mixed at the facility. The mixing process requires care so that much of the CO_2 formed during the procedure is not lost from solution; it must be used within 24 hours of mixing.

Bicarbonate concentrate is very susceptible to bacterial contamination and proliferation. Even the stabilized solution should not be used if the container has been opened more than 72 hours. All containers for mixing, holding, or dispensing "B" concentrate must be scrupulously sanitized at regular intervals. Contamination must be avoided.

One manufacturer utilizes a delivery system that accepts a closed container of dry bicarbonate onto a special holder. Warm water passes through the column, producing a saturated solution of bicarbonate that is proportioned with water and then with the "A" concentrate by a conductivity-controlled feedback system.

There are many formulations of "A" concentrate to tailor the final dialysate sodium, potassium, calcium, and magnesium to the dialysis prescription. Each brand of delivery system has its unique proportioning and mixing ratios. *Extreme care must be exercised to ensure that the concentrates selected are correct for the delivery system being used.*

What kind of water is used to prepare dialysate?

The water must meet AAMI standards for chemical content and for bacterial and pyrogen content. In most instances, this involves complex and expensive treatment of feed water. Chapter 6 gives the various processes involved to achieve "dialysis-quality water."

Water for bicarbonate dialysis must meet or exceed AAMI standards. Hydrogen ion content should be near 40 NMOL/L (pH 7.4). For high-flux dialysis, United States Pharmacopoeia (USP) standards for *water for injection* should be used. These include "less than 10 colony-forming units/ml and limulus amebocyte lysate (LAL) test of not more than 1 ng/ml (5 EMU/ml)."

What is the LAL test?

LAL is the abbreviation for *limulus amebocyte lysate*. It is an assay for endotoxin which uses a protein extract from the Limulus, or horseshoe crab. It is reported in nanograms per milliliter or in endotoxin units (1 mg/ml = 5 EU/ml).

Why is dialysate verification and monitoring so important?

Serious patient reactions and deaths have resulted from dialysate preparation errors or equipment malfunction. Dialysate must be verified for each dialysis. Each delivery system should have a function check daily.

What methods are used to check the dialysate composition?

There are two general methods, primary and secondary. A *primary* method specifically measures the concentration of one solute by a laboratory method of known reliability. Usually two solutes are determined, such as sodium by flame photometry and chloride by titration. This is particularly important for bicarbonate dialysis to ensure proper ratio of acid to bicarbonate, as well as the ratio of concentrate to water.

What secondary tests are used?

The most common test of dialysate is the total conductivity. This does not measure specific ions, but the overall conductivity contributed by *all* the ions (hence it is a secondary test). Conductivity meters must be calibrated carefully to the "normal" or "safe" range for each type of concentrate used. If two or more dialysate formulas may be used, the safe range for each must be clearly identified since each has a different ionic concentration. Most manufacturers indicate on the label of the concentrate containers the conductivity of their dialysate when it is properly mixed.

An alternative secondary check of dialysate is the measurement of total osmolality by either freezing-point depression or vapor pressure. These measure total solute in the dialysate.

How do proportioning systems correctly mix dialysate?

Liquid concentrate is required. Several systems for mixing the correct proportions of concentrate and water have been used, but those in most widespread use employ microprocessor circuitry to control the speed of proportioning pumps, based on continuous conductivity and other parameter monitoring downstream of the mixing area (Fig. 5-2). The speed of the pumps and thus the volumes of the concentrates added, is precisely controlled by the electronic feedback circuit to ensure that the dialysis fluid is properly mixed.

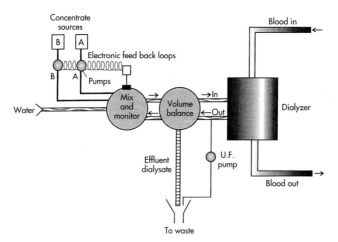

Fig. 5-2 Prototype of electronic proportioning system for bicarbonate dialysate, with volumetric ultrafiltration control.

What are disadvantages of proportioning systems?

These very complex, highly sophisticated, microprocessor-controlled electronic and hydraulic devices are quite expensive. Many functions are pre-programmed and may not be readily changed. Sensors and monitoring devices must be fail-safe and redundant. Troubleshooting is often difficult, and factory-based service personnel may be needed for repairs.

How does a sorbent regenerative supply system work?

In this system, a small volume of dialysate is recirculated through a cartridge of adsorbent materials and chemically regenerated. Metabolic waste products transferred from the dialyzer to the dialysate are removed and the electrolyte content and pH are restored (Fig. 5-3).

Fig. 5-3 Sorbent regenerative supply system.

How does a sorbent system function?

Three actions are involved: (1) conversion of urea to ammonium carbonate, (2) adsorption of creatinine and other nonionized solutes, and (3) ion exchange resins (sodium zirconium phosphate and zirconium oxide).

What is the process of urea conversion?

As dialysate enters the regenerative cartridge (Fig. 5-4), it first passes a carbon layer, which removes heavy metals and oxidants; it then contacts a bed containing urease. Urease is an enzyme that converts urea to ammonium and carbonate.

$$CO(NH_2)_2 \xrightarrow{urease} CO_2 + 2\ NH_3^+$$
$$2\ NH_3^+ + CO_2 + H_2O \rightarrow (NH_4)_2CO_3$$

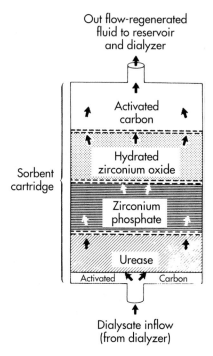

Fig. 5-4 Sorbent regenerative cartridge.

How are ammonium ions handled?

The next segment of the cartridge contains sodium zirconium phosphate, which acts as an exchange resin, taking up the ammonium ions and releasing sodium and hydrogen ions at about 1 Na^+ to 9 H^+. The carbonate ions equilibrate with hydrogen ions to yield bicarbonate ions (as $NaHCO_3$) and carbon dioxide.

$$(NH_4)_2CO_3 + 2\ H^+ \Bigg\langle \begin{array}{l} 2\ (NH_4)\ \textit{bound} \\ H_2O + CO_2 \leftrightarrow H_2CO_3 \end{array}$$

$$(NH_4)_2CO_3 + 2\ Na^+ \Bigg\langle \begin{array}{l} 2\ (NH_4)\ \textit{bound} \\ NaHCO_3 \end{array}$$

Are other ions exchanged in the column?

Yes. Calcium, magnesium, and potassium ions are also exchanged for sodium ions by the sodium zirconium phosphate. In addition, the third portion of the cartridge contains hydrated zirconium oxide, which removes phosphate ions and fluoride.

How are creatinine and nitrogenous materials removed?

The final layer of the sorbent column contains activated carbon (charcoal), which binds by adsorption creatinine, uric acid, guanidines, and other organic metabolites.

Is it necessary to replace calcium, magnesium, or potassium?

Yes. An infusion of calcium and magnesium is made just before the dialysate returns to the dialyzer to keep the desired concentration of these ions. Potassium is added, or omitted, according to the physician's desire.

What are advantages and disadvantages of the sorbent system?

Advantages include its portability and the absence of need for a special water supply or drain connections; it can be used wherever electricity is available.

Disadvantages include the somewhat expensive sorbent cartridge. There is a limit to the capacity to digest urea and to the absorption of ammonia. Ammonia may accumulate in the system and in the patient. Very large patients or those with very high serum urea values may require more than one cartridge per dialysis.

ADDITIONAL EQUIPMENT AND FUNCTIONS

Along with the dialysate mixing function, heaters, deaerators, pH and concentration monitors, dialysis delivery systems include a number of complementary functions essential to the hemodialysis procedure. These include the blood pump with an indicator for an estimate of blood flow rate, heparin infusion pump, air/foam detector, and inflow and outflow pressure sensors. On the dialysate side are temperature controls and monitors, conductivity monitors, flow rate controls, pressure sensors and ultrafiltration volume controls. An on-line urea sensor in the effluent dialysate line has potential for truly accurate quantification of urea removal. These functions are controlled by several electronic microcontrollers and programmable microprocessors with appropriate parameters displayed on video screen(s).

How is dialysate temperature controlled?

The heater and/or heat-exchanger is controlled by one or more sensors and a microcontroller circuit. Fluid temperature should hold within 0.5°C of the set point. There should be a separate sensor, independent of the heat control, for on-line monitoring with visual and audible alarms for any out-of-limits state. Accuracy should be checked regularly with a certified glass thermometer. Many ESRD patients have a body core temperature of 36° to 36.5°C. Added heat in excess of replacement causes a vasodilatory response, which may be detrimental at a time when the normal vasoconstrictive response to reduced volemia from ultrafiltration is acting to minimize hypotension. Fluid temperature over 41°C causes hemolysis of red blood cells, which can continue for several hours.

Why are deaeration devices necessary?

Water contains considerable dissolved air and microbubbles. When it is warmed, the dissolved air comes out of solution as expanding microbubbles. These have a negative effect on temperature and conductivity sensors, and flowmeters. Bubbles can reduce dialysate/membrane contact in hollow-fiber dialyzers.

Most deaeration devices use warmers along with negative pressure to bring the dissolved gases out of solution. An air trap or coalescing filter then captures the gases and vents them to the outside.

What problems are associated with dialysate flowmeters?

Solute film tends to build up with time and reduce accuracy. Calibration of the flowmeter or flow controller should be part of the routine servicing of the machine. At the bedside, actual flow can be quickly determined by a timed, measured outflow collection from the drain hose. Ultrafiltration control should be set to zero temporarily, during the measurement.

What is the importance of the dialysate pressure monitors?

If ultrafiltration is regulated by adjusting dialysate negative pressure, both inflow and outflow monitors must have high and low alarm set points, and must be accurate within +/-20 mm Hg, or 10 percent of reading. Manufacturer's directions must be followed carefully in adjusting and calibrating these monitors.

If ultrafiltration is controlled volumetrically or flowmetrically, the dialysate pressure monitors serve as a check on the ultrafiltration control and the transmembrane pressure.

How is dialysate concentration controlled and monitored?

The most suitable apparatus for this is the conductivity monitor (Fig. 5-5), which must be temperature compensated. Normal accuracy is +/- 1 to 3%. The conductivity sensor is basically an electrolytic cell, as described in Chapter 2. The electrodes of continually operating monitors are eroded by electrolytic action with a gradual loss of sensitivity over time. Most delivery systems use at least dual conductivity sensors, the readings of which must match. A confirmation test with a hand-held conductivity meter should be routine each day. Before any adjustment of the conductivity monitors, a *primary test*, such as the laboratory measurement of sodium or of chloride, should be done to verify the actual composition of the dialysate at the time.

Fig. 5-5 Conductivity monitor. (Adapted from Nosé Y: *Manual on artificial organs, vol 1: The artificial kidney*, St. Louis, 1969, Mosby.)

Is dialysate pH monitored?

There should be some type of pH verification. The usual limits are pH 6.8 to 7.6. There should be audible and visual alarms for any out-of-limits state. Sensors for pH drift with passage of time and must be recalibrated by the manufacturer's personnel.

What kinds of blood pumps are used?

A pump with internal components exposed directly to blood can present major problems in cleaning and sterilization. Peristaltic roller pumps, which work by progressively compressing special segments of blood tubing against the semicircular housing, are used almost universally.

How is blood flow rate measured?

Most blood pumps have speed indicators calibrated to show flow according to the speed of rotation. The internal diameter of the pumping segments of the tubing in use must match that for which the pump indicator was calibrated. Variations in tubing, pressure conditions in the blood circuit, and lack of linearity across the indicator scale cause discrepancies of +/- 10 to 15% between indicated and actual blood flow.

The calibration of each pump should be verified regularly, under standard conditions, with the same brand and lot of tubing used clinically. Water at 37° C should be pumped from a container, through the tubing, which is partially clamped to approximately the negative pressure between the needle and the inflow side of the pump during dialysis. The outflow should be collected in a graduated cylinder for 3–5 minutes. Volume (milliliters) divided by time (minutes) gives the flow rate. A record of each calibration should be kept on the machine, and in the central file.

How do blood leak detectors work?

Blood leak detectors are situated in the effluent dialysate line (Fig. 5-6). A beam of light is directed through a column of dialysate onto a photoelectric cell. A change in translucence and light scatter in dialysate reduces the light received by the photocell, stopping the blood pump and activating visual and audible alarms.

AAMI standards require detection of less than 0.45 ml/min of blood at hematocrit 45 over a range of dialysate flows. Particulate matter or air bubbles are frequent sources of false alarms. If a blood leak is not easily confirmed visually, the dialysate should be checked with a Hemostix. If standard maintenance procedures do not eliminate the problem, the manufacturer's representative should correct or replace the unit.

How do air bubbles in blood detectors behave?

Whenever a pump is used to propel blood through the extracorporeal circuit, some degree of negative pressure is created at the intake side. Air may be sucked into the line at connections that are not absolutely tight (as at the needle hub), through needle punctures or breaks in the tubing, or from empty fluid containers attached at the infusion sidearm. These potential air sources are especially important as pumping speed is increased in the efforts to achieve high blood flow rates. Air in blood can obstruct fibers of hollow-fiber kidneys, and if the quantity is sufficient, air may pass the venous bubble trap and go on to cause massive air embolism to the patient.

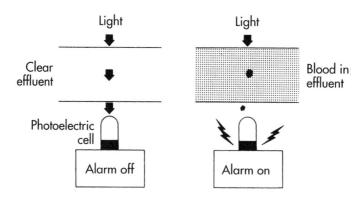

Fig. 5-6 Blood leak detector. (Adapted from Nosé Y: *Manual on artificial organs, vol 1: The artificial kidney*, St. Louis, 1969, Mosby.)

A commonly used detector employs an ultrasonic beam to identify air, foam, and microbubbles in blood (Fig. 5-7). Sound travels more quickly through fluid than through air, thus even minuscule bubbles slow the sonic beam and result in an alarm. Sonic detectors may be armed while the blood lines contain only saline; they do not respond to light or light changes in the surrounding environment.

Most air/foam detectors have no external sensitivity adjustment. The dialysis delivery system can be operated with the detector disarmed for priming and rinsing. There should be a low-level alarm, clearly discernible from a distance, to indicate the disarmed status. No patient should be permitted to dialyze with the air/foam detector in the disarmed state.

How do ultrafiltration controls work?

These devices exactly match the outflow dialysate volume with the inflow volume, plus a precisely measured extra effluent volume representing the desired (programmed) ultrafiltrate. There are two basic types of ultrafiltration controllers: (1) volumetric and (2) flowmetric (Figs. 5-8 and 5-9).

Fig. 5-7 Sonic air/foam detector.

Fig. 5-8 Volumetric ultrafiltration control. (Redrawn from Vlchek DL: Staying tuned in to the high-tech world—part 2: dialysis delivery systems, *Dialysis Transplant* 18 Aug. 1989.)

Fig. 5-9 Servo-feedback ultrafiltration control. (Redrawn from Vlchek DL: Staying tuned in to the high-tech world—part 2: dialysis delivery systems, *Dialysis Transplant* 18: Aug. 1989.)

How do volumetric ultrafiltration devices operate?

The most common system employs two diaphragm chambers to balance the inflow and outflow dialysate (Fig. 5-10). While one side of the first chamber is filling with fresh dialysate, its diaphragm is forcing out an equal volume of used fluid from the other side. Simultaneously in the second chamber, one side is filling with spent fluid from the dialyzer while the opposite side is ejecting an equal volume of fresh dialysate to the dialyzer. When the diaphragms have deflected across the width of the chambers, valves are reversed so that the side that was emptying now fills, and vice versa. The volume for ultrafiltrate is removed from the outflow dialysate channel by a metering pump before the outflow volume is matched to inflow, thus removing the desired amount of ultrafiltrate from the patient. Since the volumes in and out of the controller are precisely equalized, whatever pressure (negative or positive) is necessary will be created for the removal of the measured ultrafiltrate volume by the dialyzer.

How does the flowmetric ultrafiltrate control system work?

In a flowmetric system there are one or two very accurate flowmeters in both the inflow and the outflow dialysate pathways to measure the flow of fluid passing through these pathways. The speed of the dialysate pump in the outflow path is varied by the electronic control module so that the volume through the outflow meter is exactly equal to the volume through the inflow meter, plus the programmed amount of ultrafiltrate.

 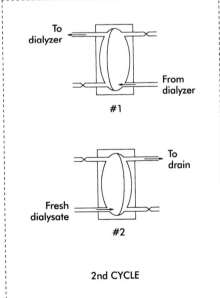

Fig. 5-10   Volumetric ultrafiltration. Matched double diaphragm chambers.

HIGH-EFFICIENCY AND HIGH-FLUX DIALYSIS

What are equipment needs for high-efficiency dialysis?

There are four requirements:
- A highly permeable cellulose membrane (ultrathin Cuprophan, Hemophan, cellulose acetate ester, etc.) with surface area 1.5 m^2 or more
- Reliable blood flow of 350 ml/min or more; dialysate flow of 750 ml/min or more
- Bicarbonate dialysate delivery system
- An ultrafiltration control system

The combination of a large area of membrane of high mass transfer capability and high Q_b and Q_d produces increased small molecule transfer. Intermediate-sized and large solute transfer rates are enhanced by the area and permeability increases.

What are the advantages of high-efficiency dialysis?

It allows reduction of time on dialysis for many patients, up to a total of 6 to 9 hours per week. This frees the patient for other activities and reduces total cost per dialysis for large facilities.

What are the system requirements for high-flux dialysis?

As with high-efficiency dialysis, in the high-flux system it is important to maintain high blood flow rate, high dialysate flow rate, and precision control of ultrafiltration volume. High-flux dialyzers use synthetic membranes of very high permeability, with convective transfer providing a major share of solute transport (see page 38). These dialyzers have ultrafiltration coefficients of 20 to 70 ml/hr/mm Hg or more.

The ultrafiltration controller precisely manages net fluid removal, but in so doing generates a dialysate pressure profile that creates reverse filtration from dialysate to blood in the distal portion of the dialyzer (Fig. 5-11). A problem of contamination of blood by pyrogenic material and endotoxin fragments is created, since high-flux membranes readily pass particles of 2,000 to 10,000 d. The LAL test (see Glossary and page 55) is used to monitor dialysate for endotoxin.

How might the problem of reverse filtration be countered?

AAMI standards require not more than 200 colony-forming units of bacteria per milliliter in water for dialysate, and not more than 2000 cfu bacteria or 5 EMU by LAL test for endotoxin in dialysate leaving the delivery system. Bacterial multiplication continues as the dialysis fluid courses through the dialyzer; pyrogenic materials increase and cross the high-flux membrane during backfiltration.

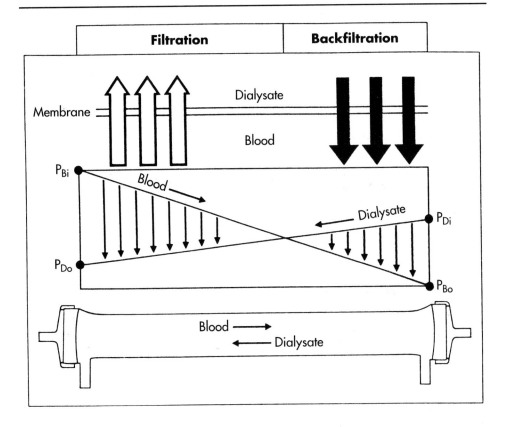

Fig. 5-11 Backfiltration and pressure distribution. (From Baurmeister U et al: Dialysate contamination and back filtration may limit the use of high-flux dialysis membranes, *Transact ASAIO* 35:21, 1989.)

Addition of a molecular filter or ultrafilter (see Chapter 6) to the dialysate path immediately ahead of the dialyzer may be necessary for high-flux dialysis. A 50,000 to 100,000 d ultrafilter will reject intact endotoxins; the 1000 to 10,000 d ultrafilter will be necessary if endotoxin fragments are the problem. Some manufacturers have a provision for ultrafilters in their delivery systems.

OTHER EXTRACORPOREAL TREATMENT MODALITIES

There are techniques other than dialysis for removing metabolic wastes, toxic materials, and/or excess water. Some of these are very useful in the Intensive Care Unit for the patient with complex problems and/or multiple organ failure.

What are some of these techniques?

There are three basic modalities in use clinically:
- Hemofiltration
- Hemoperfusion
- Apheresis

HEMOFILTRATION

What is hemofiltration?

In conventional hemodialysis, diffusion or conductive transfer accounts for the major portion of solute movement across the membrane. The natural kidney in its process of glomerular filtration actually uses ultrafiltration, or convective transfer. Convective transfer across a synthetic membrane is also used to remove uremic wastes from blood. This is the process of hemofiltration, or diafiltration.

How effective is hemofiltration?

Using membrane or hollow fibers of PAN, polyamide, polysulfone, or polycarbonate, ultrafiltration of more than 100 ml/min is possible at blood flow rates of 200 to 350 ml/min. If the blood urea nitrogen were 50 mg/dl, that amount of BUN would also be removed in one minute. The removal of creatinine, middle and large molecules, such as β_2-microglobulin far exceeds that of conventional hemodialysis.

What problems may occur with hemofiltration?

- The infusion of replacement fluid must be carefully and continually monitored to avoid under- or overhydration.
- Blood leak can be a serious hazard when negative pressure is applied to the filtrate bag to enhance ultrafiltration.
- The serum level of various beneficial medications (antibiotics, cardiac drugs, anticonvulsants) may be adversely altered.
- The essential sterile replacement fluids are expensive.

What are clinical advantages of hemofiltration?

Several low-flow modalities of hemofiltration are useful for critically ill individuals needing multisystem support.
- Hypotension is less of a problem than with hemodialysis, even though a large volume of fluid is removed.
- Dysequilibrium and other systems/findings of intracellular osmolar shift are rare.
- Large volumes of parenteral nutrition may be given, while fluid balance is maintained at a stable level.

- Improved blood pressure control in hypertensive individuals during periods between treatments has been attributed to better sodium and volume control, and improved autonomic stability.
- Hemofiltration allows removal of harmful substances of large molecular size, such as myocardial depressant factor (MDF).

These positive attributes of hemofiltration have resulted in the development of continuous renal replacement therapy (CRRT).

What is Continuous Renal Replacement Therapy?

CRRT is used primarily to treat patients in acute renal failure, particularly those with multiple organ failure. Such individuals tend to be hemodynamically unstable, to have cardiac insufficiency, and to tolerate hemodialysis poorly. Various hemofilters are available, hollow fiber or plate design, and characterized by small contained blood volume and low resistance to flow. There is increasing evidence that CRRT is improving patient survival in acute renal failure.

What are some CRRT modalities?

- CAVH: continuous arteriovenous hemofiltration.
- CVVH: continuous venovenous hemofiltration.
- CAVHD: continuous AV hemodialysis with filtration.
- CVVHD: continuous VV hemodialysis with filtration.
- CAVU: continuous AV ultrafiltration.
- SCUF: slow continuous ultrafiltration.

CAVH requires both arterial and venous access, but does not use a blood pump. If solute removal by convective transport is not sufficient, diffusive transport is added by also using hemodialysis.

CVVH and CVVHD do not require arterial access with its attending problems, but instead use double lumen catheters in major venous sites. In each person, flow is controlled with a blood pump (Fig. 5-12).

What are problems in the use of CRRT?

For those procedures requiring arterial access, such as CAVH and CAVHD, there is risk of damage to the artery itself, as well as danger of hemorrhage if a connection is faulty or a leak develops in the blood circuit. Critically ill patients are often hypotensive, with the blood flow rate inadequate for effective filtration. In addition, correction of electrolyte imbalance and/or fluid overload may be slower than desired. Clotting problems are frequent.

For systems utilizing venovenous flow, a blood pump is needed. Monitoring is required to avert air being drawn into the blood circuit and to watch for bleeding from a loose connection in the downstream side.

Fig. 5-12 Continuous renal replacement therapy (CRRT) using hemofiltration. Left: Continuous arteriovenous hemofiltration (CAVH). Right: Continuous venovenous hemofiltration (CVVH).

HEMOPERFUSION

In hemoperfusion blood is brought in direct contact with a sorbent material, packaged in a cartridge or column. Most devices use 70 to 300 g of activated charcoal coated with a polymer film to reduce embolism by tiny carbon particles and to decrease platelet and cellular element buildup.

What are the indications for using hemoperfusion?

Hemoperfusion is used primarily for drug overdose or toxic exposure of great severity. Activated charcoal binds most chemicals in the range of 100 to 20,000 d. Most medications have molecular weights of 500 to 2000 d. Hemoperfusion is more effective than hemodialysis for removal of most sedatives, theophylline, digoxin, and some pesticides and herbicides.

In association with DFO chelation, charcoal may be used to remove excess aluminum or iron from body tissue.

What are the adverse effects of hemoperfusion?

A transient decrease in platelets is frequent; it corrects within 24 hours in most instances. Some patients have a fall in white cell count. Hemolysis or red cell damage is unusual. Hypotension is frequent; the poisoned patient is already very brittle. Heavy anticoagulation is needed, and postprocedure bleeding may be prolonged.

Is there a limit to the capacity of the cartridges?

Yes, adsorptive capacity is limited and is difficult to determine in advance. The kinetics of adsorption are complex. Overall mass transfer relates to a fluid transfer rate and an intraparticle transfer rate, which depend upon microcapillary size and solute diffusion. Clearance of some solutes may decrease gradually over time until the sorbent is filled; for others, clearance may fall off rapidly even though considerable sorbent capacity remains.

APHERESIS

The term "apheresis" is a Greek expression for "taking something away." Plasmapheresis has been conducted for a number of years to separate plasma protein components using special centrifuges. Synthetic hollow fiber technology produces filters of selectively permeable capability to remove specific blood constituents, e.g., antibodies and immunoglobulins.

Plasmapheresis has been used experimentally for a variety of conditions, including transplant rejection by reducing antibody titer. The technique is of definite value in hyperviscosity syndrome, cryoglobulinemia, thrombotic thrombocytopenic purpura, myasthenia gravis crisis, Guillain-Barré syndrome, refractory idiopathic—or autoimmune—hemolytic anemia, multiple myeloma with renal failure, and Goodpasture's syndrome.

Water Treatment

Martin V. Hudson

Water is a complex and incompletely understood chemical compound. The purest form of water is freshly formed rain as it leaves the cloud. It is also a very high-energy form of water. In the journey from rain cloud to final delivery tap, much of this energy is expended in acquiring various impurities as solute or suspension.

Improved dialysis technology has made high-purity water critical for dialysis fluid preparation. Fortunately, the science of water purification has made parallel advances. Enhanced membranes for reverse osmosis, ultrafiltration (UF) devices to screen out endotoxins as well as bacteria, and improved monitoring systems are available and are being applied in the renal community.

What impurities may be present in tap water?

Three categories of contaminating substances can cause patient injury or equipment malfunction: (1) chemical solutes, (2) bacteria or bacterial products, and (3) particulate matter. Of these, the chemical and bacterial contaminants may be directly harmful to patients receiving dialysis.

How do impurities get into water?

Falling rainwater passing through the air contacts carbon dioxide and sulfur dioxide, forming carbonic and sulfuric acid in weak solution. Upon hitting the ground, this water encounters limestone and other minerals to form calcium bicarbonate and sulfate, magnesium carbonate, and other salts. Calcium carbonate is the more prevalent impurity in tap water and accounts for most of its hardness.

What other inorganic chemicals may be present in tap water?

Sodium, chloride, iron, aluminum, nitrates, manganese, copper, zinc, iodide, and fluoride are common ionic constituents. The types of mineral present in the geographic area and the time the water is in contact with them determine the content.

Trace elements that may be present include arsenic, silver, strontium, selenium, chromium, lead, cadmium, cyanide, barium, tin, and others.

Are these chemicals harmful?

Nitrates may cause methemoglobinemia, in which red cell hemoglobin cannot transport oxygen. Copper in excess may cause hemolysis. Manganese can be toxic, and iron may possibly be toxic also. Fluoride is believed to aggravate uremic bone disease; it does accumulate in bone, and it is toxic to enzyme systems. Tin has been found in significantly higher quantity in tissues of dialyzed uremic patients than in nonuremic individuals. Aluminum accumulates and is related to the dialysis-dementia syndrome, as well as to a form of anemia and osteodystrophy. Zinc causes gastrointestinal upset and may produce anemia. In areas of radioactivity, the presence of 90Sr may pose a danger.

Are there other materials in tap water?

Nonionic organic compounds, particularly nitrogenous matter such as proteins and polypeptides, phenols, indoles, and aldehydes, may be present. Solid particles of iron, sand, and silica are frequent. Suspended material, including mud, algae, plankton, bacteria, viruses, pyrogenic matter, and dissolved gases (ammonia, carbon dioxide, chlorine) are often present. The most common soluble organic compounds are chloramines from urban water treatment systems. The content of these materials as well as ionic impurities varies with the water source, season, and distribution system.

Some water supplies have identifiable amounts of pesticides or herbicides present, such as chlordane, DDT, aldrin, lindane, 2,4,4-T, and others.

Most water supplies contain various kinds of bacteria. Many are not detected by routine testing for coliform organisms. Such organisms include *Flavobacterium, Achromobacter, Serratia, Pseudomonas*, and several atypical mycobacteria.

If a water supply meets the requirements of the Safe Drinking Water Act and Environmental Protection Agency standards, is it safe for dialysis?

No. Contaminants in the water used to make dialysis fluid may enter the patient's bloodstream through the dialysis membrane. In addition, most dialysis procedures use bicarbonate as the buffer. Some delivery systems, in bicarbonate mode, will not function properly if the pH is outside the range of 6.5 to 7.8. The pH of untreated tap water may be extremely acidic or extremely alkaline.

Why is special water treatment necessary to make dialyzing fluid?

During hemodialysis the amount of water that contacts the patient's blood is more than 25 times the amount taken in by drinking. A substance present in water to only one quarter of its upper limit of safety for drinking purposes may enter the body during hemodialysis in amounts 10 to 25 times that much.

Ingested water is processed by the gastrointestinal tract before reaching the bloodstream. This selective membrane can alter the rate at which foreign substances are absorbed from ingested water. In a dialyzer system the dialyzer membrane cannot select ions to be absorbed or rejected, and they pass by diffusion. Substances that are harmless in drinking water may be toxic in dialysis water.

What methods are used to treat water for use in hemodialysis?

- Filtration
- Adsorption by activated charcoal
- Softening
- Reverse osmosis (RO)
- Deionization (DI)
- Ultrafiltration (UF)

What is accomplished by filtration?

Suspended particles (mud, sand, rust, algae) are removed by mechanical filtration through a wound filament or membrane cartridge or by tanks containing granular material that can be backflushed. These effectively filter particles down to about 5 μm in size. Submicron filters are available that screen out particles as small as 0.2 μm. Such filters will remove bacteria but require frequent replacements. Filtration does not remove *dissolved* particles or ions from the water.

Ultrafilration (UF), a process similar to reverse osmosis (see below), is highly effective for the removal of fine particles, bacteria, endotoxin and other pyrogenic matter, as well as high molecular weight organic molecules.

What is the silt density index?

The silt density index (SDI) is an indicator of the colloid and suspended particulate matter present in tap water. The measuring device indicates the pressure drop over time as the tap water crosses a 0.45 μm membrane filter. The more suspended material present, the slower the water passes. An SDI of less than 5.0 is required of feed water for most reverse osmosis systems.

How is activated charcoal used in water treatment?

Activated charcoal acts by adsorption. It will not remove electrolytes, such as calcium or sodium. It has a unique ability to adsorb chloramines, odor-producing materials, and low molecular weight (60 to 300 d) material, as well as higher molecular weight organic matter. Commonly, there are two types of carbon tanks: (a) portable exchange or (b) "permanent" portable exchange. Portable exchange tanks are "changed out" on a cycle that is developed by the facility. The vendor then replaces them with "new charcoal"-filled tanks. Permanent tanks are equipped with a control unit that allows them to be backwashed at the facility's discretion. At intervals the carbon is replaced by the vendor. Backwashing does not regenerate the carbon beds. It actually "fluffs" the carbon particles so that channels are removed and the total bed is once again available to contact water passing through it.

What does softening of water achieve?

Hardness of water is caused primarily by calcium and magnesium ions. Softening units replace these divalent ions with sodium ions from an exchange resin bed on a milliequivalent-for-milliequivalent basis. For each calcium ion removed, two sodium ions are added.

If the feed water is very hard, a softener will remove most of the calcium and magnesium before further treatment. If a deionizer is used downstream, the softener will reduce the divalent ion load presented to the deionizer resin bed and prolong its life. If the subsequent treatment is RO, the removal of calcium and magnesium by the softener may result in higher quality product water and longer RO membrane life.

What problems occur with the use of water softeners?

If the raw water is very hard, considerable sodium is substituted in the exchange for calcium and magnesium. Municipal water supplies often vary seasonably or even during a single day if multiple sources are used.

There are two types of softeners, portable exchange and permanent. Portable exchange units are provided ready-for-use by the vendor. Regeneration of the media resin is performed by the vendor at a central facility.

Permanent softeners have a concentrated brine tank and valves and controls for on-site regeneration.

There are no on-line monitors that will indicate "hard" or "soft" water, but commercial test kits for total hardness are available and are quite reliable. The degree of hardness of both source water and product water should be determined each day. This will indicate the need for the regeneration cycle, as well as any softener malfunction.

What is reverse osmosis?

Reverse osmosis (RO) represents the ultimate in ultrafiltration. RO membranes have such small "effective pore size" (under 1.0 nm diameter) that transfer of even low molecular weight solutes is retarded. High hydraulic pressure is necessary to overcome the osmotic backpressure and to move water across the membrane. The osmotic backpressure for dissolved solids is about 1 psi for each 100 mg/L, or around 15 psi for average fresh water. The "reverse" in RO is the hydraulic force needed to overcome the osmotic backpressure. Organic particles are physically screened out. Water passes through the membrane by ultrafiltration. The membrane "repels" ions near its surface. The hydraulic pressure required for a useful flow of product water ranges from 200 to 450 psi.

How does the membrane "repel" electrolytes?

This results from electrochemical tension at the water-membrane interface. It is greater for divalent than for monovalent ions. The rejection rate for divalent ions is more than 95 percent and for monovalent ions, 90 to 98 percent, depending on the particular membrane.

How are organic compounds processed by the membrane?

Organic compounds have no net charge and are not electrically repelled but are physically screened by the membrane. Almost all particles of molecular weight greater than 200 d are rejected. This includes bacteria, viruses, and pyrogens.

What types of membranes are used for reverse osmosis?

Membranes for RO use must be: (1) freely permeable to water, (2) highly impermeable to solutes, and (3) able to tolerate very high operating pressures. Desirable characteristics include tolerance to a wide range of pH and temperature and resistance to attack by bacteria and by chemicals such as chlorine.

Membranes in general use include: (1) cellulose, (2) aromatic polyamide, (3) thin film composites, and (4) high-flux, chlorine-resistant polysulfone.

- Cellulose acetate membranes have high water permeability but poor rejection of low molecular weight contaminants. Range of pH tolerance is limited; they degrade at temperatures greater than 35°C (95°F), and they are vulnerable to bacteria. They are relatively inexpensive.
- Polyamide membranes have wide pH tolerance and are more resistant to bacterial action and to hydrolysis than are cellulose membranes. They are very susceptible to degradation by free chlorine.
- Thin film composites are expensive. The supporting layer is usually a porous polysulfone. Fixed to this is a thin, dense, and solute-rejecting surface film such as polyfurane cyanurate or a polyamide. Composite membranes have better water flux and better solute rejection than cellulose acetate. They are less subject to compaction and bacterial action.
- Chlorine resistant polysulfone membranes have a very long service life. They tolerate a wide span of pH and of temperature. Water flux is high. They differ from other membranes in that if divalent ions are present in the feed water, rejection of monovalent ions is sharply reduced. Therefore, it is essential that the feed water be softened or deionized before entering the RO unit.

What configuration of reverse osmosis modules are used?

Module design must include such features as a large membrane surface area, a tolerance for very high pressure (up to 500 psi), good flow characteristics, and a low pressure drop. Configurations in use for hemodialysis water are (1) the spiral-wound or spiral-wrap (Fig. 6-1) and (2) hollow-fiber modules.

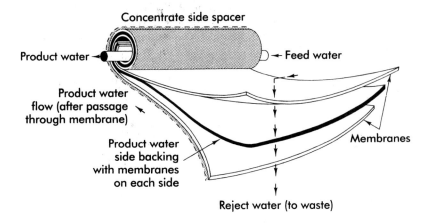

Fig. 6-1   Spiral-wrap reverse osmosis module.

Spiral-wound units consist of two layers of membrane with a fabric material fastened between, sandwich fashion. The fabric material is the product carrier. The membrane-sandwich sheet, along with a plastic mesh separator, is wrapped in a spiral around a central perforated tube in a manner somewhat similar to that of an old style coil dialyzer. Feed water under high pressure enters one end of the unit and flows along the channels provided by the plastic mesh; some water is forced by the hydraulic pressure through the membrane. The central fabric conducts this filtered water to the central tube, from which it emerges as product water.

In hollow-fiber units the membrane is formed as capillary fibers of 80 to 250 μm inside diameter. Several thousand of these fibers are bundled inside a high-pressure cylinder. Pressurized feed water surrounds and permeates the hollow fibers, forming the product water inside the capillary lumina. The small internal diameter of the hollow fibers can contribute to plugging and reduced permeate flow.

What are special advantages of RO over other types of water treatment?

There are several advantages:
- Bacteria, viruses, and pyrogen materials are rejected by the intact membrane. In this respect RO water approaches distilled water in quality.
- Available units are relatively compact and require little space. They are well suited to home dialysis.
- In average use, the membrane has a life of a little over 1 to 2 years before replacement is necessary.
- Periodic complete sterilization of the RO system with formalin or other sterilant is practical.

What are disadvantages of RO systems?

Disadvantages include the following:
- The membranes have a limited service life. For instance:
  - Cellulose acetate membranes have limited pH tolerance. They degrade at temperatures over 35°C. They are vulnerable to bacteria. They eventually hydrolyze.
  - Polyamide membranes are intolerant of temperature over 35°C. They have poor tolerance for free chlorine.
  - Thin film composites are intolerant of chlorine.
  - High-flux polysulfones require softening or deionization of feed water to function properly.
- As with hemodialysis membranes, leaks are possible. Continual monitoring of product water flow rate and conductivity is necessary.
- Product water is 25 to 50 percent of feed water. The remaining 50 to 75 percent goes to waste, a matter of economic and environmental concern.
- The membrane must be kept continually wet throughout its entire life. The flow cannot simply be stopped and the unit maintained filled with water; bacterial growth, hydrolysis of the membrane, and pyrogen production are likely to result. When not in operation, the unit should be held in a sterilant-filled state.
- Chloramines—oxidant compounds of chlorine and ammonia used as bactericidal agents in some city water supplies—are nonionic and freely cross the RO membrane. Anemia resulting from chloramine has occurred in some dialysis patients. A carbon filter should always be used ahead of an RO system to remove any chloramine.
- To meet peak flow needs in large hemodialysis facilities, a reservoir or holding tanks for processed water from the RO unit may be necessary. The water is recirculated in a continuous loop from RO unit to tanks and back to prevent stagnation. The tanks and plumbing are sites for potential microbial growth and endotoxin formation. Tank design is

important in minimizing contamination. A steeply rounded or conical tank bottom with the drain port at the extreme low point ensures complete emptying. The re-entry port should be near the top and use a special nozzle to spray the under side of the cover. This prevents water droplets from forming on the cover, and the cascade of water down the sides prevents the collection of stagnant water. The top should have a microbial filter in the air vent. This design also provides excellent sterilant contact during chemical disinfection, and complete flushing away of sterilant at "rinse-out." Chlorine or iodine may also be metered into the system between the RO unit and the tanks to control the growth of organisms (Fig. 6-2).

What is deionization?

Ion exchange resins, somewhat like those of a softener but more sophisticated, remove both cations and anions from the feed water.

How does a deionizing unit work?

There is a cation bed and an anion bed. Each bed is composed of grains of ion exchange resin about the size of fine sand, called zeolite. Zeolites are large, organic chemical molecules that have active side-chain groups attached to them. The side chain of the zeolite in the cation bed is a carboxyl ($^-$COOH) group. In the anion resin bed, there are attached substitute ammonium groups (NH_3 and OH^-). In passage through the cation bed, calcium, magnesium, sodium, and other cations in the water combine with the carboxyl radicals, with release of hydrogen ions. In the anion bed, anoins—chloride, fluoride, sulfate, nitrate, bicarbonate, and others—are exchanged for the hydroxide ion (OH^-). The released hydroxide ions combine with hydrogen ions released at the cation bed to form water chemically (Fig. 6-3).

What is the difference between two-bed, single-bed, and tri-bed deionizers?

The two-bed system has the cation-removing and anion-removing resins in separate tanks; water flows first through the cation bed and then to the anion bed. The single-bed, or mixed-bed, system has the two resins mixed together; because of the mixing, a much higher quality (purer) water is produced. The tri-bed system is the best option. The two-bed system produces water of lesser quality, but is economical to regenerate and has a relatively long service life. When used ahead of a mixed bed unit, the service life of the latter is lengthened. The mixed-bed becomes a "polisher."

Fig. 6-2 Recirculating loop water treatment system with holding tank. (Courtesy Mar Cor Services, Harleysville, PA)

CATIONS	ANIONS
Na$^+$	Cl$^-$
K$^+$	F$^-$
Ca^{++}	SO$_4^=$
Mg^{++}	NO$_3^-$

CATION RESIN BED

H$^+$	Cl$^-$
	F$^-$
	SO$_4^=$
	NO$_3^-$

ANION RESIN BED

| H$^+$ | OH$^-$ |

H$_2$O

Fig. 6-3 Schematic diagram of two-bed deionizing system.

Deionizers produce water of high ionic purity, but they do not remove bacteria or pyrogens. Indeed, deionizers often make the quality of water worse in terms of bacteria and endotoxin content; the resin bed provides an environment conductive to bacterial proliferation. It is prudent to follow deionization equipment with submicron filtration or an ultrafiltration unit. It is imperative that some type of monitor be installed to ensure the chemical quality of the product water. AAMI guidelines state that product water should not be allowed to go below 1 Megohm resistance; at that point the tanks should be exchanged (Fig. 6-4).

What problems occur with deionizers?

There are several problems to watch out for:

- An initial problem is obtaining the maximum flow rate needed. As with softeners, proper size of the DI set is critical. Peak and normal operating flow rates and operating line pressures should be determined. The user then should look at the operating specifications for a variety of tank sizes and select the size that best meets the facility's needs, taking account of the pressure drop across the DI set. Pressure indicators before and after this subsystem are advisable so that the difference in pressure can be easily determined.
- Total ion content of the feed water is a problem; only a finite quantity of ions can be removed by a resin bed of given size. Service life of the deionizer depends on water composition and volume. If a DI unit is

Fig. 6-4 Direct feed water treatment system to produce ultrapure water. (Courtesy Mar Cor Services, Harleysville, PA)

positioned ahead of an RO unit, its service life will be short. It will be processing water of high ionic content while the RO unit will serve primarily as a bacterial and endotoxin screen. If the DI unit is located downstream from the RO device, the DI then becomes a "polisher." It also increases chances of microbiologic contamination. It is recommended that a submicron filter or an ultrafilter be placed downstream.

- Resin beds tend to exhaust suddenly. A parallel bypass installation is necessary so that switchover can be made while the exhausted tanks are replaced. The water in tanks that are standing idle will be stagnant. Provision for flushing a reasonable volume to the drain should be part of the system. The volumetric capacity of deionizers (gallons of water passing through the tanks) is rated in "grains per gallon (GPG) of total dissolved solids (TDS)," expressed as calcium carbonate. (NOTE: One grain/gal approximates 17.1 mg/L $CaCO_3$.) Rated capacity of the deionizer divided by the TDS of the feed water will give an approximation of the volume of water that may be treated before the unit exhausts. On-line, continuous readout resistivity meters should be positioned to monitor the effluent water. When the resistance degrades to 1 $M\Omega$/cm, the tanks should be exchanged (an AAMI standard).

- Usually the anion and cation resins exhaust at different times. If the tanks are used to exhaustion, ions previously removed may be released, possibly in a concentration greater than that of the feed water. The water may become extremely acidic or extremely alkaline, depending on which resin exhausted first. This situation may be hazardous to patients or equipment.

What degree of water purity is required for hemodialysis?

The AAMI developed a set of water quality guidelines that is recognized as the U.S. national standard. The standard now applies not only to chemical or inorganic contaminants but to microbiologic contaminants as well. These requirements are shown in Box 6-1.

What quality of water is produced by the various methods described?

RO alone produces water of 200,000 to 600,000 Ω/cm resistance, depending on the type of membrane. The product water is free of bacteria, viruses, and known pyrogens, provided there is no membrane leak.

DI systems produce water of 200,000 to 300,000 Ω/cm resistance from two-bed units; addition of a mixed bed will give 16 to 18 $M\Omega$ water, depending on the quality of resin regeneration. Prefilters, charcoal units, and submicron post-filters must be used to remove organic material, pyrogens, and bacteria.

Box 6-1 AAMI Standards for Facilities/Users

MICROBIOLOGIC MONITORING
- Should be performed at least monthly
- Total viable microbial counts shall not exceed 200/ml in water used to prepare dialysate, or 2000/ml in proportioned dialysate exiting the dialyzer

CHEMICAL CONTAMINANTS MONITORING
- Should be performed at least yearly if prepared by DI or RO, more frequently if prepared with lesser level of treatment
- AAMI maximum levels of chemical contaminants:

Contaminant	Suggested maximum level (mg/L)
Calcium	2 (0.1 mEq/L)
Magnesium	4 (0.3 mEq/L)
Sodium†	70 (3 mEq/L)
Potassium	8 (0.2 mEq/L)
Fluoride	0.2
Chlorine	0.5
Chloramines	0.1
Nitrate (N)	2
Sulfate	100
Copper, barium, zinc	0.1 each
Aluminum	0.01
Arsenic, lead, silver	0.005 each
Cadmium	0.001
Chromium	0.014
Selenium	0.09
Mercury	0.0002

From Vlchek DL, Burrows-Hudson S: *Quality assurance guidelines for hemodialysis devices*, Washington, DC, February 1991, U.S. Department of Health and Human Services, Food and Drug Administration.

* The physician has ultimate responsibility for determining the quality of water used for dialysis.

† 230 mg/L (10 mEq/L) where sodium concentration of the concentrate has been reduced to compensate for the excess sodium in the water, as long as conductivity of water is being continuously monitored.

A combination of RO followed by the tri-bed DI system and appropriate filtration will yield microbial-free, pyrogen-free water of 18 MΩ/cm resistance. This is called ultrapure water; its electrolyte content approximates 0.00035 mEq/L of sodium.

What problems are there in handling very pure water?

As water is treated increasingly near its pure state, its energy level also increases. Such pure water very quickly reacts chemically with materials it contacts. Only pipe or tubing of medical-grade stainless steel, polyvinylchloride (PVC), or one of the new inert materials may be used to carry the product water. Tanks must be of such material. If exposed to air, ultrapure water will quickly absorb and react with carbon dioxide.

What problems are there with bacteria and pyrogens in water treatment?

The original AAMI standard was based upon dialysis fluid made with acetate concentrate and dialyzer membranes of Cuprophan. The microbial standard of 200 cfu/ml in water for preparing dialysis fluid, and 2000 cfu/ml in the proportioned dialysate exiting the dialyzer, was appropriate for such hemodialysis. While this standard has not changed, dialyzer membranes have changed significantly (see Chapter 5). New membranes are much more porous to water, solutes and suspended matter. Transmembrane movement is bi-directional, relative to pressure and solute concentration gradients. Proper prefilters with an RO unit, or DI with submicron postfiltration, will in most instances meet the standard. Bacteria proliferate on filter surfaces, carbon tanks, softener and DI resin beds, and the feed water surface of the RO membrane. A regular schedule of backflushing with an approved sterilant must be used to minimize bacterial growth in all components of the water treatment system. The sterilant must, of course, be thoroughly rinsed from the system before water is used for patients. Chemical sterilization kills bacteria but does not destroy them, and actually fixes some of the protein and polysaccharide components and endotoxins. Copious backflushing is needed to wash these debris away from the collecting surfaces.

A majority of facilities use bicarbonate-containing concentrate in their fluid-proportioning systems. Many facilities use dialyzers with high-flux membranes, along with controlled ultrafiltration devices.

Bicarbonate concentrate, when stored, supports proliferation of endotoxin-forming microorganisms. Whether these originate from the water used to prepare the concentrate or from the bicarbonate powder, it is likely that more strict microbial and endotoxin limits will be necessary. For high-flux dialysis where backfiltration poses a problem, delivery of sterile, pyrogen-free fluid from the proportioning system to the dialyzer may become necessary.

How may microbiologic contaminants be further reduced?

There are four means most commonly used:

- Ultraviolet irradiation of product water will halt proliferation of many, although not all, bacteria. Endotoxin content may actually increase because of the microbial debris. UV treatment is not highly regarded.
- Chlorine may be metered into RO product water. This is sometimes utilized in facilities that recirculate RO water through a holding tank system. However, the chlorine produces problems also.
- Submicron (0.05 μm) filters will stop passage of bacteria and viruses. Such filters must be replaced frequently and are expensive. They do not exclude all pyrogenic matter.
- UF will reject bacteria and endotoxins effectively. Initial installation is relatively expensive, but operation is economical. Sanitization is simple, and service life is good.

How is ultrafiltration used to remove bacteria and endotoxin?

UF membranes have an effective pore size of more than 0.001μm. Pores of this size do not retard the movement of osmotically active solutes, hence less hydraulic pressure is needed for the transmembrane movement of water than is needed with RO membranes.

UF membranes are often called molecular filters; they filter suspended particles of molecular size rather than dissolved substances. The larger particles do not have the osmotic effect of dissolved solutes. There is little osmotic back-pressure, compared with reverse osmosis membranes; hence, less need for high hydraulic pressure. However, these molecular filters reject bacteria, endotoxin, and endotoxin fragments that are thousands of daltons in size. Ultrafilters are available that exclude particles of 50,000 to 100,000 d; in fact, an even tighter membrane of 1000 to 10,000 d is available.

UF devices may be placed ahead of RO units to prevent bacterial growth or accumulation of particulate material on the feedwater surface of the RO membrane. When used as the final step before delivery of product water to the proportioning system, UF will ensure its microbiologic quality.

What microbiologic standards apply to dialyzer reuse?

This is defined in the *AAMI Recommended Practice for Reuse of Dialyzers (RD47)*. The water used in reprocessing should have a bacterial count of no more than 200 cfu/ml, or an endotoxin level of 1 ng/ml (5 EU) by LAL. This also may be made more strict because of the problems with bicarbonate and with high-flux dialyzers.

What kind of water processing is best for the individual dialysis unit?

This depends on the quality of available tap water and its solute content. Feed water should be analyzed on a regular basis for chemical and bacteriologic content and should meet the EPA *Drinking Water Standard*. Product water—the final purified water used to prepare dialysis fluid should meet the AAMI and other applicable standards. Components of a system to meet these requirements may include:

- Initial sediment filter(s)
- Resin-type softener (water hardness checked twice daily)
- Activated carbon filter (two in series)
- RO unit (with continuous conductivity/resistivity monitoring of inflow and outflow water)
- Deionizer (DI) unit (continuous conductivity monitoring of outflow, plus monthly bacteriologic, limulus test, and chemical analysis)

A complete system of this type will provide maximum purity water, approaching 18 MΩ/cm resistance. Thorough investigation is necessary to reach the desired purity of water in the most economic manner. Ongoing monitoring is essential to ensure its maintenance.

Where may information about available tap water quality be obtained?

State Departments of Health conduct regular and detailed analyses of public water supplies, except for Indiana and Wyoming, where the Environmental Protection Agency (EPA) has responsibility. The reports are available upon request, and often, upon request, any periodic reports will be sent to the facility. The Department of Health may do an analysis of a specific water supply on request. Manufacturers of water treatment equipment and supplies seek to tailor their equipment to each individual dialysis facility's needs. They may provide a detailed water analysis as part of their service.

Information on chemical content is usually given in parts per million (ppm). This is equal to milligrams per *liter*. To convert to mEq/L, multiply milligrams per liter times valence and divide by molecular weight. For example, for calcium:

60 ppm = 60 mg/L
mEq/L Ca^{++} = 60 x 2 (valence) = 120 ÷ 40 (molecular weight) = 3

Thus 60 ppm Ca^{++} represents 3 mEq/L.

What cost factors are involved in establishing an adequate water treatment system?

Before setting a dollar figure on how much to spend, the facility should consult with a knowledgeable designer of dialysis facility water treatment systems and reliable supplier/installer. Facility needs, current and future, should be determined. Consideration should be given to each of the following factors:

- Peak volume needs
- Desired quality of product water (minimum should exceed AAMI standards)
- Expertise of the technical staff
- Cost of feed water
- Compliance with standards
- Type(s) of therapy to be delivered
- Ease of operation
- Maintenance requirements

Components listed on page 87 should be included only to achieve a particular goal, with the final objective of meeting or exceeding AAMI standards. If the source water is of very low mineral content, it may be possible to achieve 1 $M\Omega/cm$ product water by RO alone, or by DI alone, after appropriate filtration. Only the minimum number of components necessary should be used to meet or exceed AAMI standards.

Preparation of bicarbonate dialysate and high-flux dialysis may necessitate more stringent microbial control than is required by current AAMI standards and the 1991 Quality Assurance Guidelines.

What are the FDA "Guidelines for Water Treatment Equipment"?

According to the FDA Guidelines, each premarket notification for a water purification component or system should include the information listed in Box 6-2. This helps the FDA determine whether the application has "substantial equivalence" to a water purification system already on the market. A copy of the guidelines can be obtained from the Center for Devices and Radiological Health's Division of Small Manufacturers Assistance (DSMA).

Box 6-2 Factors Included in Premarket Notification for Water Purification Products

- Device name, including both the trade or propriety name and the classification name
- Establishment registration number, if applicable, of the owner or operator submitting the premarket notification
- The generic class (class 2) in which the device has been placed under section 513 of the Federal Food, Drug, and Cosmetic Act and the appropriate panel
- A statement of the action taken by the registered manufacturer for special controls
- The Safe Medical Devices Act of 1990 (SMDA) requires all persons preparing a premarket notification submission to include (a) a summary of the safety and effectiveness information in the premarket information notification submission upon which an equivalence determination could be based, or (b) a statement that safety and effectiveness information will be made available to interested persons upon request
- Proposed labels, labeling, and advertisements sufficient to describe the water purification component or system, its intended use, and the directions for use (including maintenance, operation, cleaning, and troubleshooting), accompanied by a specific intended use statement and any warnings, contraindications, or limitations clearly displayed
- Statement comparing the water purification component or system to a legally-marketed predicate device (one which was in commercial distribution prior to May 28, 1976, or one which has been cleared for marketing in the United States under Section 510(K) of the act)
- For a device or device labeling that has undergone a change or modification that could significantly affect the safety or effectiveness of the device, the 510(K) must include any additional supporting data to show that the manufacturer has considered the effects that the change or modification might have on the safety and effectiveness of the device
- Requirements are listed for these Water Purification Components:
  - Reverse osmosis (RO)
  - Water softeners
  - Carbon absorption beds
  - Deionization (DI)
  - Sediment and cartridge filters
  - Ultraviolet (UV) disinfection unit
  - Ultrafilters
  - Auxiliary components

(continued)

Box 6-2 (cont'd)

- Additional Requirements for Water Purification Systems Applications:
  - Provide a description of the decision-making process utilized to meet the needs of the user.
  - Describe the consequences of failure for each component and the required corrective action.
  - Provide user's manuals for each component of the system, as well as guidance for the installation, start-up and maintenance of the system.
  - Label each component in the system with the name and address of the supplier.
  - Provide the results of leech testing and identify the chemical composition of any material that leeches from the system.
  - Certify that the water produced by each purification system will meet or exceed current standards and regulations.

Modified from FDA Guidelines, *Nehphrology News and Issues*, Vol. 10, No. 10, October, 1996.

Note: Thanks are expressed to Ron Wathen, MD, PhD, Environmental Water Technology, Louisville, KY, for permission to use materials on reverse osmosis and ultrafiltration.

Dialyzer Preparation and Reprocessing

James Curtis, Ronald Emerson, and Anna L. Corea

DIALYZER PREPARATION

Each dialyzer has its own specific characteristics and procedure for preparation for patient use. Manufacturers' instructions are updated frequently as alterations are made or improved techniques are developed. It is very important to read package inserts frequently to ensure adherence to current recommendations.

What are the essential parameters when a dialyzer is prepared for patient use?

- All air in the dialyzer must be removed. Any air left in the dialyzer could be dialyzed across the membrane and into the patient's vascular system. Also, air trapped in the wall of the hollow fibers will reduce the dialyzer clearance by preventing diffusion between the blood and dialysate compartments.
- Any particulate matter left in the dialyzer from the manufacturing process must be flushed out with the saline prime.
- Dialyzers must have all disinfectant used in the reprocessing procedures removed, and be free of residual disinfectant.
- Dialyzers must always be flushed and primed with a physiological saline solution (0.9 g NaCl/100 ml water) compatible with patient blood.

How is air removed from a dialyzer?

To remove the air from a dialyzer, prime normal (physiological) saline into the dialyzer from the bottom. This is accomplished by attaching the blood lines to the dialyzer, and then turning the dialyzer so that the venous end is up. Then run the saline in through the arterial blood line, through the dialyzer into the venous blood line, and into a basin. As the dialyzer is filled, the air will be forced out the top of the dialyzer. Tap the dialyzer lightly, and turn it from side to side to ensure that all of the air is removed from the header.

How much saline should be used to prime the dialyzer?

It will take from 500 to 1000 cc. The amount depends on the type of dialyzer and whether or not it has been reprocessed. A new dialyzer should have

1000 ml of prime to remove the glycerin and particulate matter remaining from the manufacturing process. A reprocessed dialyzer requires 500 ml because the prime will be recirculated with the dialysate flowing counter clockwise to remove any residual disinfectant.

Should anything be different when priming a reprocessed dialyzer?

Yes. Reprocessed dialyzers are filled with a disinfectant, and it is important that no air be introduced into the dialyzer. Once air is introduced, it is very difficult to remove. All air must be removed from the arterial blood line before attaching it to the dialyzer. This is accomplished by priming the arterial blood line with saline, making sure all the air is removed prior to attaching the line to the dialyzer. After this is done, turn the dialyzer venous end up and continue the priming procedure.

Do manufacturers make any recommendations regarding the priming of their dialyzers?

Yes, all of them do. Some dialyzers should have the blood compartment filled first, and for others the dialysate compartment is filled first. Dialysis personnel should read and follow the instructions that come with the dialyzers used in the particular facility.

What other checks should be done on the dialysis machine prior to patient use?

It is necessary to ensure that machine functions have been checked, and that they work correctly: All extracorporeal alarms should be tested to ensure that they respond appropriately. Arterial pressure, venous pressure, and air detector alarms should all cause the blood pump to stop and the venous line clamp to close. In addition, conductivity and temperature of the dialysate should be tested to ensure that they are within the proper range. These alarms must be working at all times so that if any problems arise, the dialysate will be diverted from the dialyzer and a major complication avoided. Finally, there should be an adequate amount of dialysate concentrate to complete the patient's treatment.

DIALYZER REPROCESSING

Reuse of dialyzers is safe and cost effective. The guidelines in AAMI's *Recommended Practice for the Reuse of Hemodialyzers* (RD47) must be followed, as HCFA has adopted them as standards governing the practice. Dialyzer manufacturers are now required by the FDA to label their dialyzers so that users know that they are appropriate for reprocessing. The manufacturer must also recommend appropriate reprocessing techniques.

Blood lines and other disposable items have been reused, but are regulated and restricted by the Food and Drug Administration (FDA) and are rarely reused in the United States. The Department of Health and Human Services (Health Care Financing Administration) has taken an official ESRD program position on reuse and has published specific written requirements. Some chemicals used to reprocess dialyzers are considered hazardous and are regulated by the Occupational Safety and Health Administration (OSHA).

Is cost saving the only motive for reuse?

Cost containment is the primary reason for dialyzer reuse. Dialyzer cost per treatment can be reduced as much as 75 percent in a successful reuse program. There are purported clinical advantages to the reuse of dialyzers. On rare occasions a patient may react to a new dialyzer. These reactions are believed to be caused by either bioincompatible membranes or ethylene oxide residue left in the sterilized dialyzer. A reaction may occur shortly after initiation of dialysis, and could be life-threatening. Once the dialyzer has been reprocessed for reuse, such reactions are not observed during subsequent treatments. Reprocessed dialyzers rarely develop leaks. With reuse there is significant reduction of medical waste products.

How many times can a dialyzer be reused?

Some centers arbitrarily settle on three or five reuses per dialyzer. Even these small numbers represent a significant savings. To determine cost effectiveness of reuse, divide the original cost of the dialyzer by the total cost of reprocessing. To qualify for reuse, a dialyzer must meet defined criteria: residual volume must be 80 percent or greater of original volume, it must pass a pressure-holding test, and the appearance evaluation should show no more than a few clotted fibers. After each clinical use, the dialyzer is evaluated using these criteria and must meet them to be used again for a patient.

What are the basic steps for reuse?

The basic steps in most reprocessing programs are as follows: (1) flushing the dialyzer to remove most of the blood residuals; (2) cleaning, usually done with chemicals (bleach or Renalin) and reverse ultrafiltration; (3) testing to verify that the membrane is intact and that the dialyzer will remove waste products as expected; and (4) disinfection with either a chemical or heat.

What are specific criteria used to determine if a dialyzer may be reused.

There are four main criteria for reuse:
- Total cell volume (TCV) measurement is the most widely used method to determine whether a reused dialyzer maintains adequate solute

removal capability. In this test, the dialyzer is filled with water, pumped dry, and the contained volume is measured in a graduated cylinder. This volume is the standard for that dialyzer and the value against which it will be compared after each use. If less than 80 percent of initial volume remains, the dialyzer is rejected for further patient use. A dialyzer with 80 percent of its initial volume still has 90 percent of its initial solute removal capability.

- Pressure testing of the dialyzer is performed to determine whether there are broken fibers that would lead to a blood leak during dialysis. Pressure is applied to the dialyzer and then held. If the pressure drop is too great, the dialyzer is discarded.
- Some reuse machines test the dialyzer's k_{UF} (ultrafiltration coefficient). Though this is not a test to predict dialyzer clearance, it is an indication of how "open" the dialyzer membrane may be to large molecules.
- Finally, appearance is an important criterion. A dialyzer with larger streaks of residual blood, indicating a large number of clotted fibers, is cause for immediate rejection.

To be used again, a dialyzer must meet minimum requirements of TCV and pressure tests.

Is large solute clearance affected by reprocessing?

Yes. The extent of this effect depends on the dialyzer membrane and reprocessing technique; some membranes tend to become more open when exposed to bleach cleaning. Most membrane clearance of large solutes such as Beta-2 microglobulin is decreased when Renalin is used. It is very important to understand how particular dialyzers are affected by the reprocessing technique used.

How are reprocessed dialyzers disinfected?

Renalin is the most commonly used chemical disinfectant, used by about 70 percent of dialysis units; formaldehyde (formalin) is the second most common disinfectant used. Gluteraldehyde and heat are used by some facilities to disinfect dialyzers.

What exposure time is required for Renalin and formaldehyde?

Renalin, a mixture of hydrogen peroxide, peracetic acid, and acetic acid, is a sterilant and requires a 0.5% solution for an 11-hour contact time. In contrast, aqueous formaldehyde, a high-level disinfectant, kills all microorganisms, including spores and viruses, with a minimum exposure of 24 hours and a 4% concentration of formalin at room temperature. A lower concentration, 1.5% formalin, is effective at 100°F for a 24-hour exposure.

What happens if a dialyzer is not adequately disinfected?

If there is not sufficient exposure (concentration and time), bacteria in the dialyzer will not be killed and may even multiply. This could result in a patient becoming bacteremic when the blood is exposed to the dialyzer during a subsequent treatment.

What information should be verified before using a reprocessed dialyzer for a patient?

Several checks must be completed. The most important is to verify that the dialyzer is being used for the correct patient. Other requirements include ensuring that the dialyzer contained an adequate level of disinfectant before it was rinsed, and that all of the disinfectant was removed during the rinsing process. Finally, the dialyzer must pass all reuse testing such as TCV and pressure tests.

What precautions are necessary when using chemical disinfectants?

The use of protective gear—including eye shield, gloves, and a waterproof gown—is necessary. Adequate ventilation (in adherence to OSHA Guidelines) is also required. Any splashes on skin or eyes should be flushed with copious amounts of water and appropriate medical care should be sought.

Note: OSHA requires that personnel be well informed about these hazardous chemicals and their potential toxicity. Every dialysis facility must have printed OSHA requirements and regulations related to the use of disinfectants.

Are these chemicals stable over time?

No. Renalin is broken down fairly rapidly by temperature greater than 80°F, exposure to light, and exposure to organic matter (such as blood). Time is another factor: once diluted, Renalin has a relatively short shelf life. It is very important to test each dialyzer for Renalin potency just prior to preparing it for patient use. Formaldehyde is quite stable for long periods of time.

How should the dialyzer be prepared before the next run?

After the dialyzer is filled with disinfectant at the end of the reprocessing procedure, it is necessary to document the presence of the disinfectant by an appropriate chemical test. This helps to confirm that the dialyzer is stored with the disinfecting chemical. Before the next clinical use, the disinfectant must be removed. The blood lines are connected to the dialyzer, and sterile saline is rinsed through the blood side of the dialyzer. Usually 250–500 ml of saline is run through the dialyzer and discarded. The arterial and venous blood lines are then connected to establish a closed loop. The blood pump is started, and the recirculation of saline, with ultrafiltration, should remove any residual chemical left in the system. Essentially, the disinfectant is simply dialyzed out of the system.

Just before use, the recirculating saline in the dialyzer is sampled using the test appropriate for the disinfectant used. After the test is performed, the absence of the disinfectant must be documented. Only after a negative test has been confirmed is the dialyzer considered safe for patient use. Many dialysis units and some state agencies require two persons to verify that the dialyzer is correct for a specific patient and has a negative disinfectant test before using the reprocessed dialyzer.

When Renalin is the disinfectant used, is there a specific order in which the compartments are primed?

Yes. Renalin is a strong acid, so it is important to prime the blood compartment with normal saline before attaching the dialysate lines. If the dialysate compartment is primed first, reaction between the dialysate and Renalin will cause some of the CO_2 to come out of solution as a gas. These bubbles can be trapped in the fibers, creating an air gap between the blood and dialysate, with poor diffusion.

Are there circumstances in which reuse is inappropriate for a particular patient?

Yes, patients with systemic infections or with sepsis are generally excluded from reprocessing programs. Patients with infectious diseases are usually excluded also, including (but not limited to) Hepatitis B, HIV and methicillin-resistant *Staphylococcus aureus* (MRSA).

Are patients required to give their consent for reuse of dialyzers?

Yes, HCFA requires that patients give consent in writing. The consent must be made part of the patient's clinical record. If the patient does not give this written consent, reuse is not permitted.

ACCESS TO THE BLOODSTREAM

Susan C. Vogel

HISTORICAL BACKGROUND

Effective hemodialysis became a reality in the 1940s. Each treatment required a surgical cutdown. Hollow tubes (cannulas) of glass or metal were inserted into an artery and a vein. The glass and metal tubes were later replaced with cannulas of polyvinyl chloride or other plastic materials. During the 1950s, attempts were made to leave the cannulas in place for more than one treatment. Different methods of maintaining patency were tried. These attempts, at best, lasted only a few treatments.

In 1960, Scribner, Quinton, and Dillard at the University of Washington, devised a cannula that could be left in place much longer. It consisted of Teflon tubes, one placed in an artery, and one in a vein. These tubes were connected externally, allowing for continuous rapid flow of blood through the device. This technique was improved in 1962 with the use of Silastic (silicone rubber) for the external shunt loop, and Teflon for the vessel tips. This allowed for greater flexibility of the tubing and increased comfort for the patient. This innovation was not only effective for a single hemodialysis but also offered a method for repeat treatments.

Another major development came in 1966 when Cimino, Brescia, and coworkers developed the forearm internal arteriovenous fistula. This was created by performing a surgical anastomosis between a forearm artery and vein. The subsequent flow of arterial blood into the vein permitted percutaneous puncture of this vessel that offered adequate flow for hemodialysis.

Use of internal synthetic graft materials began in 1974. Today, the most common type of synthetic graft is polytetrafluorethylene (PTFE). A "button" needle-free form of vascular access was developed in 1980. The "button" needle-free worked, but not as well as the other internal synthetic graft material. These new synthetic grafts and devices offered new possibilities for patients who did not have adequate vessels for a Cimino fistula.

Shaldon described temporary access for hemodialysis via cannulation of the femoral vein in 1961. Uldall, in 1979, devised a special catheter for temporary access in the subclavian or internal jugular vein. When the dual lumen catheters were introduced, this further enhanced a means of temporary access, by allowing one catheter to function as both the inlet and outlet ports.

Vascular access, as used for hemodialysis in the early '60s, has evolved considerably during the last thirty years or more. However, maintaining patent access with adequate blood flow remains one of the major problems in the chronically hemodialyzed patient. (Fig. 8-1).

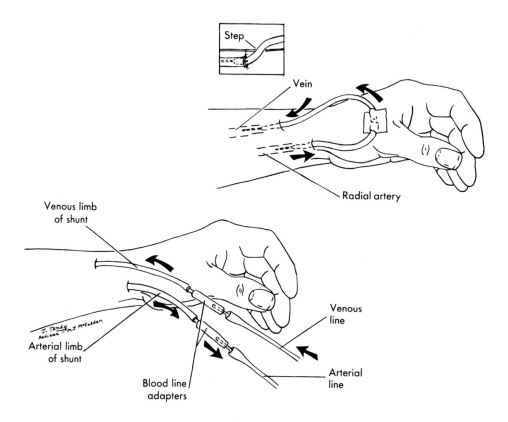

Fig. 8-1 A, Quinton-Scribner shunt with connector in place between dialysis runs. **B,** Shunt arms separated and connected to dialyzer blood lines. From Larson E, Lindbloom I, Davis KB: *Development of the clinical nephrology practitioner,* St. Louis, 1982, Mosby.

INTERNAL ARTERIOVENOUS FISTULAS

What is an internal fistula?

In an internal fistula, a small (5 mm) opening is created surgically in an adjoining artery and vein, and the two vessels are joined at this opening, creating an arteriovenous fistula. The diversion of arterial blood causes the veins to become enlarged and prominent, allowing placement of large-bore needles to provide adequate blood flow for dialysis (Fig 8-2).

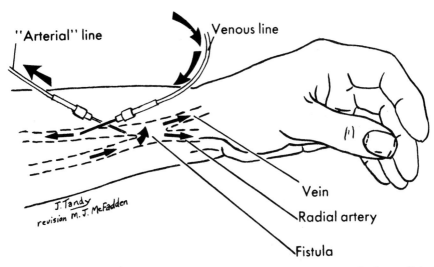

Fig. 8-2 Brescia-Cimino AV fistula (side to side) with needles in place for hemodialysis. From Larson E, Lindbloom L, Davis KB: *Development of the clinical nephrology practitioner*, St. Louis, 1982, Mosby.

What is a graft arteriovenous fistula?

A biologic, semibiologic, or prosthetic graft is implanted subcutaneously and one end is attached to an artery, the other end to a vein. The synthetic graft is used most often in patients who do not have adequate vessels to create an internal AV fistula.

What are the advantages of an internal AV fistula for access to the bloodstream?

Because it is under the skin, or internal, the AV fistula is less susceptible to infection and/or blood loss.

What are special care needs and potential problems with use of AV fistulae for access to the bloodstream?

Needle insertions are necessary for each hemodialysis. With repetitive venipunctures, scar tissue forms over the fistula, making insertion of needles more difficult and painful. Furthermore, if a needle becomes accidentally dislodged and passes through a vessel wall, bleeding into the tissues may result in formation of a painful hematoma. Use of the fistula may be difficult or impossible until swelling decreases.

At the end of each hemodialysis treatment, after the needles are withdrawn, firm pressure must be applied over the puncture area for 10 to 20 minutes to prevent persistent bleeding.

Are there special problems with an internal AV fistula?

Size and location of arterialized veins are important. It is often a matter of weeks, and sometimes months, before the veins become sufficient in size that large-bore needles may be inserted without difficulty. In women this process takes longer than in men. The veins of the forearm vary in their pattern and distribution. The location of easily accessible vessels may be limited, so that a few sites must be repeatedly used for insertion.

Occasionally, the desired blood flow is difficult to obtain through the inlet needle. This problem may result from the size of the vein or from branches that divert the flow. Occasionally the needle must be placed very near the anastomosis to obtain sufficient flow (the needle tip should never be closer than 2 cm from the anastomosis). Sometimes with side-to-side AV fistulas, most of the dilation of the veins occurs over the back of the hand, and the arm veins do not become prominent. Surgical revision may be required to correct the flow of the blood.

A third problem is spasm of the vessel, which is common. This usually occurs at the beginning of hemodialysis, causing decreased arterial blood flow. Spasms occur when attempting to maintain high blood flows in an immature fistula. The lumen of the needle sucking against the vessel wall can cause spasms. This is painful and is accompanied by a fluttering sensation at the needle. The use of back-eye needles may help.

On the return-flow side, resistance may be high secondary to venous stenosis in the outflow vessel above the anastomosis. Other mechanical causes of return flow resistance include position of the extremity and placement of the needle against the vessel wall. Repositioning of the needle may be necessary.

A fourth problem is accidental tearing of the vessel during venipuncture. This may result in formation of a large hematoma, making the vessel difficult or impossible to use for many days. The same type of accident may occur if the patient suddenly moves or thrashes about during dialysis.

In addition, the "radial artery steal" syndrome may develop. A few patients develop ischemic changes of the fingers. This is manifested by coldness, poor function, and even gangrene and necrosis of tips of the fingers. The "steal" is caused by low arterial pressure at the fistula site, resulting from diversion of radial artery blood to the vein. Since the radial artery distal to the fistula normally connects with the ulnar artery, the pressure gradient causes ulnar blood to be diverted from the arteries to the fingers and flows instead toward the fistula. If recognized early, the syndrome may be corrected by surgically tying off the radial artery distal to the fistula.

Infections, thromboses, and aneurysms are three additional potential AV fistula problems. Infection of the fistula can occur secondary to poor personal hygiene or poor aseptic technique during cannulation. This local infection can lead to thrombosis or sepsis if not treated. Signs and symptoms include redness and swelling of the access and/or pain and fever. Diagnosis is confirmed by culturing the drainage and/or doing blood cultures. Antibiotic therapy is employed.

Thrombosis is the most common complication of AV fistulae. In addition to infection, it can be caused by hypotension or stenosis of the fistula. Thrombosis can also be secondary to compression of blood flow, either by the use of tight bandages or a fistula-needle–holding device, by the patient sleeping on the fistula arm, or from hematoma formation.

Finally, aneurysms (outpouchings of the vessel wall) can occur from repeated cannulation of the same site and from infection. Large aneurysms limit available cannulation sites.

What types of grafts are available?

Synthetic grafts are the most common grafts currently in use. Many synthetic materials (Dacron, PTFE) are available in various diameters and lengths. A newer form of PTFE allows for needle insertion immediately after placement, although the manufacturer recommends waiting 5-7 days (Fig. 8-3 displays two types of placement for synthetic grafts).

What are the advantages of a graft fistula?

Graft fistulas can be used sooner than AV fistulas, usually after two weeks. Maturation time for the vessel to enlarge is not required. The larger vessel size allows for easier cannulation.

What are the disadvantages of a graft fistula?

The disadvantages are the same as for AV fistulas.

How does one assess the internal fistula for patency and blood flow?

Assessment involves several steps:
- Visibly observe the fistula, noting any signs of infection.
- Palpate the fistula. A "thrill" will be felt over the entire length.
- Listen with the bell of a stethoscope for a bruit. This should be clearly audible over the entire length of the fistula.
- The person initiating the treatment assesses access prior to dialysis.
- Teach the patient to assess the access daily.

What is the proper aseptic preparation for cannulation of a graft?

An antiseptic solution, such as povidone iodine, should be used to cleanse the skin over and around the fistula. Apply the antiseptic in a circular motion away from the puncture site until a circle of two inches in diameter has been covered. Be sure to follow the antiseptic manufacturer's directions for effective

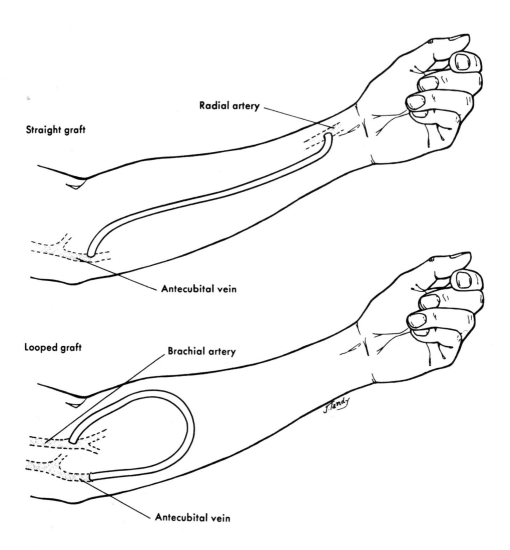

Fig. 8-3 Two types of subcutaneous AV grafts. *Top*: Straight graft, radial artery to cubital vein; *Bottom*: Loop graft, brachial artery to cubital vein. From Larson E, Lindbloom L, Davis KB: *Development of the clinical nephrology practitioner*, St. Louis, 1982, Mosby.

disinfection. The povidone iodine must be allowed to dry on the epidermis before needle insertion. If the patient is allergic to povidone iodine, isopropyl alcohol may be used, but needle insertion must be performed while the epidermis is wet.

What types of needles are used for puncturing the AV fistula?

Large-bore, thin-wall, back-eye needles are preferred. The larger bore needle is used for the high blood flows necessary for high-flux or high-efficiency dialysis. Blood flows of 400–500 ml/min may be attained with 14-gauge needles. Smaller bore,17-gauge needles are used with children, or infants to accommodate their small vessel size and decreased blood flow rate requirements.

Are there particular points to be observed in placing the needles?

The inlet (arterial line) needle should be placed nearest the anastomosis but at least 6 cm away from the site. The return needle (venous line) should be located so that the point is at least 8 to 10 cm away from the inlet needle. It should always be directed toward the heart.

Why is this positioning of the needles important?

Placing the arterial needle near the anastomosis will achieve the best blood flow. The tip should not be closer than 2 cm from the fistula, to lessen damage to the intima and decrease the risk of thrombosis. Placement of the needle toward or away from the anastomosis depends on the optimal blood flow. Usual practice is to place the arterial needle point with the flow.

Finally, spacing the needles 8 to 10 cm apart minimizes recirculation of blood that may result in an inadequate dialysis.

What conditions favor recirculation?

A fistula with a low blood flow rate leads to recirculation. The low flow can be caused by stenosis at the arterial end, or more commonly, by stenosis at the venous end. It is usually associated with an increase in venous pressure and, if the recirculation is sufficiently great, may result in the "black blood" syndrome.

What is the "black blood" syndrome?

When recirculation is severe, the blood becomes acidotic, and the red cells cannot carry oxygen. The pH of this blood is usually below 7.0, and the blood appears very dark.

How is occurrence of recirculation determined?

The concentration of any substance (urea or creatinine) should be the same in the arterial blood line going into the dialyzer as in the patient's systemic circulation. If the arterial concentration is less, the substance may be diluted by venous blood returning from the dialyzer so that some blood is going through the dialyzer more than once without returning to the systemic circulation. To calculate the percentage recirculation, three blood samples are obtained simultaneously. One represents the systemic circulation (peripheral blood or P). Also necessary is a specimen from the inflow line just before it enters the dialyzer (arterial blood or A), and the outflow line just after it leaves the dialyzer (venous blood or V). Calculate the estimated recirculation as follows:

$$\text{Percent recirculation} = \frac{P - A}{P - V}$$

Example: P = 100, A = 90, V = 25

$$\text{Percent recirculation} = \frac{100 - 90}{100 - 25} = \frac{10}{75}$$

$$10 \div 75 = 0.13$$

$$0.13 \times 100\% = 13\%$$

Given a good fistula and use of two well-placed needles, the percentage of recirculation should be less than 10 percent. With double-lumen catheters, recirculation commonly may be as high as 15 percent. Recirculation greater than 15 percent is excessive and should be investigated and corrected.

How is the peripheral (P) blood sample obtained?

Peripheral veins are no longer used. The peripheral sample is obtained from the inflow line before the dialyzer, using the slow/stop flow technique for measuring access recirculation. See Box 8-1.

What other techniques are available to measure access recirculation?

Newer techniques allowing for real-time measurement of access recirculation include the HD01 hemodialysis monitoring system (Transonic Systems, Ithaca, NY, USA) and the Crit-Line instrument (In-Line Diagnostics Corporation, Farmington, Utah, USA).

Box 8-1   Revised Slow/Stop Flow Technique for Measuring Access Recirculation

1. Perform test after approximately 30 minutes; turn off UF.
2. Draw arterial (A) and venous (V) line samples.
3. Immediately reduce BFR to 120 ml/min.
4. Turn blood pump off 10 seconds after reducing BFR.
5. Clamp arterial line above sampling port.
6. Draw systemic or peripheral blood sample from arterial line port.
7. Unclamp line and resume dialysis.

Revised slow/stop flow technique for measuring vascular access recirculation. From Sherman R, et al. Recognition of the Failing Vascular Access: A Current Perspective, *Seminars in Dialysis* 10(1): 1-4, 1997.

How do these devices measure recirculation?

The Transonic Systems device uses flow dilution sensors placed on the arterial and venous blood lines. Saline is injected through the venous drip chamber or a port in the venous tubing. A laptop computer preloaded with dilution measurement software measures the volume flow through the blood lines and the changes in the ultrasound signal velocity and calculates the percentage of recirculation. The Transonic Systems device also measures cardiac output.

The In-Line Diagnostics device uses a disposable blood chamber placed between the end of the arterial blood tubing and the arterial port of the dialyzer. An optical sensor is placed on the blood chamber and is attached to the In-Line Diagnostics device. The In-Line Diagnostics device calculates the percentage of recirculation based on changes in hematocrit following micro-infusions of saline. This instrument also measures hematocrit, oxygen saturation and blood volume change (see Fig. 8-4; also see Chaper 9, page 126, for a discussion of the Crit-Line instrument).

May the venous needle be placed in another extremity?

Occasion may arise when two needles cannot be placed in the fistula extremity (usually because of hematoma formation or infiltration upon needle insertion). Often a vein in the opposite extremity can be found that will accommodate the outflow from the machine.

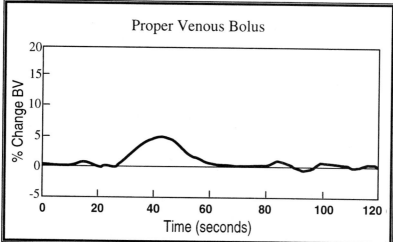

Fig. 8-4   A, Proper arterial bolus. The peak height should be at least 15%. **B**, Proper venous bolus. The screen now displays a smaller bolus. If recirculation is occurring, Crit-Line will calculate the area under the curve. (Crit-Line manufactured by In-Line Diagnostics Corporation, Farmington, UT)

Can anything be done to cause the veins of an arm with an AV fistula to enlarge more quickly?

Nothing should be attempted for 4 or 5 days after the fistula is created. A tourniquet or blood pressure cuff may be placed around the upper arm, snug enough to cause distention of the veins; it may be left in place for a half hour and may be repeated several times each day. Hand exercises, such as squeezing a rubber ball while the tourniquet is in place, may help. Warm compresses or soaks several times a day may speed up the venous distension.

What care is required for the fistula arm between dialyses?

An arm with a new fistula should be elevated on a pillow between treatments to decrease swelling in the extremity. It is important to maintain adequate pressure, either by hand or with a tight pressure dressing, over the puncture sites for 10 to 20 minutes after the needles are removed. Most patients still have some heparin effect at the end of dialysis, and bleeding can be a serious problem. Even oozing under the skin can cause hematoma and scar formation, which eventually makes the vessel difficult to use. After the bleeding has stopped, plastic bandages are sufficient to protect the puncture sites. If bleeding continues from the puncture site more than 20 minutes after removal of needles, the heparin dose should be evaluated and readjusted. Activated clotting times should be monitored during dialysis to ascertain optimal heparin requirements for each patient. Daily cleaning with soap is advised. Some people like to use an ointment to keep the skin soft.

SINGLE-NEEDLE TECHNIQUE

Kopp developed the single-needle device in 1970 for use with the internal AV fistula and the single-lumen catheter. Single-needle dialysis has not been practiced in the United States for several years; however, it is popular in Europe.

What is the principle of operation of single-needle dialysis?

A Y-type hub is connected to a single needle or catheter. As blood is drawn into the dialyzer, a clamp simultaneously occludes the outflow line. Then the inflow line is occluded while the outflow is released to return blood from the dialyzer to the patient. In Europe two blood pumps are used; one for the arterial blood line and one for the venous blood line. High-flux dialysis, with its need for high blood flow rates, and the popularity of dual-lumen catheters have minimized the use of single-needle devices outside of Europe.

TEMPORARY VASCULAR ACCESS

What veins are used for temporary access?

The subclavian, internal jugular, and femoral veins are used (Fig. 8-5A). Vessels are accessed using double lumen catheters (Fig. 8-5B).

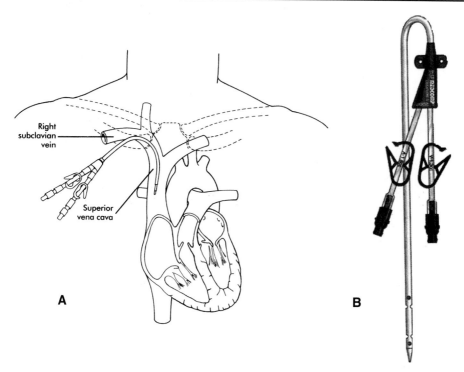

Fig. 8-5   A, Temporary vascular access using subclavian dual-lumen venous catheter, **B**, Dual-lumen temporary catheter. Courtesy MEDCOMP Corporation, Harleysville, PA.

What are the indications for using a subclavian or jugular catheter?

These are used in patients requiring urgent hemodialysis. For example:
- The ESRD patient whose fistula or graft needs time to mature
- Patients on peritoneal dialysis requiring temporary hemodialysis because of peritonitis
- Acute renal failure patients
- Patients undergoing plasmapheresis
- Patients receiving venovenous continuous renal replacement therapy.

It should be noted that prolonged use of subclavian vein catheters will result in subclavian vein stenosis.

What are the contraindications for using subclavian or jugular catheters?

Subclavian or jugular catheters should not be used on the following patients:
- Patients with acute respiratory distress who cannot be positioned either supine or in the Trendelenburg position
- Patients with known subclavian vein stenosis

How is the subclavian or jugular catheter placed?

The physician uses strict aseptic technique. The patient lies supine in the Trendelenburg position with the head turned to the opposite side. The skin around the area is cleaned and covered with sterile drapes. With local anesthesia, the catheter is inserted and sutured into place. Verification of correct placement by chest x-ray examination is required before the catheter may be used.

What complications can occur?

Immediately after the insertion, pneumothorax, hemothorax, or air embolism may occur. Bleeding is another complication, if the artery is inadvertently punctured during insertion.

What are indications for using a femoral catheter?

A femoral catheter is used in the following types of cases:
- The acutely ill patient confined to bed
- The ESRD patient whose access is clotted, but who requires urgent dialysis
- Continuous renal replacement therapy
- Patients who may have subclavian vein stenosis

What complications can occur?

- Retroperitoneal hemorrhage from puncture of the vein during insertion
- Bleeding at the insertion site

Is special nursing management necessary with these catheters?

Aseptic technique when initiating and when terminating dialysis is of utmost importance. All catheters are prone to infection. The caps and ports should be wrapped in a 4x4 dressing soaked in povidone iodine for 5 minutes, before initiating or ending dialysis. The exit site should be cleaned with peroxide and povidone iodine after every treatment, and a sterile dressing should be applied. The appearance of the exit site, especially if there is redness or drainage, must be documented.

Heparin is instilled into the port(s) of the catheter following dialysis. This heparin must be removed before the next dialysis to avoid the patient's receiving a bolus. Do not attempt to instill saline into a clotted catheter; this might force the clot into the vascular system.

What technical problems can occur with these catheters, and how are they best combatted?

The main problem, poor blood flow, can be corrected by:
- Lowering the patient's head, or turning the patient's head to the opposite side from the catheter, if using a subclavian or jugular vein
- Keeping sterile dressing intact until the end of the treatment
- Applying external pressure to the exit site
- Rotating the catheter shaft 180 degrees if the catheter has wings
- Reversing the lines, using the arterial port for venous return (as a last resort)

The other difficulty that commonly occurs is clotting. Proper heparinization of the catheter after dialysis, according to the manufacturer's directions, will help to alleviate this problem. Fibrinolytic agents, such as urokinase, may be prescribed if the catheter is clotted or to prevent clotting.

Are there dual-lumen catheters available for permanent use?

The permanent catheter is becoming more widely used. A silicone rubber catheter is inserted intraoperatively. The catheter has a subcutaneous dacron graft that impedes infection. These catheters are usually placed in the internal jugular vein and a subcutaneous tunnel is created that allows the catheter to exit through the chest wall (Fig. 8-6A). Permanent catheters are also placed in the subclavian, mammary and femoral veins. A newer type of permcath, modified by Tesio® (Fig. 8-6B), uses two single-lumen catheters placed side-by-side in the same vein. This allows for customized catheter placement with increased blood flow rate. Permcaths are useful in pediatric patients whose small arteries and veins prohibit placement of an AV graft.

What continuous quality improvement issues are important with vascular access?

Greatest concern surrounds issues of assessment, clotting, and venous pressure. In assessment, documentation on the treatment record should include absence or presence of a bruit and thrill with fistulas and shunts. A decrease in thrill may denote graft stenosis and impending graft clotting. Note the appearance of the access, including redness, swelling, and any drainage. It is important to document the ease or difficulty of cannulation.

Second, adequate blood flow is important to prevent clotting of the lines and dialyzer, resulting in unnecessary loss of blood. Clotting occurs most often with catheters. Increased bleeding from the needle sites after dialysis may indicate venous stenosis.

Finally, increasing venous pressure is often a sign of stenosis. Venous pressure is measured immediately after initiation of hemodialysis at a blood flow rate

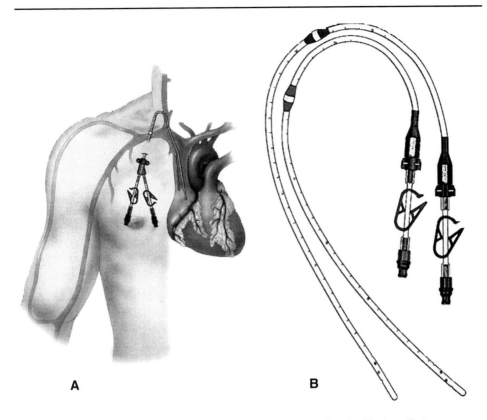

A   **B**

Fig. 8-6 A, Internal jugular permanent vascular access using the Tesio catheter, **B,** Permcath modified by Tesio. Courtesy MEDCOMP Corporation, Harleysville, PA.

(BFR) of 200 ml/min. With 16-gauge needles, the venous pressure should be <150 mm Hg. With 15-gauge needles, the venous pressure should be <100 mm Hg.

What are the DOQI guidelines for vascular access?

The Dialysis Outcomes Quality Initiative (DOQI) guidelines, formulated by the National Kidney Foundation in 1997, advocate both early placement of an AV fistula predialysis and avoidance of temporary catheters. The guidelines also emphasize that the AV fistula should be the first access attempt. DOQI guidelines also suggest that the percent of AV fistulae should be increased. To follow these guidelines, each dialysis unit should have an aggressive CQI access program. Copies of the DOQI Vascular Access guidelines can be obtained from the National Kidney Foundation. (See page 333 for additional information on NKF-DOQI.)

What are some of the newer trends in blood access?

Innovative locations are used for arteriovenous graft and permcath placement when usual sites are no longer available. Examples include the axillofemoral or the mammary artery to mammary vein graft. Research continues, in hopes of devising a graft that doesn't clot.

In summary, when the Scribner shunt was developed in 1960, the impact it would have on prolonging the life of the patient with end stage renal disease was unforeseen. Currently, over 220,000 patients in the United States are on maintenance hemodialysis, and there are many people in acute renal failure whose care is facilitated by technological advances in vascular access. Experimentation with new devices is ongoing. The future portends innovations that will enhance the care and the quality of life of the patient with renal failure.

Patient and Machine Monitoring and Assessment

Anna L. Corea, Sandra Smolka-Hill,
Linda S. Christensen, and Susan C. Vogel

Initial and ongoing assessment of the patient and continuous monitoring of dialysis equipment are among the most vital functions of dialysis personnel. Both registered nurses and patient care technicians (PCTs) have defined roles and responsibilities. State boards of nursing regulate the practice of nursing, including the direct supervision of non-professionals to whom specific tasks may be delegated. Readers are advised to review the regulations guiding practice in the states in which they practice.

In some states, only registered nurses are allowed to perform assessment as described by the Nursing Practice Acts. Several states, however, have special laws that allow the unlicensed dialysis patient care technicians (PCT) to perform certain tasks. In California, PCTs are certified by the state to infuse normal saline IV for priming and hypotension, inject subcutaneous xylocaine prior to insertion of 14- or 15-gauge needles into the vascular access and to administer IV heparin for anticoagulation per protocol or physicians' orders. These tasks are allowed under the direct supervision of a registered nurse.

In this chapter *assessment* refers to the *nurses'* role. *Monitoring* or collection of data is the role of the *PCT*. After data are collected, the nurse and the PCT work together to initiate changes in the dialysis treatment per physicians' orders or protocols.

What is patient monitoring?

Patient monitoring is a series of repeated or continuous observations and documentation of the patient's physiologic state and response to dialysis. Machine monitoring is continuous and includes the following: arterial and venous pressures, blood flow rate, transmembrane pressure (TMP), ultrafiltrate removed, dialysate temperature, dialysate flow and conductivity, and remaining treatment time. Dialysis personnel are responsible for reading, documenting and evaluating these parameters. Vital signs are measured at least every hour or more frequently in unstable patients. Assessments determine the appropriate dialysis intervention to attain the goals of treatment.

What are dialysis treatment outcome standards?

The National Kidney Foundation—Dialysis Outcomes Quality Initiative (NKF-DOQI) provides guidelines with indicators for outcomes. Four different clinical practices guidelines (hemodialysis adequacy, peritoneal dialysis adequacy, treatment of anemia, and vascular access) are used to assess and improve the outcome of each dialysis. Additional guidelines for pediatrics and nutrition are being developed. (See page 333 for additional information on NKF-DOQI.)

What are the different types of hemodialysis assessment?

Types of assessment include the following: physical assessments, laboratory data analysis and interpretation, first dialysis assessment, intradialytic assessment (predialysis, postdialysis, and monitoring of hemodialysis procedure), and the multidisciplinary team assessment using the NKF-DOQI clinical practice guidelines.

GENERAL ASSESSMENT PARAMETERS

Assessment involves collecting data through interviews, physical examination, performance of laboratory tests, and interpretation of patient observation. These data directly affect the patient's care.

What does physical assessment include?

Physical assessment consists of the following: assessing weight, blood pressure (BP), temperature, pulse, respiratory rate; evaluating respiratory effort, extent of edema; auscultating for quality of heart sounds and breath sounds; comparing apical and peripheral pulses; assessing skin integrity, skin color, jugular vein distension (JVD); and evaluating vascular access.

When are patients weighed?

Dialysis patients are weighed before and after each dialysis treatment. Some patients follow their weights at home to guide the adjustment of their fluid intake between dialyses.

Why is measurement of weight important?

Weight is a good indicator of how well the patient is controlling fluid balance between dialyses. Predialysis weight indicates how much ultrafiltration is required during the treatment. Postdialysis weight is the best indication of how much ultrafiltration occurred during the hemodialysis procedure.

What is meant by the patient's dry weight?

Dry weight is the *ideal* postdialysis weight after the removal of all or most excess body fluid. Patients who are at dry weight are usually normotensive. If the postdialysis weight suggests volume status is too high, the patient may be on the borderline for fluid overload and may be hypertensive. If postdialysis weight is too low, the patient may be hypovolemic and at risk for hypotension and clotting of the vascular access.

How much weight gain is permissible between dialysis treatments?

Weight gained between dialysis procedures is due to fluid retention. Most dialysis units encourage patients to limit their weight gain to 0.5 kg (or 1 lb) per day. Refer to Chapter 12 for further discussion and calculation of fluid restrictions.

Why is blood pressure (BP) measurement important?

Blood pressure is often volume-related. Hypertension may indicate volume overload. Hypotension may indicate dehydration. Blood pressure is measured while the patient is sitting and standing to evaluate orthostatic changes requiring intervention.

What is normal blood pressure?

Normal BP is an individual matter. In the ESRD patient, blood pressure is analyzed for trends, rather than absolute values. A systolic value greater than 170 mm Hg or less than 90 mm Hg or a diastolic value greater than 100 mm Hg should be reported to the physician.

Where can the cuff be placed for blood pressure measurement?

The upper arm is the most common cuff placement site. Two alternative placements are: (1) A large thigh cuff can be applied around the mid- thigh area. The pulse is audible via a stethoscope at the popliteal space. (2) A regular cuff may be applied above the ankle with auscultation over the posterior tibial or dorsalis pedis artery. This usually yields an audible BP, but the readings obtained will be 20 to 40 mm Hg higher than arm pressures. A notation should be made on the patient's chart whenever leg pressures are taken.

Why are temperature, pulse, and respiration (TPR) monitored?

TPR observations serve as a baseline at the start of dialysis. Temperature elevation suggests infection or complicating illness. An elevated temperature is often a sign of vascular access infection. Fever during dialysis may be caused by high dialysate temperature or by a pyrogen reaction. A rapid pulse may result from anemia or fluid overload. Irregular heart rate (arrhythmia) may indicate cardiac complications, including those associated with serum potassium levels. An increase in pulse rate during dialysis may be associated with falling blood volume (from ultrafiltration) and may occur just before a drop in BP. Increased respiratory rate may indicate excessive fluid gain. Any unexpected findings should be reported to the physician.

What is edema?

Edema is the excessive accumulation of fluid in the tissue spaces. Excessive weight gain between dialyses results in edema. Edema appears in different areas of the body in different patients. It may present at the ankle or sacrum, facial or periorbital areas or peripherally. The jugular veins are often distended when the patient is fluid-overloaded. Fluid status assessment determines the amount of ultrafiltration required during dialysis.

Are there other physical assessments?

The predialysis assessment includes a subjective analysis of the patient's health since the previous dialysis treatment. Ask whether he or she has experienced symptoms such as headaches, hypotension, bleeding, or diarrhea. Dialysis personnel can assess changes in mentation, speech, or thought processes while patients describe their health and any problems between dialysis sessions.

LABORATORY DATA ANALYSIS AND INTERPRETATION

Important laboratory values include electrolytes (sodium, potassium, chloride, carbon dioxide), blood urea nitrogen (BUN), creatinine, hemoglobin, hematocrit, white blood cell count, reticulocytes, platelets, iron, and iron-binding capacity, ferritin, calcium, phosphorus, magnesium, albumin, total protein, glucose, alkaline phosphatase, transaminase (ALT, AST), cholesterol, PTH, aluminum, and hepatitis panel are important laboratory tests used to monitor the dialysis patient.

What are normal laboratory values and how are they interpreted in the ESRD patient?

Review of the laboratory reports are included in the overall patient assessment. Any deviations from normal should be further evaluated for what is acceptable value for a dialysis patient. For example, creatinine and blood urea nitrogen (BUN) values may not fall within the range of normal because of ESRD. However, dialysis personnel should follow a protocol that defines when the BUN and creatinine values exceed the acceptable range for a person on dialysis and take appropriate action. Deviations from the acceptable range of laboratory values should be reported to the dialysis physician for appropriate intervention. Interventions may include a change in the dialysis prescription and/or medication(s). More detailed discussions of laboratory values and interventions can be found in Chapters 14 and 17.

What is the BUN-creatinine ratio?

The usual BUN-to-creatinine ratio is 10:1.

What causes an abnormal elevation of the BUN-creatinine ratio?

Some factors that elevate BUN out of proportion to creatinine include the following: internal bleeding, bruising, steroids, dietary indiscretion, sepsis, and loss of muscle mass.

What is the importance of the calcium-phosphorus product?

Maintaining the calcium-phosphorus product between 40 and 60 is essential in avoiding bone disease.

What is the function of oral calcium as a phosphate binder?

Oral calcium (usually as calcium carbonate), when taken immediately after a meal, binds phosphorus in the stomach so that it passes out with the stool, thereby not contributing to raising the serum phosphorus. This helps control the calcium-phosphorus product. If the calcium is taken too long after eating or on an empty stomach, it may contribute to making the patient hypercalcemic. If a high serum phosphorus with a low serum calcium is left untreated, the parathyroid glands become stimulated and result in loss of calcium from the patient's bones. This condition is known as renal osteodystrophy.

What are the indications for administering Vitamin D analogue 1, 25-dihydroxyvitamin D₃ (calcitriol)?

Calcitriol is used to treat hypocalcemia in patients receiving chronic dialysis. It increases calcium levels and has been shown to reduce elevated PTH levels, preventing secondary hyperparathyroidism and improving renal osteodystrophy.

How and when is calcitriol administered?

Calcitriol in the intravenous form, Calcijex, is administered during a hemodialysis treatment as an intravenous bolus. An oral form of calcitriol, Rocaltrol, is available.

Are there any adverse effects of treatment with calcitriol?

Hypercalcemia can result from calcitriol treatment. Serum calcium and phosphorus must be evaluated on a regular basis to avoid hypercalcemia that could lead to generalized vascular calcification and soft tissue calcification (eyes, skin, heart).

When is calcitriol withheld?

Hold the calcitriol (Calcijex) when the serum calcium is between 10.5 and 12.5 mg/dL and the product (calcium mg/dL times the phosphorus mg/dL) is greater than 70. Conversely, hold the calcitriol if the serum calcium is greater than 12.5 mg/dL, *even if* the product is less than 70.

What is Zemplar (Paricalcitol injection)?

Paricalcitol is a recent synthetic analog of vitamin D for treatment of secondary hyperparathyroidism. Zemplar is given IV to ESRD patients to decrease PTH with minimal effect on calcium and phosphorus. It is an aggressive treatment of secondary hyperparathyroidism.

When is erythropoietin administered?

Epoetin is administered IV during hemodialysis to stimulate red cell production. A predialysis hematocrit is used to monitor anemia and determine epoetin administration. Each dialysis unit should follow its own protocol. The amount of epoetin required is determined by hematocrit, hemoglobin and individual patient response. Adequate iron stores and folic acid are required for erythropoietin to be effective. (A serum ferritin of 300–500 ng/ml is considered optimal per NKF-DOQI guidelines.)

When is iron therapy required?

The need for iron therapy is determined by two things: First, the serum iron value is divided by the total iron binding capacity, times 100. This is called the transferrin saturation or TSAT and correlates with the amount of iron available for erythropoiesis. (Optimal TSAT is 25–35%. Less than 20% indicates absolute iron deficiency; over 50% indicates risk of iron overload, according to DOQI guidelines published by the National Kidney Foundation.) Second, if the serum ferritin level is less than 100 ng/ml, iron therapy is prescribed, usually by the intravenous route.

How is iron administered?

Iron is administered orally and/or intravenously. Oral iron should not be taken with phosphate binders, which diminish its effect. When oral iron is prescribed, the patient should be instructed to always take the medication with food to avoid gastrointestinal distress. Patients will usually need to supplement oral iron with the intravenous form at intervals to maintain adequate stores for erythropoiesis. Intravenous iron is given during hemodialysis. The dosage is determined by the patient's starting hematocrit and TSAT. If TSAT is less than 20% and serum ferritin is less than 100 ng/ml, NKF-DOQI guidelines recommend 50 to 100 mg of iron IV once per week for 10 hemodialysis treatments. However, each facility should follow its own policy. Intravenous iron should be held if the TSAT is greater than 50% or serum ferritin is greater than 800 ng/ml in accordance with NKF-DOQI guidelines.

When should serum glucose be monitored in the diabetic patient?

A serum glucose (Chemstick or Accucheck) assessment should be performed at the beginning of the dialysis. Unstable diabetics need more frequent checks. A serum glucose value below 50 mg/dL may require a bolus of 50 ml of 50% dextrose to prevent hypoglycemic shock. An elevated glucose may require a dose of regular insulin to prevent diabetic coma. (See Chapter 17, "Diabetes").

When is deferoxamine mesylate used?

Deferoxamine mesylate (Desferal) is a chelating agent used to remove excessive metals from the bloodstream. It was originally formulated to treat iron overload. However, it has been found to be useful as an aluminum chelating agent in dialysis patients, and acts to remove aluminum from the tissues so it can be dialyzed out or adsorbed by a special cartridge. The usual dosage is 500 mg intravenously in 200 ml normal saline infused during the last 2 hours of the dialysis treatment 3 times a week. Desferal should be held for 2 weeks after infusion of intravenous iron.

FIRST HEMODIALYSIS ASSESSMENT

Why is the first hemodialysis procedure so important?

The first hemodialysis is critical because it sets the atmosphere for all future treatment procedures. The first dialysis is usually performed in the hospital. The patient may be unstable and feel sick. The information the nurse gives the patient during this first dialysis is often forgotten or misunderstood. Therefore, the nurse and dialysis personnel must reiterate teaching instructions regarding medications or access care again and again. Written manuals and instructions are helpful so patients have a reference as needed. Sometimes the first dialysis is performed in an outpatient dialysis facility. When this is the case, it is imperative that the dialysis personnel be cognizant of the emotional status of the new patient. The patient may be fearful because of the myths he or she has heard, or because of the equipment's appearance. These fears, combined with the fact that he or she is chronically ill, are strong reasons for the patient to be in emotional shock and to not recall instructions given during that first dialysis. The dialysis nurse and personnel must make the first dialysis as smooth and uneventful as possible.

What procedures take place before the first hemodialysis?

The physician evaluates and prescribes the dialysis orders for the new patient. The nurse reviews the orders, determines the proper dialyzer, and (after the fluid composition and machine settings are programmed), starts predialysis assessment. Prior to the first meeting with the patient, medical records should be reviewed. This information will be helpful during the physical assessment. After introductions, a brief tour around the facility should be conducted. The first visit should be as simple and as pleasant as possible. Remember that instructions will have to be repeated many times.

Make certain that a signed consent for the dialysis treatment is completed and retained in the patient's medical records. The physical assessment begins with the patient's weight, blood pressure, temperature, pulse, and respiratory rate. A general assessment of the patient's fluid status and overall well-being follows. Is there edema? Is the patient in any respiratory distress or experiencing any pain? Any bleeding or bruising? Is there residual renal function? Are bowel movements regular? Are there sleep problems? These are some questions that should be asked. Many units have assessment forms that offer guidelines to the caregiver.

During this first procedure, some of the dialysis parameters will be set: for example, heparin requirements, tolerance of fluid removal, arterial and venous pressure readings, saline requirements, tolerance to the dialyzer, and the dialysate composition. Because the first dialysis is so critical, the physician usually prescribes a slow blood flow and only two hours of dialysis. If the patient is very fluid-overloaded, has a high BUN, or is a child, the physician may order mannitol to prevent hypotension and to avoid a complicated first dialysis. This helps prevent the occurrence of the dialysis disequalibrium syndrome.

PREDIALYSIS ASSESSMENT

What is predialysis assessment?

Before initiation of hemodialysis, the patient and machine are both evaluated. The patient's physiologic status is assessed to ascertain the need to adjust dialysis orders or prescribed medications. The machine parameters are assessed to ensure that the prescribed procedure is implemented correctly.

What is included in the patient's preassessment?

Preassessment includes the following:
- Fluid status (respiratory rate/effort, JVD, heart sounds, breath sounds, presence of edema)
- Weight
- Blood pressure, sitting and standing
- TPR, including apical/peripheral pulse evaluation
- Skin color, temperature, turgor, and integrity
- Vascular access patency and freedom from bleeding and infection
- Interpretation of physical assessment and laboratory data for appropriate intervention and medication administration

What is included in machine preassessment?

Preassessment includes the following:
- Dialyzer membrane check for patency and integrity
- Blood tubing intact without leaks
- Appropriate prescribed dialyzer
- Dialysate fluid composition as ordered and within safe limits (12.8 to 14.8 mhos) as read by a Myron-L meter
- Appropriate prescribed dialysate potassium and calcium
- Temperature within limits (35–37° C)
- Correlation of machine conductivity with an external meter reading of dialysate (Myron-L or Western)
- Dialysate delivery system free of sterilant or disinfectant agents
- Extracorporeal blood circuit free of air
- Blood pump properly occluded
- Physician's orders reviewed to ensure adherence to dialysis prescription
- All alarms programmed and set within limits
- Dialysis quality water evaluated for chloramines

What is sodium modeling/variation and when is it applicable?

Sodium variations allow the dialysis treatment to be modified by increasing the concentrate-to-water ratio slightly, resulting in a rise in dialysate sodium. This feature allows the dialysis staff to initiate hemodialysis with a high dialysate sodium concentration and use progressively lower sodium-containing dialysate, decreasing to the original baseline level in a programmed time and profile. These maneuvers are intended to reduce the incidence of hypotension and cramping. There are several machines available to perform this treatment function. The Fresenius 2008H has three sodium variation system profiles. They are step decrease, linear decrease, or exponential decrease. Figure 9-1 illustrates these systems. The baseline is determined by the basic setting of the mechanical acid/acetate and bicarbonate concentrate pumps. With this method of sodium modeling, there is a significant variation in the dialysate potassium level. If the dialysate sodium is increased from 140 to 160 mEq/L (about 14%), the dialysate potassium concentration will also increase by 14%. If the baseline concentrate has 3 mEq/L of potassium and is increased by 14%, the new potassium concentrate would be 3.4 mEq/L. If there is a decrease in the dialysate sodium to 120 mEq/L (decrease of 14%) the new potassium concentrate will be 2.6 mEq/L. Increasing sodium in the dialysate has assisted many patients in the prevention of hypotension, cramping, and disequilibrium syndrome during dialysis.

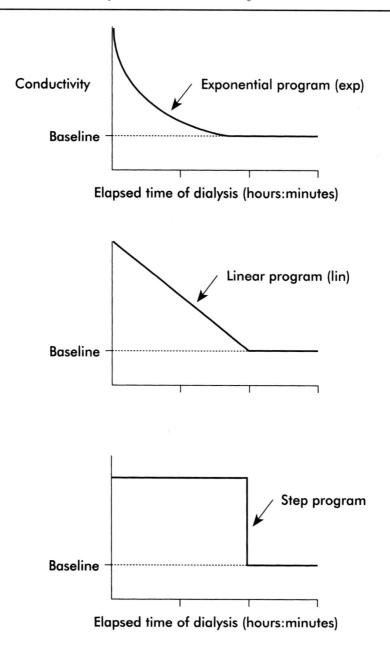

Fig. 9-1 Sodium variation system profiles. The exponential program causes the conductivity to decrease toward the baseline over the programmed time in a smooth curve. The linear program is a straight line reduction from the program maximum to the baseline level. The step program allows for a single large step to be performed. (From Gotch FA, Heineken F, Keen M, Evans M: Measurement of whole body ultrafiltration on urea mass transfer coefficients: implications for Na+ urea modeling in dialysis, Presentation at the American Society of Nurses, 1984.)

Why is it necessary to do such a thorough assessment of the patient and the machine before initiation of the dialysis treatment?

The accuracy of assessment and the appropriateness of the interventions directly affect the patient's outcome and will ensure that the goal of adequacy of dialysis is achieved.

What is ultrafiltration?

Ultrafiltration is the removal of fluid during dialysis. Ultrafiltration is the result of hydrostatic force across the dialysis membrane. The difference in hydrostatic pressure, blood to fluid, is the transmembrane pressure, or TMP. The rate of ultrafiltration is the sum total of positive and negative pressures plus the filtration factor, known as the ultrafiltration coefficient (k_{UF}), of each individual dialyzer. The k_{UF} ranges from 0.5 to 80 ml/hr/mm Hg, depending upon specific dialyzer characteristics. (See Chapter 4.)

What information does one need to calculate ultrafiltration?

All of the following questions must be answered:
- What is the patient's dry weight?
- What weight loss is needed (in kilograms)?
- What is the target post-dialysis weight?
- How much fluid will the patient receive orally and/or intravenously during the treatment?
- What is the ultrafiltration coefficient (k_{UF}) of the dialyzer?
- How much saline will be infused to rinse the blood circuit?
- What is the length of time the patient is to be dialyzed?

How is fluid removal calculated?

The following steps are taken in calculating fluid removal:

1. Add   Amount of weight to be removed in milliliters
               Amount of fluid intake in milliliters during treatment
     +   Amount of IV fluid to be removed in milliliters

               Total amount of fluid to be removed in milliliters

2. Divide $\dfrac{\text{Total amount of fluid to be removed in milliliters}}{\text{Number of hours of dialysis}} = \text{ml/hr}$

3. Divide $\dfrac{\text{Total from Step No. 2}}{\text{Ultrafiltration coefficient (}k_{UF}\text{) of dialyzer}} = \text{TMP}$

An example of how to calculate fluid removal is as follows:

Dialyze for 3 hours, remove 2.3 kg, conventional dialyzer k_{UF} equals 4.

1. Add	Weight to be removed in millimeters	2300 ml
	Oral intake	600 ml
+	Saline rinsed back	100 ml
	Total amount of fluid to be removed	3000 ml

2. Divide $\dfrac{\text{Fluid to be removed (3000 ml)}}{\text{Number of hours of dialysis (3 hr)}} = 1000 \text{ ml/hr}$

3. Divide $\dfrac{\text{Total from No. 2 (1000 ml)}}{\text{Ultrafiltration coefficient } (k_{UF}) = 4} = 250 \text{ TMP}$

In a conventional dialysis delivery machine, the TMP must be set manually. Many systems now provide a programmable function for controlled ultrafiltration. This controlled ultrafiltration allows the machine to adjust and control the fluid removal.

What is high-efficiency dialysis?

High-efficiency dialysis is performed with a special dialyzer with a large surface area. This dialyzer has a permeable membrane that allows solutes in the low to middle molecular weight and up to 5000 daltons to be removed. The k_{UF} ranges from 5 to 15 ml/hr/mm Hg. With this higher k_{UF}, an ultrafiltration control system is essential to control fluid loss. In addition, cardiovascular instability becomes more of a problem because of the rapid fluid removal and accompanying hypotension. Therefore a bicarbonate delivery system is imperative to allow for fluid removal while maintaining cardiovascular stability. Blood flow rates are from 300 to 500 ml/hr and dialysate flow is from 500 to 1000 ml/hr.

What is a high-flux dialysis?

High-flux dialysis is performed with a special dialyzer with a synthetic, highly permeable membrane that allows small and large molecular weight solutes to be convected across the membrane. The major difference in high-efficiency and high-flux dialysis is the membrane. High-flux membranes have solute clearance in the molecular weight range of 5000 daltons (insulin) to 12,000 daltons (β_2-microglobulins, B_2M). The membrane surface area ranges from 0.6 to 2.0 square meters. Water permeability is much higher in high-flux than in high-efficiency membranes and much higher than with conventional membranes, thus resulting in possible backflow of dialysate. The k_{UF} for high-flux membranes ranges from 20 to 80 ml/hr/mm Hg. A fluid delivery system with ultrafiltration control is required. High-flux dialysis requires a blood flow rate of 300 to 500 ml/min. Bicarbonate dialysate is required for cardiovascular stability. Usually dialysate flow is at 1000 ml/min. Since the membrane is so permeable, very stringent water quality is imperative (see Chapter 5 on dialyzers, Chapter 6 on water treatment, and Chapter 7 on dialyzer preparation and reprocessing). The equipment and bicarbonate dialysate containers must be disinfected on a regular basis.

INTRADIALYTIC ASSESSMENT AND MONITORING

What is intradialytic monitoring?

Intradialytic monitoring is the ongoing assessment of the patient and equipment during the hemodialysis treatment. The patient and the machine are monitored every hour by the caregivers. Monitoring is done more frequently in unstable patients. The vital signs and machine monitors are assessed. Machine parameters are listed in the box below.

Machine Parameters

Arterial pressure
Venous pressure
Fluid removal
Dialysate flow
Blood flow
Visual check of the dialyzer, blood tubing, and connections
Visual check of the machine monitor setting
Heparin pump
Visual check of the air/foam alarm status

These parameters are adjusted as needed in accordance with the treatment goals. All assessments are logged on the dialysis flow records. In computerized fluid delivery systems, the machine parameters are automatically monitored and recorded on the dialysis flow sheets.

What are potential hemodialysis complications?

During the hemodialysis procedure many potential complications can occur to both the patient and the equipment. These complications may result from the process itself or from complex interactions between the patient and the dialysis procedure.

What is the most common complication during the hemodialysis treatment?

The most common complication is hypotension related to rapid decrease of circulating blood volume caused by ultrafiltration. Lack of vasoconstriction caused by antihypertensive medications or other cardiac factors are other causes of hypotension.

How is hypotension prevented and treated intradialytically?

Sodium modeling, discussed earlier in this chapter, is an excellent method of preventing severe hypotension. Blood pressure monitoring, with careful observation and/or the use of an in-line hematocrit monitor (such as a Crit-Line; see Chapter 8) is also helpful in reducing hypotensive episodes. If hypotension is treated early by placing the patient in the Trendelenburg position, by decreasing the ultrafiltration pressures, or by giving replacement fluid, more serious complications may be avoided.

What is the Crit-Line instrument?

The Crit-Line monitor is an arterial in-line medical instrument that provides continuous measurement of absolute hematocrit, percent blood volume change, and oxygen saturation in real time. It measures blood volume change based on the hematocrit since these two values have an inverse relationship. As fluid is removed from the intravascular space, the blood density increases. This is displayed in percent of blood volume change on a grid-like graph on the Crit-Line screen. (See Fig. 9-2.) With this device, it is possible to maximize ultrafiltration safely and prevent hypotension, cramping and other intradialytic complications associated with volume depletion. A disposable blood chamber is attached to the arterial side of the dialyzer and a photo-metric technology is utilized. This device will also measure access recirculation. The Crit-Line is CLIA exempt.

What are other serious complications during hemodialysis?

Other complications that can occur are hemolysis and air embolism.

What is hemolysis?

Hemolysis is the lysis (break up) of the red blood cells resulting in the release of intracellular potassium. The blood in the extracorporeal circuit appears transparent and "cherry pop" in color. Hemolysis results when the patient's blood is exposed to hypotonic or hypertonic solutions, agents such as formaldehyde and bleach, improperly mixed dialysate, dialysate temperature over 42° Centigrade, or from a maloccluded blood pump. Monitors should detect a hypotonic dialysate solution or high dialysate temperature; however, machines are not infallible. Careful monitoring by dialysis personnel is essential to avoid this potentially life-threatening complication.

$$Hct = \frac{RCV}{BV} \times 100$$

Fig. 9-2 (A) Absolute hematocrit. (B) Percent of blood volume change. Courtesy In-Line Diagnostics, Farmington, Utah.

What should be done if hemolysis occurs?

If hemolysis occurs, stop the blood pump, clamp the lines and do not return the hemolyzed blood to the patient. Returning hemolyzed blood could cause hyperkalemia. Notify the physician and follow instructions; these usually include checking the patient's serum potassium and hematocrit levels, changing the dialyzer, and restarting the dialysis.

Describe an air embolism.

Air embolism occurs when air or a large amount of foam (microbubbles) is introduced into a patient's vascular system. Air embolism can occur when arterial or venous lines become disconnected or when blood or saline infusion bags run dry. The resultant vacuum causes microbubbles or foam. Dialysis personnel are responsible for setting and monitoring the air detector throughout the entire dialysis procedure.

What action is taken if a patient receives an infusion of air or complains of chest pain, and air is discovered in the lines of the dialysis circuit?

When a patient receives air, treatment must be immediate. The blood lines are clamped and dialysis is stopped. The patient is placed on the left side in the Trendelenburg (head down) position. This position decreases the movement of air to the brain and traps air in the right atrium above the tricuspid valve. This minimizes foaming, which occurs primarily in the right ventricle of the heart. The patient must be moved as little as possible and must be maintained in the Trendelenburg position. It takes several hours for all of the air, particularly the nitrogen, to be totally reabsorbed. A chest x-ray examination should be done to evaluate the amount of air present in the heart.

Are there other complications associated with hemodialysis treatment?

Yes. Table 9-1 outlines complications and their relationship to hemodialysis treatment.

Are any other patient assessments done during dialysis?

An important one, not subject to numerical recording, is the general condition and response of the patient during the procedure. Nausea, apprehension, shortness of breath, restlessness or agitation, irritability, itching, flushing, twitching, irrational behavior, sensation of faintness, and complaints of pain are some of the many signs or symptoms that can occur. A person on regular dialysis has an individual pattern of response, and any change in the pattern is significant. Acute dialysis patients must be evaluated more often because of their less stable condition and unknown response to therapy. All observed clinical condi-

Table 9-1   Complications During Hemodialysis

Complications	Relationship to Hemodialysis Treatment
Hypotension	Ultrafiltration Dialysate composition Extracorporeal blood volume Bioincompatibility of membranes Medications
Cramps	Ultrafiltration
Dialysis disequilibrium syndrome	Diffusive clearance
First-use syndrome/blood membrane interaction	IgE-mediated reactions Bioincompatibility of materials (complement activation)
Arrhythmias and angina	Composition of dialysate Ultrafiltration
Hypoxia	Dialysate composition Bioincompatibility of materials
Hypoglycemia	Dialysate composition Concomitant drug administration
Hemorrhage	Anticoagulation Dialyzer leak
Iatrogenic complications Air embolism Hemolysis	Air in extracorporeal circuit Dilute dialysate Copper contamination Chloramine, nitrate, or formaldehyde contamination
Contaminated dialysate	Overheated dialysate Bacterial contamination Trace elements or compound contamination

From Jacobson HR, Striker GE, Klahr S: *The principles and practice of nephrology*, ed 2, Philadelphia, 1995, BC Decker.

tions are documented on the chart and reported to the physician. Sometimes reactions or complications are reported to the Continuous Quality Improvement (CQI) committee for the purpose of ongoing monitoring or corrective action.

What are potential hemodialysis equipment problems?

Hemodialysis equipment is designed to protect the patient from complications that may occur during the treatment. However, machines are not infallible and will periodically malfunction. A malfunction of the temperature control device can cause hyperthermia, resulting in hemolysis. If not detected, this condition could cause death. Its opposite, hypothermia, can also occur; this condition can cause extreme chills and violent shaking.

Are there other equipment complications?

Yes. Other complications may occur when dialyzers and bloodlines become disconnected, leak, or clot. Most machine complications can be prevented by careful monitoring. Machine maintenance also plays an important role in the prevention of machine-related accidents. Chapter 5 discusses the equipment and its preventive maintenance.

What is arterial pressure?

Arterial pressure is a measurement of the extracorporeal blood circuit pressure between the patient's needle site and a site proximal to the blood pump. It is not the equivalent of the systemic arterial pressure but the *negative pressure* created by the blood pump. Arterial monitoring guards against excessive suction on the vascular access. For example, if the patient's arterial pressure has been reading (-) 100 mm Hg and it suddenly increases to (-) 200 mm Hg, this could indicate a clotted or dislodged needle, a drop in the patient's systemic BP, or a kink in the arterial line. If the arterial negative pressure either increases or decreases, as long as the monitor is properly set, the alarm will be activated and the blood pump will shut off. This audible and visual alarm alerts the caregiver of a dialysis complication and always requires immediate attention. The alarm will remain activated, and the blood pump will not work until the abnormality is corrected.

What is venous pressure?

Venous pressure is a measurement of the extracorporeal blood circuit pressure at some point after the dialyzer and before the blood reenters the patient's body. The monitoring line is usually attached to the top of the venous bubble trap. Venous extracorporeal pressure measures the resistance of the blood returning to the patient via the venous needle. For example, if the patient's venous pressure reading suddenly increases from 50 mm Hg to 150 mm Hg, this increase would indicate that the venous line may be kinked, the bubble trap may be clotted, the venous needle may be clotted or malaligned, or the vascular access may be in danger of failing. If, however, there is a sudden and dramatic decrease in venous pressure, the venous needle may have been pulled out, the transducer may be wet, or the arterial chamber may be clotted. The venous pressure alarm is similar to the arterial pressure alarm in that once activated, the abnormal condition must be corrected before the machine will allow the blood to continue through the blood circuit.

Note: All alarms must be set properly at the initiation of dialysis. This ensures that if any complication occurs, an audible and visual alarm will be activated and alert caregivers to a potential problem.

What effect does the dialysis solution (dialysate) flow rate have on the dialyzer clearance?

Dialysis solution flow rate affects clearance of small solutes such as urea. The usual dialysis solution flow rate is 500 ml/min, although some types of dialysis equipment (e.g. sorb system's Redy 2000®) use 250 ml/min. The slower flow rate leads to slightly lower dialyzer urea clearance. Dialysis solution flow rates of greater than 500 ml/min are used to increase clearance for high-efficiency dialysis. Higher dialysate flow rate can be used to enhance urea clearance when the blood flow rate is reduced for any reason. According to Nissenson, "little clinical benefit is achievable using presently available equipment at blood flow rates greater than 500 ml/min. There is a point where the relationship between dialysis solution flow rate and dialyzer clearance levels off with the higher dialysis solution flow rates."

Why should ESRD patients control their food and oral fluid intake during dialysis treatment?

There are several reasons for controlling intake. First, the amount of fluid removed by ultrafiltration is the net change in weight from the predialysis to the postdialysis weight. If the patient consumes large amounts of food and drink, this net weight change does not reflect a realistic fluid loss. The quantity of food or fluid ingested during dialysis should always be taken into consideration when calculating how much fluid to ultrafiltrate during the dialysis procedure. If it is permissible for patients to eat during dialysis, it is best to limit this to very small snacks. Food in the digestive tract causes pooling of blood and may cause hypotension and vomiting and increased risk of aspiration. Still, with more efficient dialysis and removal of fluid, ESRD patients have fewer restrictions with respect to oral intake then formerly. See Chapter 12 for more on nutrition.

What about the consumption of ice chips as a water substitute?

Ice has two advantages: (1) its coldness and (2) the time required for it to melt in the mouth. These factors make it more effective in alleviating the sensation of thirst. A 200-ml glass filled with ice chips yields about 150 ml of water. Therefore the patient will consume less fluid by eating ice chips than by drinking water.

POSTDIALYTIC THERAPY ASSESSMENT

What is postdialytic assessment?

Postdialysis assessment is the total evaluation of the patient, the treatment, and an interpretation of the predialysis goals. Factors to be included are listed in the box below.

Patient Parameters Evaluated After Dialysis

Patient's weight and weight loss
Vital signs, e.g., TPR and BP
Resolution/improvement of problematic predialysis parameters (improvement of fluid status)
Total of infusions given; both saline and blood
Patient's subjective physical assessment, e.g., any pain or complaints
Access assessment
Bleeding status

Are there other postdialytic assessments?

The dialysis prescription plan is assessed for any changes that will be implemented in the next dialysis. Finally, the date for the next dialysis is scheduled.

MONTHLY ASSESSMENTS

What is the purpose of monthly assessments for ESRD patients?

Each patient's prescription should be evaluated monthly to review his or her status and determine the adequacy of dialysis treatment. See the box below.

Items for Monthly Evaluation of ESRD Patients

Nutritional status, dry weight control, diet and fluid control
Kt/V and/or URR-dialyzer, blood flow, hours of treatment
Chemistries-dialysate K and Ca
Vital signs and BP-sodium modeling
Access-complications, aneurysm
Any bleeding in relation to heparin dose
Physical assessment
Bowel habit changes
Sleep habits
Sexuality
Medication review
Psychosocial review for general problems (social or financial)

In summary, there are multiple types of assessment in the treatment of the ESRD patient. Each assessment is used to improve patient outcomes and decrease the mortality and morbidity. The National Kidney Foundation-DOQI has established guidelines to enhance and promote the assessment of the ESRD patient for improved patient outcome.

10 Anticoagulation and Heparin Administration

Susan K. Hansen, Jo Anne Strutz

Blood, when it encounters any surface that is not the lining of a normal blood vessel, tends to clot. This mechanism is vital to preserving the life of the individual. Thus, blood will clot soon after entering the extracorporeal circuit of the hemodialysis system, rendering treatment impossible, unless the ability to clot is interrupted. There are several methods to prevent coagulation of the extracorporeal circuit—each with advantages and drawbacks for patient and/or practitioner. It is essential that the dialysis practitioner be familiar with more than one method, in order to safely and effectively meet the needs of each individual hemodialysis patient.

What is anticoagulation?

Anticoagulation is the blocking, suppression, or delaying of clotting of the blood. Clot formation occurs when blood contacts "foreign" surfaces, such as it does when it enters the bloodlines and dialyzer. Normally, blood does not clot within the vascular system. However, clots can form under certain conditions, most commonly after an injury, when the clot serves to seal the damaged vessel and prevent further blood loss.

What causes blood to clot?

Clotting is a part of a complex body process called hemostasis. This process involves: (1) retraction and contraction of the injured vessel, (2) the ability of blood platelets to stick to the injured area, and (3) a complex interaction of coagulation factors resulting in a formed clot. These coagulation factors are present in normal blood and are identified by Roman numerals I to V and VII through XIII.

Platelets are damaged by contact with a foreign surface. Platelet factor III is released, causing platelets to stick and start the clotting process. Plasma factors XI and XII are also activated by contact with a foreign surface and contribute to clotting.

Why doesn't blood clot within the normal vascular system?

The lining of the blood vessels, the endothelium, is smooth, allowing the blood to flow freely through the vessels. The other surfaces of cells—vascular endothelial cells, platelets, and red cells—are gelatinous and hydrophilic, with a high water content. They have low interfacial tensions and have little tendency to adhere when intact.

Why is anticoagulation needed during dialysis?

Blood coagulates when it comes into contact with foreign surfaces such as dialyzers and blood lines. To avoid this, anticoagulants are used. The first anti-coagulant was hirudin, obtained from the heads of medicinal leeches. In 1916, McLean found an anticoagulant in the liver of animals. This extract he called heparin, but it was not purified for human use until 1936. Its potency was finally standardized in the United States in 1966.

What is the nature of heparin?

Heparin is an acid mucopolysaccharide and is neutralized by strong basic compounds such as protamine sulfate, toluidine blue, and quinidine, causing it to lose its anticoagulant properties. Heparin for clinical use includes a number of fractions, with molecular weights (MWs) ranging from 8,000 to 14,000 daltons. Heparin composed only of low MW (4000–6000 daltons) is becoming available in the United States and, while more expensive, has the benefit of single-dose administration, less bleeding risk, and less effect on circulating lipases, poten-tially resulting in lower triglyceride and cholesterol levels in long-term hemodial-ysis patients. This latter factor may be significant, since high triglyceride and cholesterol levels are associated with cardiovascular disease.

How does heparin prevent coagulation?

Heparin combines with a blood protein fraction called heparin cofactor (antithrombin III). The complex of heparin-antithrombin III combines with and inactivates thrombin, activated factor X, and activated factor XI, thus preventing clotting at all three stages of coagulation (Fig. 10-1). Peak anticoagulant activity is reached 5 to 10 minutes after injection. The half-life is about 90 minutes for doses usually used in dialysis. The mechanism of heparin inactivation is not completely clear; it is metabolized by the liver and is also taken up by the retic-uloendothelial system.

Are there different kinds of heparin?

Most heparin is derived from pork intestinal mucosa or from beef lung. Pork-mucosal heparin is more abundant, less expensive, and most commonly used. The United States Pharmacopoeia (U.S.P.) unitage—i.e., units of activity per ml—for both forms is the same, but there is a difference in their anticoagu-lant actions on a weight basis—that is, 1 mg of porcine heparin has more antico-agulant activity than 1 mg of beef-lung heparin. The rare patient who develops a

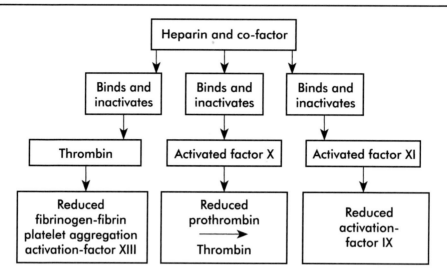

Fig. 10-1 Schematic diagram of heparin effect.

sensitivity to pork mucosal heparin may need to be switched to heparin derived from beef lung.

What is the unit measurement of heparin?

The official U.S.P. unit is that quantity of heparin that prevents clotting of 1 ml of sheep plasma for 1 hour under specified conditions.

The heparin concentration commonly used in dialysis is 1000 units/ml. The same number of units of either lung or mucosal heparin produces an equivalent degree of anticoagulation. It should be noted that the International Unit values used in Britain and Europe differ slightly from the U.S.P. unit in anticoagulant activity.

How is the effect of heparin measured clinically?

Heparin effect is estimated by the increase in the length of time necessary for a clot to form. There are several laboratory methods for this, including Lee-White clotting time, activated partial thromboplastin time (APTT or PTT), and the activated clotting time (ACT), discussed on the following page. The clinician should be aware of the impact of CLIA (Clinical Laboratory Improvement Act,1992). Although CLIA was intended to apply to non-certified employees doing lab tests in doctors' offices, its broad wording encompasses all lab tests done by non-laboratory-certified personnel in any setting. Thus, CLIA effectively prohibits dialysis staff from performing clotting time determinations on acute and chronic hemodialysis patients unless provision is made for appropriate staff and equipment certification.

Which tests are best for clinical hemodialysis?

Normally, one of three tests is used for monitoring clotting times during dialysis.

The first of these is the Lee-White clotting time, which is performed by putting 0.4 ml of blood into a tube and inverting the tube every 30 seconds until the blood clots. Because of the long clotting times involved, poor standardization, and poor reproducibility, it is the least desirable method to use during dialysis. Normal clotting times with this test are 6 to 17 minutes.

The second test is the PTT. This test must be performed in the laboratory and is reliable only at lower levels of anticoagulation.

The third test is the ACT. It is similar to the PTT but uses siliceous earth in the tube to hasten the clotting process. The test is done by an automated method that has excellent reproducibility. Evaluation of heparin effect can be done in 180 to 275 seconds. Because of this, the ACT test was easily used in dialysis units. Blood samples were drawn from the "arterial" line before the infusion of heparin, reflecting the status of the patient circulation rather than the extracorporeal circuit. The box below gives a protocol for clotting time using the ACT method.

Protocol for Activated Clotting Times

Regular control	150–180 sec
Moderate control	105–150 sec
Tight control	90–120 sec

How is heparin given during dialysis?

There are two techniques: intermittent infusion and continuous infusion.

Describe the intermittent intravenous heparin technique.

An ACT test is first performed. Normal is about 60 to 90 seconds. An intravenous priming dose of heparin is given at the beginning of dialysis, and smaller doses are repeated intermittently throughout the procedure. The usual objective is to maintain the ACT at about 3 times the baseline. In acute dialysis, when the patient could have a problem with bleeding, heparin dosage is set to give a clotting time between 150 and 180 seconds. Alternatively, given the CLIA limit on performing clotting times, the circuit can be rinsed at 30- to 60-minute intervals with about 100 ml of saline, the fibers and air-blood interface of both drip chambers inspected for signs of early clotting, and the heparin dose adjusted as needed. Naturally, the UF goal must be increased to remove this extra fluid infusion.

The priming dose, most often around 25 to 50 units/kg of body weight, is given either through the venous side of the vascular catheter or via the last needle placed, if the patient has a graft or fistula. The latter method is intended to prevent any oozing of blood or hematoma formation if there is any difficulty with the initial needle insertion. In the few minutes before the patient is attached to the dialyzer, the entire blood volume will become anticoagulated. This is "systemic heparinization."

Describe the continuous infusion technique of intravenous heparin.

A priming or "loading" dose of heparin is given as previously described. Heparin is then slowly injected into the extracorporeal system at a constant rate by an infusion pump. This is continued throughout the dialysis, usually at a rate of 1000 to 2000 units/hr. Clotting is evaluated at intervals, usually by saline flushes and visual inspection of drip chambers and/or dialyzer fibers, and the heparin infusion rate is adjusted accordingly. The infusion is normally stopped 30 minutes to 1 hour before the end of the treatment to allow the clotting time to begin its return to normal, especially for those patients from whom needles must be removed post-dialysis.

What is the danger of bleeding when heparin is used for hemodialysis?

There is always a danger of bleeding when heparin is used. Uremic patients tend to bleed easily. One must be particularly concerned about any patient who has had surgery within the preceding 24 to 48 hours or is scheduled for surgery immediatly post-dialysis, who has recently been injured, has pericarditis, or may have a hemorrhagic lesion of the gastrointestinal tract or uterus.

Are there special techniques for using heparin in hemodialysis when there is danger of bleeding?

Three approaches have been used for this situation: regional heparinization, low-dose or "tight" systemic heparinization or no-heparin/saline flush techniques.

What is regional heparinization?

In regional heparinization, an anticoagulant is infused continuously into the inlet (arterial) line of the dialyzer while simultaneously neutralizing it by infusing an antidote into the outlet (venous) line before the blood returns to the patient.

In the past, heparin was used as the anticoagulant and protamine sulfate, a low molecular weight protein derived from salmon sperm, was infused into the venous line. Protamine, a strongly basic protein, bound the acidic heparin and thus neutralized its effect on the coagulation system. However, because of a number of difficulties—precise balancing of dosage of each infusion, a tendency toward rebound anticoagulation several hours post-dialysis, and protamine-induced anaphylaxis—this method is rarely used today.

An alternative method of regional anticoagulation involves the use of sodium citrate. Regional citrate anticoagulation works by binding the ionized calcium present in the extracorporeal circuit; calcium ions are essential for clot formation. This technique involves infusing trisodium citrate into the arterial line. A calcium-free dialysate must be used. Since returning blood with a decreased ionized calcium to the patient would be dangerous, the process is reversed by the infusion of calcium chloride into the venous line as close as possible to the vascular access connection.

The major disadvantages of this technique are that frequent laboratory tests must be done to check the patient's total calcium level as well as clotting times. Metabolism of the citrate produces bicarbonate. Plasma level of bicarbonate will increase, occasionally to significantly alkalotic levels. (An alternative version uses a large volume of dilute sodium citrate, normal dialysate and no calcium infusion. The disadvantages are minimized, but UF goals must be adjusted to remove the extra fluid.)

Both types of regional anticoagulation require a high level of experience, skill and attention to detail. With the low-dose /"tight" systemic and heparin-free techniques available today, regional methods are generally reserved for the most critically ill acute dialysis patients.

What is low-dose or "tight" heparinization?

Low-dose or "tight" heparinization consists of monitoring the patient with frequent clotting times and administering only enough heparin to keep the clotting time at 90 to 120 seconds by ACT. Low-dose or "tight" heparinization is usually the most practical technique for managing the patient who is at risk for bleeding. A baseline clotting time is drawn through the first dialysis needle inserted, and this acts as a guide to the size of the priming dose and maintenance heparin requirements. After the administration of the minimal priming dose, usually 10 units/kg, heparin dosage is adjusted to provide an ACT of 110 +/- 10 seconds.

In some centers, low-dose or "tight" heparin is used for the patient's first dialysis treatment. After several treatments a consistent dose of heparin can be established. However, due to CLIA restrictions, anticoagulation methods which require the use of clotting time determinations present a problem.

Can patients be hemodialyzed without heparin?

Heparin-free dialysis has become the method of choice when treating actively bleeding patients and in those with an increased risk of bleeding, pericarditis, coagulopathy, or thrombocytopenia.

Several techniques can be utilized, but most commonly the following are used:

- The blood lines and dialyzer are rinsed with saline containing 3000 units of heparin/l. The saline priming dose with the heparin is then discarded. No heparin is used for the saline prime of dialyzers for patients who are at very high risk of bleeding (e.g., patients with liver disease).
- The blood flow rate is set as high as possible, 350 to 450 ml/min if it can be tolerated.
- The dialyzer is rinsed with 100 to 200 ml of saline as often as every 15 minutes but at least every hour. This is done by occluding the "arterial" line and infusing the saline rapidly. The dialyzer is visually inspected if possible for clotting during the rinse. The extra saline should be added to the UF goal unless the patient needs the extra fluid volume.

Can blood be transfused into at-risk patients during heparin-free dialysis?

Blood transfusions can complicate heparin-free dialysis, especially since they commonly involve packed RBCs. The transfused blood increases the viscosity of the blood in the dialyzer and may infuse clinically significant amounts of normal (i.e., non-uremic) clotting factors. A modification of the standard method for blood transfusion involves the use of a large-bore three-way stopcock inserted between the patient's access and the tip of the venous bloodline (Fig. 10-2). The stopcock is positioned to run three ways simultaneously so that the transfused blood enters the flow of dialyzed blood returning to the patient; the blood bag is either elevated 1 meter above the patient or fitted with a pressure bag inflated to 300 mm Hg. The other parameters—saline flushes, blood flow rate, etc.—remain the same as used in heparin-free dialysis.

How can vascular catheter patency be protected between treatments?

Although the anticoagulation methods need not be altered for use with vascular catheters, the method used for the "heparin lock" to preserve catheter patency between treatments has significant clinical implications. It is essential to keep sufficient heparin within the catheter lumen to prevent clotting, yet prevent any of the heparin from entering the circulation of an at-risk patient. The following method should be used. After dialysis, flush each lumen (side) of the catheter with 10 ml normal saline to clear it of blood cells, then rapidly instill a volume of 5000 u/ml heparin sufficient to exactly displace the saline in the catheter lumen and clamp the lumen immediately. The key is to inject precisely the volume of 5000 u/ml heparin that the catheter can hold so that there is no excess to go into the patient and, to inject it fast enough so that it does not mix with the saline and become diluted. This volume can be determined by noting the individual volume printed on each vascular catheter and injecting exactly that amount.

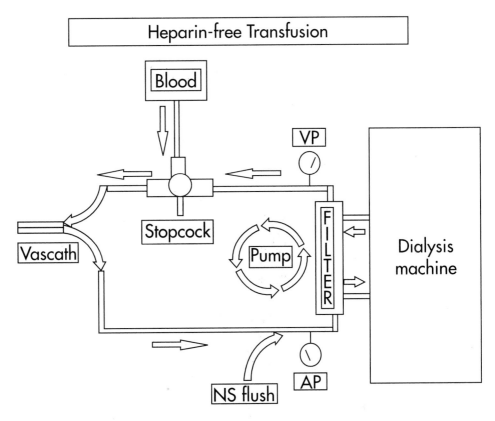

Fig. 10-2 Transfusion and dialysis circuit showing direction of transfusion and blood flow. Sepulveda S, Davis L, Schwab S: Blood transfusion during heparin-free hemodialysis. *Kidney International* (1997) 51:2018–2021.

What are contributing factors that prevent hemorrhage during hemodialysis?

Success in preventing hemorrhage during the dialysis procedure rests on the general management of the patient and the care with which the dialysis is done. The bleeding tendency of uremic patients is correctable with adequate dialysis. The technique used for anticoagulation during dialysis is an important part of the process, as any coagulation in the extracorporeal circuit will impair treatment outcome. Thus the timely institution of an adequate dialysis program is an important initial factor in the prevention of hemorrhage, but subsequent success is dependent upon careful and continuous attention to all of the factors related to optimal treatment adequacy.

Medication Problems and Dialysis

Ginette A. Pepper

Dialysis patients routinely take an average of ten different medications and experience adverse drug reactions at least three times more frequently than the general population (Jick, 1977; St. Peter et al., 1997). To optimize drug outcomes health professionals must be prepared to recognize and manage problems associated with medication use. Table 11-1 lists several problematic reactions to medications that clinicians encounter in providing care to patients on dialysis and other patients with renal impairment. Corresponding responsibilities of dialysis personnel are also outlined in the table.

All of these problem areas are complex and require consideration of multiple factors unique to each situation, including patient characteristics (e.g., severity of renal impairment, acuity or chronicity of renal failure, comorbidities, age, nutritional status), drug properties (e.g., pharmacokinetics, pharmacodynamics, dose, route), and the dialysis procedures (e.g., type, equipment, duration). The purpose of this chapter is to emphasize the pharmacologic principles common to managing these problem areas and overview each problem area briefly.

How do drugs cause renal impairment?

The rate of drug-induced nephrotoxicity ranges from a fraction of 1 percent in the general population to as high as 90 percent in at-risk patients (Bailie, 1995). There are several reasons the kidneys are particularly vulnerable to damage by drugs. The kidneys only constitute 0.4 percent of body weight, but receive 20 to 25 percent of total blood flow. This disproportionate blood flow exposes kidneys excessively to drugs in the blood. In addition, drugs are concentrated as the tubular filtrate passes through the nephron and water is reabsorbed. Tubular transport systems further concentrate drugs in the filtrate. Enzymes in the kidney may metabolize drugs to metabolites that are nephrotoxic. In renal insufficiency, the remaining functional nephrons are even more susceptible to nephrotoxins.

Drugs contribute to nearly 30 percent of acute renal failure in hospitalized patients (Davidman, Olson, & Kohen, 1991). The most commonly implicated pharmacologic nephrotoxins are antibiotics (aminoglycosides, cephalosporins, pentamidine, amphotericin B), radiocontrast agents used for radiologic studies, cyclosporine, cisplatin, amphotericin B, ACE inhibitors, and nonsteroidal antiinflammatory drugs (NSAIDs). Because of the development of new agents (e.g., lower osmolar radiocontrast agents), changing drug use patterns (e.g., decreased

Table 11-1 Problem Areas Involving Drugs

Problem Area	Corresponding Responsibility of Dialysis Personnel
Drugs can damage kidneys, initiating or worsening renal failure.	Monitor renal function of patients on drugs or drug combinations that can damage kidneys. Identify patients at high risk for renal damage from drugs. Avoid or use extreme caution with drugs that damage renal function in high risk patients and those with existing renal disease. Initiate hydration and other documented measures to minimize nephrotoxicity.
Pharmacologic activity of drugs is altered by renal failure.	Adjust dosages to compensate for altered pharmacokinetic and pharmacodynamic activity. Monitor for therapeutic failure, adverse effects, or toxicity of all drugs used. Anticipate more adverse effects in patients with renal impairment.
The amount of medication removed from the body during dialysis varies, depending on the characteristics of the drug and dialysis conditions.	Using references and formulas, estimate how much drug is removed by dialysis. Calculate dosage adjustments and/or post-dialysis replacement dosages. Monitor clinical response to calculated doses and alter the dosage as indicated.
Some poisons or drugs taken in overdose can be removed wholly or in part by dialysis.	Know which poisons and overdosed drugs can be removed by various dialysis procedures. Implement dialysis to treat poisoning and overdose, providing appropriate supportive care and observation during the procedure.
Medications may increase risks associated with the dialysis procedure.	Know what medications the patient is taking. Monitor for excess effects of the medication.

use of aminoglycosides), and the shift of care from inpatient to outpatient settings, nonsteroidal anitiinflammatory drugs (NSAIDs) and angiotensin-converting enzyme (ACE) inhibitors are increasingly predominant causes of transient acute renal failure. In chronic outpatient settings, end stage renal failure can occur due to combination analgesics—which consist of either aspirin or an NSAID combined with acetaminophen, caffeine and/or codeine. While the agents specifically cited here are the most frequent causes of renal damage, numerous other medications from diverse drug categories cause renal damage. Whenever a patient evidences renal impairment, a careful analysis of the drug profile for potential drug nephrotoxicity should be conducted. Nephrotoxins should be avoided in patients with renal insufficiency or used with appropriate dosage adjustments and meticulous monitoring.

Describe the mechanisms by which these drugs usually cause renal damage.

Several mechanisms of renal damage by drug nephrotoxins have been identified (Zarama & Abraham, 1997), but most nephrotoxins damage the kidneys through more than one. *Hemodynamic mechanisms* involve inhibition of regulatory and compensatory processes, nonspecific renal vasoconstriction, or altered colloid oncotic pressure. A primary example of hemodynamic mechanisms for nephrotoxicity includes transient acute renal failure from inhibition of the renin-angiotensin-aldosterone system by ACE inhibitors in patients with renal artery stenosis. A second example is the inhibition of prostaglandin-dependent renal blood flow by NSAIDs in patients with conditions associated with decreased renal blood flow (e.g., volume depletion and congestive heart failure). Renal vasoconstriction is a hypothesized mechanism of renal damage from propranolol, mannitol, combination of triamterene and indomethacin, and the initial months of cyclosporine therapy. Dextran-40 can elevate oncotic pressure and impair glomerular filtration.

Another mechanism of damage is *renal vascular alterations,* such as thrombotic microangiopathy, that may result from oral contraceptives, cyclosporine, mitomycin C, cisplatin, and quinine. *Glomerular alterations* that result in nephrotic syndrome and glomerulonephritis are more often immune than toxic effects. The most common drug-induced glomerular alteration is membranous nephropathy that occurs with oral and parenteral gold therapy and penicillamine. Less common glomerular toxicities include the following: minimal change nephrotic syndrome associated with NSAIDs, ampicillin, rifampin, phenytoin, and lithium; focal segmental glomerulosclerosis secondary to heroin abuse; and membranoproliferative glomerulonephritis from hydralizine, interferon-alpha, and interleukin-2. Toxic drug effects resulting in *acute tubular necrosis* are most often caused by aminoglycosides, radiographic contrast media, cisplatin, amphotericin B, pentamidine, and foscarnet. *Tubulointerstitial disease* takes several forms and is commonly manifested as one of the following conditions: an acute allergic interstitial nephritis from antibiotics (e.g., penicillins, cephalosporins, tetracyclines, sulfonamides, fluoroquinolones), NSAIDs, diuretics, and anticonvulsants; chronic interstitial nephritis from lithium and cyclosporine; and papillary necrosis from analgesics (e.g., NSAIDs, aspirin, and acetaminophen used alone or in combination) or high-dose dapsone therapy.

Obstructive nephropathies from drugs include uric acid nephropathy during chemotherapy; rhabdomyolysis from phencyclidine, adrenergic drugs including terbutaline, cocaine, vasopressin infusion, erythromycin, and systemic cholesterol-lowering drugs , especially HMG CoA reductase inhibitors (e.g., lovastatin, atorvastatin, simvastatin); and urinary tract outflow obstruction from anticholinergic drugs (e.g., tricyclic antidepressants, disopyramide), cyclophosphamide, and methysergide.

How can renal damage from such drugs be minimized or avoided?

Naturally, drugs with potential to cause renal damage should be avoided or used cautiously in patients with high risk for renal impairment. Conditions that predispose to renal damage by drugs include use of multiple nephrotoxins, sodium or fluid depletion, preexisting renal disease, and low renal blood flow in patients with diseases like congestive heart failure and cirrhosis (Davidman, Olson, & Cohen, 1991; Zarama & Abraham, 1997). Often drug-induced renal damage is reversible if the drug is discontinued and supportive care initiated before permanent effects occur. Giving saline intravenously may decrease damage by some nephrotoxins such as cyclosporine and cisplatin by diluting the concentration of the drug in the renal tubule. Misoprostol, a prostaglandin analogue, may prevent NSAID nephropathy. Drugs with the least nephrotoxic potential should be selected. For example, acetaminophen, aspirin, nonacetylated salicylates, sulindac, or nambumetone may have less nephrotoxicity than other NSAIDs. Finally, drugs should be given in the lowest effective doses for the shortest possible duration.

How does renal failure itself alter response to medications?

The changes that accompany renal failure can alter drug response by two major mechanisms: pharmacodynamics and pharmacokinetics. Medications chemically interact with receptors on cell membranes or on enzymes to cause their effects. This interaction is known as *pharmacodynamics* and can be thought of as what the drug does to the body. Adverse effects (also called side effects or toxic effects) occur when a drug or metabolite acts at receptors other than the target receptors or when excess drug is present at the target receptor. Uremic substances in the blood or altered electrolyte concentrations resulting from renal failure can modify the drug-receptor interaction, resulting in altered drug effect. Altered receptor sensitivity is thought to be responsible for increased central nervous system effects of narcotics, sedatives, and hypnotics, as well as for the resistance to effects of epinephrine and other catecholamines that occurs in uremic patients. Altered electrolyte and acid-base balance also affect the response to such medications as antiarrhythmics, digoxin, phenothiazines, and antidepressants.

The magnitude and persistence of drug action depends on the duration and concentration of the drug in proximity to the receptor. This relationship of time and drug concentration is known as *pharmacokinetics* and can be thought of as how the body acts on the drug through the processes of absorption, distribution, metabolism, and excretion. How renal failure affects pharmacodynamics is not well understood. On the other hand, many of the effects of altered pharmacokinetics in patients on dialysis have been sufficiently studied to develop mathematical formulas for calculating drug dosage. Decreased renal excretion is the most obvious alteration in pharmacokinetics resulting from renal dysfunction, but each of the other pharmacokinetic processes may also be altered.

What are the pharmacokinetic parameters that reflect alterations caused by renal failure?

There are several measurement parameters that can be computed for each drug to represent its pharmacokinetic profile. These include *bioavailability*, *volume of distribution*, *clearance*, and *elimination half-life*. *Bioavailability*, which is abbreviated *F* for fraction, is the measure of drug absorption. Bioavailability is the percentage of the administered dose that gets absorbed into the systemic circulation.

Each drug has a unique pattern of distribution throughout the body, represented as its *apparent volume of distribution (V_d)*. Volume of distribution is the hypothetical volume that would be required to contain the dosage of drug at its concentration in the plasma. For example, if 500 mg of a drug were administered to a patient and an hour later the concentration of the drug in a sample of his plasma was 0.001 mg/ ml, the V_d would be 500L. Stated another way, if each ml of plasma had 0.001 mg in it, 500 L would be required to contain 500 mg. Although V_d is an abstraction, it can be interpreted to reflect the distribution characteristics of a drug. If the V_d is 5 L (0.06 L/kg), it is likely most of the drug stays in the intravascular space. If the V_d is more than 46 L (0.7 L/kg), the drug is sequestered in the peripheral tissues, usually dissolved in fatty tissues or bound to tissues. Drugs with large volumes of distribution are poorly dialyzable because most of the drug is outside the bloodstream and therefore is not exposed to the dialysis membrane. V_d is used in the calculation of loading doses.

The two modes of elimination, metabolism and excretion, are measured as drug *clearance (CL)*. Clearance is defined as the rate of removal of a drug in proportion to its concentration in the plasma. Clearance is reported as the volume of plasma cleared of the drug per unit of time. Therefore, if the plasma concentration of a drug is 0.002 mg/ml and the body eliminates 2 mg per hour, the clearance is 1 L/hr or about 17 ml/min. (This is because, in such cases, 1000 ml or 1 L of plasma is needed to contain 2 mg at a concentration of 0.002 mg/ml.) Like volume of distribution, clearance is a useful abstraction, rather than a concrete reality. CL is useful for calculating the maintenance dose of a drug. In the patient with renal impairment and lower clearance, lower maintenance doses are needed.

Elimination half life ($t_{1/2}$) is an indicator of how long a drug stays in the body. It is the time required for half of the drug to be eliminated and is manifested clinically as the time required for the concentration in the blood to decline 50 percent. Half-life is prolonged by large V_d or by slow CL, which are both pharmacokinetic changes common in renal failure. The relationship among half-life, volume of distribution, and clearance is:

$$t_{1/2} = 0.7 \times \frac{V_d}{CL}$$

What factors affect absorption of medications in patients with renal failure?

In uremia the breakdown of urea in the gastrointestinal tract may raise pH and slow absorption of acid drugs, such as aspirin, iron preparations, and diuretics. Gastroparesis and gastrointestinal responses to uremia (nausea, vomiting, and diarrhea) may significantly alter the absorption of oral medication. Antacids, commonly used to bind dietary phosphate in ESRD, diminish absorption of drugs by forming unabsorbable compounds with drugs like digoxin, iron preparations, and some antibiotics (e.g., tetracyclines and fluroquinolones). Drugs used to suppress gastric acid secretions such as H_2 blockers (e.g., cimetidine, ranitidine, famotidine), antacids, and proton pump inhibitors (omeprazole, lansoprazole) affect the absorption of some drugs. For example, ketoconazole, which requires an acid environment for absorption, would have decreased bioavailability in patients taking drugs that suppress gastric acidity, while oral penicillins, which are inactivated by gastric acid, would have improved absorption when patients take these agents.

Orally administered drugs pass through the liver before reaching the main circulation, and large portions of a dose of drugs like morphine, propranolol, and codeine are metabolized during this "first pass" through the liver. Because the first past effect reduces the bioavailability (F) of orally administered morphine, the oral dose of morphine must be much larger than the injected dose to achieve the same amount of pain relief. In uremia, the fraction of drug metabolized by this first-pass effect may be decreased, unchanged, or increased because some metabolic byproducts of uremia change the activity of liver enzymes.

Thus, bioavailability of drugs is highly variable in renal failure.

Drugs are absorbed across the peritoneum when administered into the dialsylate. Antibiotics are frequently given via this route, which results in high concentrations at the site of a peritoneal infection. Some patients have experienced improved diabetic control with intraperitoneal administration of insulin. Administration of drugs by the peritoneal route will result in a different plasma profile than oral or parenteral administration, usually with delayed onset, decreased peak plasma concentration, and prolonged duration of action. Presence of peritonitis will alter the bioavailability of drugs administered peritoneally.

What factors affect distribution of medications in patients with renal failure?

Once a drug is absorbed into the blood, some molecules bind to proteins in the plasma. Drugs that are highly bound to plasma proteins in the blood usually have small V_d because most of the drug molecules are attached to plasma protein, which normally cannot exit the blood vessels. Drugs that predominantly exit from the blood and bind to muscles or dissolve in fatty tissue in the periphery have large V_d. In general, drugs with small V_d have short half-lives because they are mostly in the plasma, which frequently passes through the liver and kidney (and dialysis machine) where they are eliminated. Conversely, drugs with a large V_d have longer half-lives and less susceptibility to removal by dialysis. Edema and ascites often increase V_d and will increase the half-life of drugs that normally have small distribution volumes.

Plasma protein binding of acidic drugs to albumin may be decreased in renal failure as a result of either decreased concentration of albumin or decreased capacity of the albumin to bind to drugs. Changes in protein binding can alter V_d and the drug effect, since only the free drug is pharmacologically active. Decreased albumin binding is thought to contribute to the central nervous system toxicity of acid drugs like theophylline, phenytoin, penicillin, phenobarbital, and salicylates in uremia. Some alkaline drugs (e.g., lidocaine, phenothiazines, propranolol, quinidine, and tricyclic antidepressants) that bind to glycoprotein also undergo increased or decreased binding in renal disease, but the clinical relevance of these changes are not as well studied as albumin binding. Although changes in V_d and plasma protein binding theoretically could have substantial effect on drug response, current research suggests the effects of altered V_d in renal disease are usually minimal. There are a few exceptions, in which these changes require modification in the approach to patient care. An example is decreased protein binding of phenytoin during renal failure, which must be considered in clinical management. Measured serum concentrations of phenytoin which reflect total (bound + free) drug concentration in the plasma often are reported in the subtherapeutic range in patients with renal failure. This is because the amount of phenytoin bound to albumin is decreased, but the fraction of unbound drug is increased. Since the unbound drug is the active portion, lower drug concentrations of phenytoin are desirable for patients in renal failure to achieve the desired effect (Aweeka, 1995). In some centers both free and total phenytoin drug concentrations are measured to avoid toxicity. In patients without renal disease, protein binding is about 90 percent of the total drug, whereas in ESRD binding of phenytoin ranges from 65 to 80 percent. Another approach to interpretation of phenytoin levels in ESRD patients is to use a correction formula that adjusts the reported phenytoin plasma concentration for albumin level, renal function, and decreased affinity of phenytoin for albumin in ESRD (Liponi et al., 1984).

What factors affect elimination of medications in patients with renal failure?

Some drugs are cleared almost exclusively in their original chemical form by renal excretion; these drugs are said to be excreted unchanged. Other drugs undergo alteration of chemical structure by enzymes, a process called biotransformation or metabolism. Most drugs are cleared by a combination of hepatic metabolism and renal excretion. Metabolites (form drugs take after chemical alteration by metabolism) are usually more water soluble than the original drug and are usually eliminated by the kidneys. Active metabolites retain the ability to bind to a receptor and elicit the same effect as the original drug. Inactive metabolites are usually insignificant because they do not stimulate the target receptor. Toxic metabolites are those that cause an adverse effect at a site different from the target receptor.

When a drug that is normally cleared unchanged by the kidneys is repeatedly administered to a patient with renal insufficiency, it begins to accumulate in the blood and may cause adverse effects. Increased portions of the drug may be eliminated by alternate routes such as hepatic metabolism or through the lungs, bile, or sweat glands. Metabolites of drugs accumulate in renal insufficiency, and active or toxic metabolites contribute to adverse effects. An example is normeperidine, a metabolite of meperidine, which causes stupor or seizures when it accumulates. Table 11-2 includes examples of drugs with active or toxic metabolites that may accumulate in renal failure. If viable alternatives exist, drugs with active or toxic metabolites are avoided in patients with renal failure. When drugs with active or toxic metabolites are used in renal failure, decreased dosages may be required and clinical monitoring must be vigilant. For example, patients with renal impairment taking allopurinol for gout or cancer require lower dosages than those with normal renal function because an active metabolite of allopurinol can cause exfoliative dermatitis when it accumulates in the body. Although far less important than active metabolites, inactive metabolites may also have consequences. For example, the accumulation of inactive metabolites may cause interference with laboratory tests.

Table 11-2   Examples of Drugs With Active or Toxic Metabolites

acetaminophen	levodopa
allopurinol	meperidine
amiodarone	metronidazole
azathioprine	methyldopa
buspirone	nitroprusside
cefotaxime	procainamide
cimetidine	propoxyphene
diazepam	quinidine
enalapril	triamterene
fluoxetine	verapamil
glyburide	

Impaired renal function may also affect liver metabolism, decreasing elimination of some drugs (e.g., morphine, clonidine) and increasing metabolism for a few others (e.g., phenobarbital and phenytoin). Renal impairment alters metabolism through accumulation of uremic substances that can induce (speed up) or inhibit (slow down) drug-metabolizing enzymes in the liver. Insulin is metabolized by enzymes in the kidney, so it is more slowly cleared in severe renal disease. Liver metabolism is dependent upon genetic inheritance, diet, environmental pollution, and concurrent administration of other medications; thus the effects of renal dysfunction are likely to be highly variable from drug to drug and person to person. Effects on renal elimination are more predictable: the greater the proportion of drug or its active metabolites eliminated by the kidneys, the more likely that altered dosing will be required for patients with renal impairment and those on dialysis.

How does dialysis affect pharmacokinetics of drugs and poisons?

The kidneys eliminate drugs through several processes. Although dialysis is not a substitute for all these renal processes, some drugs are removed by dialysis. Dialysis may also affect other pharmacokinetic parameters. For example, changes in total body water from pre- to postdialysis will affect the V_d of some drugs. Characteristics of drugs that promote removal by dialysis are: (1) small molecular size, (2) small V_d, (3) water solubility, and (4) low protein binding. If protein binding exceeds 90 percent, the drug will be negligibly eliminated by dialysis. Drugs are more likely to be removed when the dialyzer membrane is highly permeable and its surface area is large and the blood flow rate and dialysate flow rate are high. Peritoneal dialysis generally provides little drug removal since dialysate flow rate is slower than with other methods, although a greater amount of protein-bound drug can be removed due to large protein losses seen with this mode. Continuous therapy with hemofiltration or continuous hemodialysis for critically ill patients can remove substantial fractions of drugs. Removal of drugs by hemofiltration procedures are determined by the ultrafiltration rate and degree of protein binding. Treatment of drug overdose and poisoning involves application of these principles to decrease serum concentration of the toxic drugs or substance (Winchester & Kriger, 1995). Similarly, poisons with high protein binding or large V_d are not dialyzable. Although many standard references classify a drug as dialyzable or not dialyzable, dialyzability is not an all-or-nothing characteristic. Some drugs are virtually entirely removed by dialysis; others have negligible removal. Many drugs fall somewhere in the middle. The type of dialysis equipment and length of dialysis will greatly influence whether a drug is removed. Classification of dialyzability as *yes* or *no* is based on an expert's opinion of whether removal is clinically significant—that is, sufficient to remove an overdose—or whether the patient will require dosage replacement.

How should drugs and dosages be selected for the patient with renal impairment or ESRD?

Drug selection for the patient with renal impairment requires consideration of the impact of the drug on kidney function, electrolyte balance, and uremia. Agents that will worsen the disease state or increase metabolic load (Table 11-3) are avoided or used with caution. A drug that increases metabolic load burdens the failing kidney with chemicals that accumulate in renal disease, such as urea, sodium, potassium, or acids. For the patient with ESRD these substances must be removed by dialysis and may affect well-being or cause serious adverse effects, such as cardiac arrhythmia from hyperkalemia. Drugs with nephrotoxic properties are also used with caution in patients with renal impairment. Meticulous monitoring should be incorporated into the patient care plan for patients with renal impairment taking medications that are nephrotoxic or increase metabolic load. Medications should be avoided for self-limiting conditions and those that can be managed by nonpharmacologic methods. Whenever possible, a single agent that can manage several conditions should be selected. For example, in the absence of contraindications such as renal stenosis, an angiotensin-converting enzyme inhibitor would be a prudent choice for the patient with both hypertension and congestive heart failure. Well-studied established agents are usually preferred over newly marketed drugs. All other therapeutic considerations being equal, drugs with reliable laboratory assays for drug level are advantageous because the drug level data can enhance clinical monitoring.

Table 11-3   Examples of Drugs Producing Metabolic Loads

Sodium load	Magnesium
ampicillin (IV)	laxatives
azlocillin (IV)	antacids
antacids	
carbenicillin (IV)	**Urea**
cephalothin (IV)	dexamethasone
moxalactam (IV)	prednisone
polystyrene sulfonate (Kayexelate)	tetracycline
ticarcillin (IV)	
	Acid
Potassium load	acetazolamide
blood transfusion	aspirin
neuromuscular-blocking drugs	methenamine mandelate
potassium penicillin G (IV)	
salt substitutes	**Alkali**
spironolactone	antacids
triamterene	carbenicillin

The need for and extent of dosage modification in renal impairment depends on the pathophysiology of the disease process and its severity, as well as the pharmacology of the drug. Guidelines for dosage reduction of many drugs can be found in standard drug references such as the *Physicians' Desk Reference*, drug handbooks, and package inserts. Many nephrology textbooks and other sources provide summary tables that include pharmacokinetic parameters in ESRD (e.g., V_d, CL, $t_{1/2}$), recommended dosage adjustments for various levels of renal function, and guidelines for postdialysis replacement doses. An example of a reference table format is shown in Table 11-4. Most of these data and guidelines are based on studies in patients with stable chronic renal failure on maintenance dialysis and may not apply to the unstable acute renal failure patient. Each of the following 5 steps of dosage selection will be defined and discussed in subsequent sections:

1. Assessment of relevant patient variables
2. Determination of loading dose
3. Determination of maintenance dose
4. Determination of postdialysis replacement dose
5. Monitoring of drug levels and clinical response

What are the unique assessment requirements related to drug dosing in renal failure?

In addition to the standard assessment of drug allergies, previous drug history, comorbidities, concurrent medications, and baseline laboratory and clinical findings that precedes initiation of a new drug in any patient, patients in renal failure require estimation of residual renal function and determination of ideal body weight. Because weight may fluctuate between dialysis procedures and because daily dosage requirements usually correspond to lean body weight rather than actual weight in obese or edematous patients, ideal weight is calculated for men as 50 kg plus 2.3 kg for each inch in height over 5 feet. For women, ideal body weight is 45.5 kg plus 2.3 kg for each inch over 5 feet (Arnoff & Erbeck, 1994). Renal function can be determined in the stable patient by laboratory determination of creatinine clearance or estimation of creatinine clearance (CL_{cr}) using the Cockroft and Gault formula:

$$CL_{cr} = \frac{(140 - \text{age in years}) \, (\text{lean body weight in kg})}{72 \, (\text{serum creatinine in mg/dl})}$$

For women the estimate of CL_{cr} is 85% of the calculated value, so the results of the equation above is multiplied by 0.85 to estimate creatinine clearance in women. The Cockroft-Gault formula yields artifactual results for patients on dialysis, so it is not a reliable estimate in these patients.

In addition to assessing residual renal function, the efficiency of extrarenal mechanisms for drug elimination, especially liver function, should be evaluated, since concurrent hepatic impairment may necessitate more stringent dose reduction.

What is a loading dose and when is it indicated?

Loading doses are indicated when it is necessary to attain therapeutic plasma concentrations rapidly. Even in patients with normal renal function, loading doses can be dangerous, so this approach should be reserved for serious or life-threatening situations. This technique is most commonly employed in critical care settings. Loading doses are listed in references for some drugs or can be calculated as the product of the desired plasma concentration or "blood level" (Cp) and the volume of distribution of the drug (Swan & Bennett, 1997):

$$\text{Loading dose (mg/kg)} = V_d \, (\text{ml/kg}) \times Cp \, (\text{mg/ml}).$$

The computed dose in mg/kg is then multiplied by the patient's ideal weight.

Table 11-4   Sample Reference Chart for Pharmacokinetic Parameters, Dosage Adjustment, and Dialyzability

Drug Name	Vd, L/kg	Half-Life hr		Cl (ml/min)		% Excreted Unchanged	Protein bound %	Dialyzable	Dosage Modification in Renal Disease*			
		Normal	ESRD	Normal	ESRD				Method	GFR ml/min		
										>50	10-50	<10
Antimicrobials												
amphotericin B	0.46	24	40	15	9	5	95	no	—	24	24	24-36
cephalozin	0.14	1.8	27	60	5	85	80	yes	—	8	12	24-48
erythromycin	0.57	2	5	310	90	15	80	no		unch	unch	unch
fluconazole	0.71	32	98	-	-	80	10	yes	—	24	24-48	48-72
gentamicin	0.24	2	60	95	2	85	<10	yes	—	8-12	12	12-24
penicillin G	0.18	0.7	13	205	10	80	65	yes	D	unch	75	25-50
tetracycline	1.5	9	80	131	14	55	50	-	—	3-12	12-24	24-48
Cardiac Drugs												
captopril	3	1.9	3.5	1277	69	50	30	yes	D	unch	75	50
clonidine	3.2	8	40	315	65	50	25	no	D	unch	unch	50-75
digoxin	7.1	36	100	160	35	>90	25	yes	—	24	36	48-96
hydralazine	1.6	3	>16	430	<80	10	87	no	—	8	8	8-16
propranolol	3	3.5	3.5	695	695	0	93	no	—	unch	unch	unch

CNS Drugs: Antiseizure, Analgesics, Hypnotics

acetaminophen	1	2	2	400	400	2	15	yes	I	unch	6	8
pentazocine	-	2	2	-	-	10	65	-	D	unch	75	50
phenytoin	0.57	18	9	25	125	5	90	no	-	unch	unch	unch
phenobarbital	0.75	70	100	9	6	50	55	yes	-	unch	unch	12-16
secobarbital	1.42	25	-	4.6	-	variable	70	no		unch	unch	unch
valproate sodium	0.3	12	-	10	-	variable	95	no		unch	unch	unch

Anticoagulants, Miscellaneous

glipizide	0.16	3-7	-	52	-	7	95	-		unch	unch	unch
heparin	0.06	1	1.5	50	30	50	>90	no		unch	unch	unch
warfarin	0.11	33	30	3	3	<1	97	no		unch	unch	unch

*D = dosage adjustment indicated as percent of usual dose; I = interval extension as hours between doses; (-) = data are not available; unch = unchanged from usual dose and interval

Sources: Arnoff & Erbeck, 1994; Aweeka, 1995; Bennett, WM, et al, 1994; Brater, 1995; Cutler, Forland, & Hammer, 1995; Golper & Bennett, 1995; Swan & Bennett, 1997.

What is a maintenance dose and how is it determined?

Maintenance doses are given regularly, usually one or more times daily, but possibly less often in renal failure. Maintenance doses replace the drug eliminated since the previous dose and sustain therapeutic plasma concentrations. If no loading dose is given, plasma concentrations take four half-lives of repeated maintenance dosing to reach steady state. Steady state occurs when the amount of a drug absorbed and the amount eliminated per unit of time are equal. Before steady state, peak plasma concentrations increase with each subsequent dose. At steady state, the mean plasma concentration levels off after four half-lives and peak and trough concentrations are effectively equal from dose to dose at steady state. Generally, dosages should not be adjusted upward until steady state. Because of prolonged half-life for many drugs in renal failure, it may take days to weeks for drugs to reach steady state in these patients. Because the purpose of a maintenance dose is to replace eliminated drug, the decreased drug clearance in renal impairment requires reduced maintenance doses for agents eliminated unchanged by the kidneys and for agents with active metabolites eliminated by the kidneys. There are three main approaches to dosage reduction: (1) decreased amount of drug given at usual intervals, (2) usual dose of drug with extended time between doses, and (3) a combination of decreased amount and interval extension (Swan & Bennett, 1997). Extension of the time interval between doses causes wide fluctuations between peak and trough levels and is not indicated for drugs with a narrow therapeutic range or where a low serum concentration at the end of the dosing interval may be dangerous. The dosage reduction or combined approach is indicated when more constant serum concentrations are desirable. On dialysis days the recommended dose, as well as replacement doses, should be administered after the procedure is completed. For drugs removed by peritoneal dialysis, the additional dose is added to the usual daily maintenance dose.

Recommended maintenance doses are included in standard references, usually by level of creatinine clearance (or glomerular filtration rate), as illustrated in Table 11-4. These tables offer little individualization of dosage for the patient in renal failure since wide ranges of creatinine clearance are grouped together and the dosage recommendations may be the same for patients with tenfold differences in creatinine clearance. The wide variety of formulas used to calculate individualized maintenance doses include the following:

- *Ratio method.* Ratio methods involve the derivation of a dosage adjustment factor based on the ratio of some parameter in the patient with renal impairment compared to that of a person with normal renal function. One approach uses the ratio between the half-life in normal renal function and the half-life in renal impairment. For a drug with a half-life of 3 hours with normal renal function and 6 hours with renal failure, the ratio would be 3/6 or 1/2. Multiplying the usual dose by this ratio or dividing the usual interval by this ratio derives the therapy for renal failure: A drug usually given 300 mg every 12 hours would be given 150 mg every 12 hours or 300 mg once per day in renal failure. The ratio of creatinine clearance of the patient to normal creatinine clearance can also be used to determine dosage (Brater, 1995). The dosage adjustment factor Q can be computed as follows (Matzke & Frye, 1997):

$$Q = 1-[f_e(1-KF)]$$

where f_e is the fraction of the drug eliminated unchanged by the kidneys, and KF is the ratio of the patient's creatinine clearance to normal creatinine clearance. The usual dose is multiplied by Q to derive an individualized dose for a particular patient with renal impairment. It is also possible to derive the dosage adjustment factors from nomograms. Nomograms are graphs showing relationships among variables. Standardized nomograms have been developed and published for determining dosage in renal failure.

- *Pharmacokinetic method.* The pharmacokinetic method involves measurement of pharmacokinetic parameters for a particular patient. After the patient receives one or more doses, blood samples are taken from which the V_d, $t_{1/2}$, and CL are derived. These parameters are individualized to the patient and provide the most accurate indications of that patient's drug disposition. From these parameters, the maintenance dose can be computed using the following formula (Brater, 1995):

$$\text{Maintenance dose} = CL \text{ (L/hr)} \times C_p \text{ (mcg/ml)} \times \tau \text{ (hrs)}$$

where CL is the patient's drug clearance, C_p is the desired plasma concentration, and τ is the dosing interval. The pharmacokinetic method is often paired with therapeutic drug monitoring, which involves determination of the plasma concentration of the drug at steady state to validate the dosage selected, and at regular intervals thereafter. Therapeutic drug monitoring can also be used with the other dose calculation methods. Although the pharmacokinetic method yields the most accurate and individualized results, it is useful only when a reliable assay is available for the drug. It is commonly used with drugs with narrow therapeutic margins such as gentamycin, digoxin, and antiarrhythmic drugs.

- *Drug-specific method.* Another method to determine maintenance dose is based on studies on individual drugs published in the literature. The studies establish the relationship between pharmacokinetic parameters (e.g., V_d, total body clearance) and some continuous index of renal function, such as creatinine clearance. For example, the relationship for total clearance and clearance for gancyclovir has been reported as (Sommadossi et al., 1988):

$$CL \text{ (ml/min/1.8 m}^2) = 1.25 \text{ (CL}_{cr}) + 8.57$$

Using the creatinine clearance (CL_{cr}) for the patient, the total clearance of gancyclovir can be estimated with this formula. The result of this calculation is then used to calculate the maintenance dose of gancyclovir, using the formula listed above in the pharmacokinetic method.

How is postdialysis replacement dosage determined?

Standard references and texts include recommendations for average postdialysis replacement for drugs that are substantially removed during dialysis. These recommendations vary by procedure, because peritoneal dialysis and hemodialysis remove different amounts of drug. For example, for the beta blocker nadolol, which is renally excreted, a 40-mg dose is recommended following hemodialysis, but no supplementation is needed for peritoneal dialysis. Much of the data on which these reference tables were based was collected before recent advances in dialysis equipment affecting membrane function and blood flow rates, so it is likely that standard references underestimate the amount of drug removal during dialysis. Hemofiltration also removes different amounts of drug compared to other dialysis procedures, but research on dosage replacement after this procedure is limited. For drugs with long half-lives, regular maintenance doses may not be needed if the postdialysis replacement dose includes the drug eliminated between dialysis treatments, as well as that removed during the procedure.

For some drugs, the dialysis clearance values have been studied and published in the literature. These drug-specific values can be used to compute the replacement dose. Differences in dialysis equipment (type of membrane, surface area, blood flow rate, length of procedure) must be considered in determining replacement doses from these published values. For patients who have authorized reuse of dialysis filters, dialysis drug clearance may be lower when the filter has had multiple uses (Matzke & Frye, 1997). For increased accuracy dialysis clearance rates can also be individually calculated based on laboratory measurement of dialysate and serial plasma concentrations. Other procedures base calculations of dialysis clearance on measures of drug concentration in the blood going into the filter and blood leaving the filter.

What are considerations for monitoring drug levels?

All of the methods for determining dosages include physiologic and mathematic assumptions that may not reflect an individual patient's unique and changing physiologic status, so the formulas and guidelines should be considered beginning estimates of dosage requirements to be followed by dosage titration based on patient response. For drugs with valid and reliable laboratory assays, determination of plasma concentration (i.e., therapeutic drug monitoring) can be a useful tool for dosage adjustment. This is often called *blood levels*, which is an inaccurate term since the test is not run on whole blood, but rather on plasma or serum, and the concentration of the drug is not level, but fluctuates throughout each dosing cycle. Therefore, it is very important that blood samples for drug levels be collected at the correct time. For peak concentrations, blood is usually drawn 1 to 2 hours after an oral dose or 30 to 60 minutes after a parenteral dose, although timing may vary depending upon the characteristics of the drug and route of administration. Trough concentrations are based on blood drawn immediately before the next dose. For some drugs, such as aminoglycosides, both peak and trough values may be collected, since the peak value corresponds to therapeutic effect and the trough value may reflect risk of adverse effects with these agents.

Plasma concentrations are interpreted by comparing the patient's measured value to the published therapeutic range for a drug. However, there are several pitfalls in interpreting plasma concentrations. Not all patients get therapeutic or toxic response at the same concentration. It has been estimated that up to 50 percent of elderly with digoxin concentrations in the therapeutic range are actually experiencing toxic effects and that many elderly are adequately treated with concentrations in the subtherapeutic range. In addition, decreased serum protein binding common in renal disease may also complicate the interpretation of laboratory reports of drug concentration. Laboratories generally report concentrations of total drug, including both bound and free fractions. A change in the ratio of bound-to-free drug can result in a reported normal serum concentration, when the concentration of free (active) drug is actually at toxic levels. Conversely, a patient may be adequately treated even though the reported serum concentration is subtherapeutic, because the portion of unbound active drug is increased. Some physicians order both total and free drug concentrations and compare the published reports of the normal percentage of drug binding to that reported for an individual patient.

Therefore, even when data on serum concentration are available, clinical data such as the patient's subjective information, physical exam findings, and laboratory results should be used to regulate dosage. Interference with laboratory results by drugs and drug metabolites can be enhanced when drugs accumulate in renal insufficiency. Drug interaction with the laboratory test should be considered when reported laboratory values are inconsistent with the clinical presentation. Table 11-5 shows examples of drug-test interactions relevant to dialysis patients. The mechanism of these interactions is an interference by the drug or its metabolites with one of the reagents used in the laboratory test. When an abnormal value for one of these common tests is reported, intervention based on the laboratory result should not be initiated until the patient's drug therapy is reviewed for interacting drugs. The laboratory director should be consulted about the resolution of the drug-test interaction, since an alternate assay methodology could circumvent the interaction.

The importance of clinical monitoring and observation cannot be overstated. Knowledge of the usual pattern of responses of the patient enables the clinician to recognize at an early stage deviations that suggest the need to evaluate the drug regimen.

Table 11-5 Example of Drugs That Interfere with Laboratory Tests

Serum creatinine	**Urinary protein (dipstick method)**
ascorbic acid	acetazolamide
aspirin	aspirin
cefoxitin	cephalosporins
cimetidine	contrast media
levodopa	penicillins
methyldopa	sulfonamide antibiotics
trimethoprim	tolbutamide
Serum uric acid	
ascorbic acid	
acetaminophen	
aminophylline	
levodopa	
methyldopa	
salicylates	

Sources: Golper & Bennett, 1995; USPDI, 1998.

Can drugs affect the dialysis procedure?

Several drug groups can affect the dialysis procedure. Many patients on dialysis take antihypertensive medications, which can contribute to hypotension during the dialysis procedure. Epoetin therapy is associated with a decrease in the prolonged bleeding time seen in some patients with ESRD and may increase heparin requirement during dialysis in some patients. Vascular access thrombosis may be more frequent in those on epoetin, but there is no evidence of increased thrombosis with native arteriovenous fistula (St. Peter et al., 1997).

Nutrition Management

Susan E. Weil

Nutrition plays a critical role in the management of renal disease. The diet will vary considerably depending on the type and stage of renal disease as well as on patient and treatment modality-specific factors. A "renal diet" that can be applied to all patients does not exist. Each situation must be evaluated individually. There are certain commonalities that may apply to patients with chronic and acute renal disease.

Why is diet important for people with renal disease?

Diet therapy offers the following potential benefits:
- It may be helpful in delaying the need for dialysis.
- Diet can help attenuate many of the complications of renal disease, e.g., phosphorus restriction to aid in prevention of bone disease.
- Adequate protein and calorie nutrition can influence morbidity and mortality in patients with renal disease.
- Quality of life for people with ESRD may be improved by individualization of diet to suit lifestyle, ethnic, and socioeconomic variables.

What is the role of the registered dietitian?

The registered dietitian assesses each patient's needs and makes recommendations to the nephrologist as to the diet prescription. Patient and family are taught specifics of the diet by the dietitian, who monitors nutrition-related parameters and reevaluates needs. The dietitian is responsible for the primary diet education, and functions as a member of the interdisciplinary team. Communication between the dietitian, nurses, technicians, physician, and social worker as to changes in a patient's medical condition, dialysis treatment, medications, psychosocial situation, and nutritional status is critical to providing optimal patient care.

What are the diet concerns before initiation of dialysis?

Before the initiation of dialysis, the diet is constructed to achieve several goals. One goal is to delay the need for dialysis by slowing the decline of renal function. At present, studies are inconclusive as to whether protein or phosphorus restriction can help slow the progression of renal disease. In addition to possible delay in the progression of renal disease, protein restriction, when employed with an adequate caloric intake, can be helpful in minimizing nitrogenous wastes and can aid in the control of uremic symptoms. Diet management can often be effective in delaying the need for dialysis until the glomerular filtration rate (GFR) falls below about 5 ml/min, at which time some type of renal replacement therapy is necessary. Preservation of nutritional status by the provision of adequate calories to maintain or achieve a desirable body weight and avoid endogenous protein catabolism is of prime importance during this period.

Phosphorus control, by limitation of high phosphorus foods and/or the use of phosphate-binding medications, is often necessary when the GFR falls below 20 ml/min. Phosphorus control will be discussed later in this chapter.

Another diet concern before the initiation of dialysis is sodium control for the patient who is edematous or hypertensive. On the other hand, potassium restriction is generally not necessary until urine output falls below 1000 ml/day; therefore restriction may not be necessary until after dialysis is initiated.

What are the diet modifications for hemodialysis?

The need for dietary modification once hemodialysis begins is highly individualized depending on such factors as height, weight, nutritional status, the level of residual renal function, laboratory data, intercurrent illnesses, and prescribed medications. Maintenance of good nutritional status, as evidenced by adequate anthropometric measurements and biochemical indices, is critically important during this period. Achieving and maintaining a normal serum albumin level is the number one goal of nutrition therapy for the hemodialysis patient. Various studies have demonstrated that the primary biochemical predictor of mortality in hemodialysis patients is a low serum albumin. In the absence of proteinuria or significant liver disease, albumin levels can be maintained with provision of adequate protein and calories. Although the diet is highly individualized, certain diet commonalities do apply to most patients on hemodialysis.

What amount of protein is appropriate for hemodialysis patients?

Protein requirements, as suggested by current research, are thought to be 1.2 ± 0.2 g/kg/day, with the upper end of the range for protein malnourished patients. In general, at least 50 percent of this protein should be derived from high biological value protein sources such as meat, fish, or poultry. Such protein sources contain a full complement of essential amino acids. Examples of low biological value protein would be fruits, vegetables, and grains; however, a carefully planned vegetarian diet can be used without compromise of nutritional status. The protein needs of hemodialysis patients are higher than those of the general population, in part because of the loss of 5–10 gm of amino acid during each hemodialysis treatment.

What calorie level is advisable?

Energy requirements for hemodialysis patients are not well defined, although they are generally accepted to be 35 kcal/kg/day for maintenance. With stress or malnutrition, calorie needs may be as high as 40 to 45 kcal/kg. For the obese patient, 25 to 30 kcal/kg may be appropriate.

What about potassium control?

Almost all foods contain potassium, and certain fruits and vegetables are particularly rich sources. Once urine output falls below 1 L/day, and in some cases *before* this happens, potassium should be controlled in the diet. An intake of approximately 70 mEq or 2730 mg of potassium is a safe intake for most hemodialysis patients. The specific dietary potassium intake depends on the size of the patient, the level of potassium in the dialysate, and other factors that may affect the serum potassium level. Factors other than dietary indiscretion may contribute to hyperkalemia, including severe acidosis, constipation, catabolism, insulin deficiency and the use of certain medications such as β-adrenergic blocking agents and ACE inhibitors.

How much sodium is acceptable?

An intake of approximately 87 mEq or 2000 mg/day of sodium is appropriate for most hemodialysis patients. Adjustments can be made depending on blood pressure, urine output, and the presence or absence of edema. Hypertension in ESRD patients is largely volume related, and dry weight should be constantly reassessed in the hypertensive patient. Renin-mediated hypertension is present in a small percentage of dialysis patients. Appropriate antihypertensive medications, rather than further sodium and fluid restriction, are necessary for this subgroup.

What level of fluid intake is acceptable?

Generally, the recommended fluid intake is an amount equal to urine output plus approximately 500 to 700 ml/day. Fluids contained in foods such as fruits and vegetables are not usually counted in this total. Foods that are liquid at room temperature, such as popsicles and ice, are counted in the daily fluid allotment. The volume of fluid in solid foods, approximately 500 to 800 ml, is roughly equivalent to insensible fluid losses; therefore remaining "visible" fluid intake will correlate with interdialytic weight gain. An acceptable interdialytic weight gain is 1.5 kg, or less than 3 percent of body weight. Excessive fluid contributes to high blood pressure and results in left ventricular hypertrophy.

What about phosphorus and calcium intake?

Phosphorus intake should be limited to 600 to 1200 mg/day. Since phosphorus content of the diet correlates with protein intake, it may be necessary to include some high phosphorus food to achieve an adequate protein intake. Phosphorus is also controlled by the intake of phosphate-binding antacids such as calcium carbonate or calcium acetate. Aluminum-containing antacids should be avoided to minimize risk of aluminum bone disease. The calcium-containing antacids are given with meals and snacks, and ideally are titrated to the phosphorus content of the diet. Calcium content in the diet is typically low because foods high in phosphorus also tend to be rich sources of calcium. Calcium supplements, aside from that in the phosphate-binding antacids, may not be necessary to maintain calcium balance when either oral or intravenous 1,25 (OH)2D3 is used. Calcium requirements vary considerably depending on the phosphate intake, use of vitamin D, the calcium content of the dialysate, and the presence of hyperparathyroidism. This is discussed further in Chapter 14.

Are vitamin supplements necessary?

Patients on dialysis may be at risk for deficiencies of certain water-soluble vitamins because of poor nutrient intake, drug-nutrient interactions, altered vitamin metabolism, and dialysis losses. Although evaluation of specific requirements and recommendations is ongoing, supplementation with USRDA amounts of vitamins B_1, B_2, B_{12}, biotin, pantothenic acid, niacin, as well as 800–1000 mcg folic acid and 10 mg pyridoxine(B_6) daily, is reasonable. The recommendations for folic acid, B_{12}, and B_6 continue to be reevaluated in light of information concerning the amino acid intermediate, homocysteine. Elevated levels of homocysteine have been demonstrated to be a risk factor in cardiovascular disease and can be present in patients with end stage renal disease. High doses of folic acid, and in some studies B_6 and B_{12}, have been shown to normalize homocysteine levels and therefore may have a cardioprotective effect. The efficacy of high-dose supplementation of these B vitamins and the appropriate dosages are yet to be determined in the dialysis population. Vitamin C supplementation is limited to 60 mg/day. Higher doses of vitamin C should be avoided to prevent accumulation of oxalate, an ascorbic acid metabolite. Supplemental vitamin A should be avoided because of potential toxicity related to decreased renal degradation of retinol-binding protein in renal failure.

What about the need for trace minerals?

Trace mineral requirements are not well defined for the dialysis patient, and at present routine supplementation is not appropriate. Zinc deficiency may be present in some patients on dialysis, although the best method of measuring stores is yet to be determined in this population. In a patient who exhibits signs of zinc deficiency—such as hypoguesia (loss of sense of taste), delayed wound healing or alopecia—a time-limited trial of zinc supplementation may be reasonable. Selenium is another trace metal undergoing investigation into the possible role of selenium deficiency in promoting comorbid conditions such as cardiovascular disease and cancer in the dialysis population. The optimal method of assessing selenium status and appropriate dosing remains to be defined.

How is iron deficiency assessed?

Iron deficiency is a common finding in dialysis patients receiving human recombinant erythropoietin and concomitant utilization of iron for erythropoiesis. Before the use of erythropoietin, iron overload was common in this population as a result of multiple blood transfusions (each unit of transfused blood contains approximately 200 to 250 mg iron). Routine assessment of iron stores by serum ferritin and percent transferrin saturation (iron divided by total iron-binding capacity) should be included in any erythropoietin therapy protocol.

A low mean corpuscular volume may be a late indicator of iron deficiency. If a deficiency is present, intravenous iron administration or oral iron supplementation is warranted. Increasing the iron content of the diet generally does not provide adequate replacement once iron deficiency is identified. Various oral forms of iron are available but may cause gastrointestinal upset. Guidelines for administering intravenous iron therapy are described in Chapter 9. Erythropoietin therapy is discussed further in Chapters 9 and 14.

Do people on dialysis have to control fat intake?

Dyslipidemia, typically seen as hypertriglyceridemia, combined with low high-density lipoprotein (HDL) cholesterol and normal total serum cholesterol, is the most common lipid abnormality found in dialysis patients. Some patients may present with elevated serum cholesterol, defined as serum cholesterol greater than 200 mg/dl. For these people, it may be appropriate to prescribe a low-cholesterol, low-fat diet.

Obesity may exacerbate hypertriglyceridemia. Therefore, in the obese dialysis patient, weight control may be of benefit in helping to control triglyceride levels. A regular aerobic exercise program may also be of benefit in helping control both cholesterol and triglyceride levels. Carnitine, which will be discussed later in this chapter, and fish oil supplements have also been shown to help lower triglyceride levels.

What about sugar and carbohydrates?

Restriction of sugar and carbohydrates is not appropriate or necessary for most people on dialysis. Exceptions are diabetics or those who are overweight, or who have hypertriglyceridemia that may respond to total calorie restriction. Often sugars and other carbohydrates need to be increased to provide adequate calories in the diet.

How is nutritional status monitored?

One category of assessment tools is anthropometric measurements, which include height, weight, ideal or desirable body weight, weight changes, and other measurements such as triceps skin fold (to assess fat stores) and mid-arm muscle circumference (to measure somatic protein stores). A second category is biochemical data. Serum albumin correlates with protein nutriture in stable hemodialysis patients in the absence of a nephrotic syndrome or liver disease, although levels are influenced by volume status. Data from the U.S. Renal Data System indicates that low serum albumin, as indicative of overall nutritional status, is associated with increased mortality in patients on hemodialysis. Serum albumin appears to be a less reliable indicator of nutritional status in patients on peritoneal dialysis and does not correlate well with mortality risk in these patients. Other biochemical parameters such as serum transferrin, serum IGF-1 concentration, pre-albumin levels and low serum creatinine with low creatinine kinetics have been used to assess nutritional status, although each parameter has limitations.

Subjective data such as food diaries or diet recall obtained by a skilled interviewer can provide valuable information. A method called Subjective Global Assessment (SGA) has been used to quantify nutritional status and includes physical assessment, functional impairment, gastrointestinal symptoms, as well as anthropometric indices.

What is urea kinetic modeling (UKM)?

Urea kinetic modeling is a tool used to prescribe and monitor dialysis therapy and to assess protein intake. Although optimal methods for performing UKM and determining results are not agreed on in the dialysis community, formal UKM has become a standard of practice for both hemodialysis and peritoneal dialysis programs. UKM is usually performed using a computer because the mathematical computations are elaborate. Data entered into the computer are BUN levels from before and after a given dialysis treatment (some methods also include predialysis BUN from the subsequent dialysis treatment), and for patients who urinate, residual urea clearance is included. Information about the dialysis treatment (blood flow, dialysate flow, dialyzer clearance data, length of treatment, and interdialytic interval) and patient-specific data (pre- and postdialysis weights, height, sex, hematocrit) are also incorporated in the calculations.

What do the results mean?

One result derived from UKM is the Kt/V, which refers to:

K = clearance of dialyzer for a given dialysis treatment and, if applicable, a measurement of any residual urine urea clearance

t = length of time for a given dialysis treatment

V = volume of distribution of urea for a given patient that equates with total body water.

The goal for delivered Kt/V is thought to be at minimum 1.2 for thrice-weekly dialysis for both adults and children. Goal Kt/V for twice-weekly dialysis is undefined. Levels below 1.2 may indicate inadequate dialysis and are associated with increased morbidity and poor prognosis on dialysis. Whether or not Kt/V can be too high and whether higher levels of Kt/V improve morbidity and/or mortality remain to be evaluated.

What other methods are available for estimating adequacy of dialysis?

Percent urea reduction or urea reduction ratio (URR) is another method used to assess dialysis adequacy. A reduction of BUN of 65% during a given dialysis treatment roughly correlates with a Kt/V of 1.2 for patients on dialysis 3 times a week. URR is not a substitute for formal UKM because it does not reflect the contribution of residual renal function, does not reflect protein catabolic rate (PCR), and does not provide a means of evaluating the validity of results.

How is urea reduction ratio calculated?

$$\% \text{ urea reduction (URR)} = 100 \times (1 - C_t / C_o)$$
$$\text{where } C_t = \text{postdialysis BUN}$$
$$C_o = \text{predialysis BUN}$$

What is the PCR?

PCR refers to a given patient's protein intake expressed in grams of protein per kilogram normalized body weight, assuming the patient is stable—that is, neither anabolic nor catabolic. The goal PCR is between 0.8 and 1.4 grams of protein per kilogram and is probably optimal at the upper end of the range.

What is the basis for interpreting the results of UKM?

Interpretation was based originally on the National Cooperative Dialysis Study (NCDS) published in 1983, in which an attempt was made to correlate patient outcome with amount of dialysis delivered. Both hospitalization and morbidity increased with high BUN levels in the presence of inadequate protein intake. The NCDS data later underwent a mechanistic analysis by Gotch and Sargent, from which the concept of Kt/V was derived. Since that time the generally accepted goals for Kt/V have continued to be reevaluated and revised upward.

What about UKM for peritoneal dialysis?

Studies comparable to the NCDS are not available in the peritoneal dialysis population. Guidelines are available for determining urea clearance and weekly creatinine clearance as well as PCR for this treatment modality. For CAPD, the delivered dose of PD should be a Kt/V of at least 2.0 per week and a total creatinine clearance (Ccr) of at least 60 L/week/1.73m^2. For NIPD, the weekly delivered dose should be a total Kt/V of at least 2.2 and a weekly total Ccr of at least 66 L/1.73m^2. For CCPD, Kt/V of at least 2.1 and Ccr of at least 63 L/1.73m^2 should be used.

Peritoneal equilibration testing (PET) is performed to assess the clearance capabilities of a given patient's peritoneal membrane and determine the optimal peritoneal dialysis regimen. See Chapter 16 for further information about PET.

What can be done for the patient who is unable to eat?

The first step in helping a patient who is unable to eat is to determine why he or she cannot eat and how to correct it. This can often be best addressed by a team approach including nurse, dietitian, technician, physician, and social worker. Among the possible causes are underdialysis/uremia, gastroparesis, depression, intercurrent illness, poor dentition, constipation, side effects of medications, depression or socioeconomic factors that influence the ability to obtain, prepare, or store foods. These are but a few causes of poor nutritional intake. Inadequate intake and poor nutritional status should not be accepted as "normal" for dialysis patients. Each problem should be assessed and investigated since there will often be an etiology that can be remedied.

Once the identifiable causes of poor intake have been alleviated, certain strategies can be employed to augment nutrient intake. Commercially available supplements or homemade equivalents may be appropriate for some patients. The dietitian can evaluate the need for such supplements and recommend an appropriate type. Eating five or six small meals per day instead of two or three large ones may improve intake for some patients. The social worker can be helpful in enrolling a patient in a program such as Meals on Wheels or in involving the family in promoting food intake. Specific cultural habits and preferences are also incorporated in formulating a nutrition care plan. Medications to augment appetite have been used safely and effectively in patients with cancer and AIDS. These medications have not been well studied in the dialysis population but may be used when other strategies to augment oral intake have failed. Enteral nutrition via nasogastric, percutaneous endoscopic gastrostomy or jejunostomy tubes should also be considered as an alternative method of providing support in the patient who is unable to eat but has a viable gastrointestinal tract. If, despite these efforts, a patient continues to deteriorate nutritionally, intradialytic parenteral nutrition may be appropriate.

What is intradialytic parenteral nutrition (IDPN)?

IDPN is a form of nutrition support by which protein, fat, and carbohydrate can be given during the dialysis treatment. Typically, a 1 L solution of amino acids, lipid solution, and dextrose is infused during a dialysis run through the venous drip chamber. This provides 800 to 1000 calories and 60 to 90 grams of amino acids. The advantage is that nutrients can be provided with a concomitant removal of volume, and a central line is not necessary since the dialysis access serves as the line of administration. Although this method cannot meet a patient's entire nutritional needs, it can provide supplemental nutrition for patients who are unable to take adequate intake by mouth, for whom enteral feeding is not an option, and for whom a central line is contraindicated. Approximately 90 percent of the amino acids infused are retained during this process. Potential side effects include hyperglycemia and reactive hypoglycemia.

Is there a comparable method of administering nutritional support for patients on peritoneal dialysis?

Amino acid dialysate (AAD) has been used in patients on peritoneal dialysis, in which amino acids are substituted for a portion of dextrose in peritoneal dialysis solutions. It is typically given during one exchange in a 24-hour period and serves as both an osmotic agent as well as a protein source. It has been shown to improve protein nutritional status in patients on this modality; however, increased BUN concentrations and metabolic acidosis have been described as potential side effects. Cost factors may prohibit its widespread use.

What can be done for constipation?

Constipation is a common problem for people on dialysis and is often related to medication taken for phosphate binding. The usual recommendations for this problem given to people not on dialysis, such as increasing fluid intake, consuming relatively large amounts of bran products, and eating foods such as prunes and other fruits and vegetables, may not be appropriate for dialysis patients. Medications such as stool softeners or substances such as sorbitol, which draws fluid into the intestinal tract, may be necessary to alleviate constipation. In chronic renal failure, stool output is a major route of potassium excretion, allowing for 30 to 40 mEq of potassium excretion each day. In a patient with hyperkalemia that cannot be easily accounted for by increased potassium intake, constipation should be considered as a possible etiologic factor.

How does the diet differ for patients on peritoneal dialysis (PD)?

The diet for patients on continuous ambulatory peritoneal dialysis (CAPD), continuous cyclic peritoneal dialysis (CCPD), and other peritoneal dialysis modalities differs from that of patients on hemodialysis in several ways.

Protein. Protein needs are higher for patients on PD as a result of dialysate protein losses that average about 9 g per 24 hours. Levels of 1.2 to 1.5 g of protein per kilogram of body weight are prescribed and are often difficult to achieve, although there is evidence that some patients maintain positive nitrogen balance on lower protein intakes. As with hemodialysis, the general recommendation is that at least 50 percent of the protein should be derived from high biological value sources; however, it is possible to maintain good protein nutriture with a carefully planned vegetarian diet. Protein supplements may be used when needs cannot be met by high protein foods alone.

Calories. Although calorie needs are the same for both hemodialysis and peritoneal dialysis patients, those on peritoneal dialysis absorb 150 to 1000 calories per day from the dextrose in the dialysate. This may provide a particular advantage in the patient who has energy malnutrition or may be problematic in the obese or hypertriglyceridemic patient.

Sodium/fluid. Typically, dietary sodium and fluid can be liberalized for the PD patient as compared to the same patient on hemodialysis, since the dextrose content of the dialysis solution can be adjusted with each exchange to remove varying volumes of fluid. A sodium intake of 4 g, and a fluid intake as guided by thirst, can often provide acceptable fluid management, provided that dialysis can be adjusted to maintain euvolemia.

Potassium. Potassium control tends to be less of a problem in patients on peritoneal dialysis in part because the constant glucose infusion combined with endogenous insulin production drives potassium intracellularly. Supplemental potassium may be indicated in approximately 10 percent of peritoneal dialysis patients. Hyperkalemia may be present in others.

Phosphorus. Control of serum phosphorus presents a challenge for patients on PD. An obligatory higher phosphorus intake is often necessary to achieve an adequate dietary protein intake, as foods that are high in protein tend to be high in phosphorus. Requirements for phosphate binding medications may therefore be higher.

Vitamins and other minerals. Needs for these other nutrients are generally thought to be the same as for patients on hemodialysis.

What is the diet for acute renal failure?

There is no set diet for acute renal failure because nutritional requirements vary considerably depending on comorbid conditions, degree of renal compromise, and presence of anuria or oliguria.

High mortality rates continue to be associated with acute renal failure, and protein-calorie malnutrition is thought to be one predictor of outcome. Although aggressive nutritional support has yet to be demonstrated to improve outcome, protein and calorie intake should be provided to meet increased needs associated with hypercatabolism. Protein requirements may be 1.5 grams protein per kilogram per day or higher and can be determined using nitrogen balance studies. Both essential and non-essential amino acids should be used in most situations requiring parenteral nutrition. Calorie requirements vary considerably and can be best determined in the intensive care unit setting using indirect calorimetry.

Do the various treatment modalities influence the provision of parenteral nutrition?

Yes. The use of continuous arteriovenous or venovenous hemofiltration with or without dialysis allows for provision of large volumes of fluid necessary in order to give adequate amounts of parenteral nutrition in the hypercatabolic acute renal failure patient. Renal replacement therapy, however, also contributes to the catabolic state because of loss of nutrients (amino acids) and high-flux membranes increase these losses, in comparison with low-flux membranes. In addition, membrane characteristics, in particular bioincompatability, may further enhance catabolism.

What is carnitine and should it be routinely supplemented in patients on dialysis?

Carnitine is synthesized in the body from the essential amino acids lysine and methionine and plays a role in transporting long-chain fatty acids into the mitochondria. Although methods of measuring carnitine in various metabolic pools in the body are imprecise, free plasma carnitine and muscle carnitine concentrations may be low in patients on dialysis. Carnitine has been used to lower triglyceride levels, help with muscle cramps and muscle weakness, and decrease red blood cell fragility in patients on dialysis. The question of optimal dose and whether or not supplementation should be routine remains to be addressed.

What about the needs of pediatric patients?

The basic concepts of diet management apply to pediatric patients with chronic renal failure with one key exception: meeting the needs of protein, calories, and other nutrients to facilitate growth and development. For further reading on specific recommendations, see References and Recommended Readings, beginning on page 321.

In summary, dialysis therapy, for the patient with either acute or chronic renal failure, can provide optimal patient outcomes when combined with effective and appropriate nutrition management. Although diet management is ultimately the responsibility of the patient or caretaker, members of the interdisciplinary team play a vital role in educating and reinforcing diet information that is tailored to the individual and monitored for effectiveness.

Acute Renal Failure and Dialysis

Christy A. Price, Julia Starr, Anna L. Corea, and Mary Ann Wierszbiczki

Dialysis is often necessary for the treatment of acute renal failure. The most common indications include uremia, hyperkalemia, acidosis, fluid overload, and drug overdose.

What is acute renal failure?

Acute renal failure (ARF) is the rapid deterioration of renal function. It is usually reversible if diagnosed and treated early. Signs and symptoms of ARF are a urine output of less than 400 ml/day (oliguria), or less than 20 ml/hr for an adult, as well as an increase in BUN and creatinine, hyperkalemia, and acidosis.

What are the types of acute renal failure?

Acute renal failure is divided into three categories: prerenal, intrarenal, and postrenal (see Chapter 3).

Prerenal. Prerenal renal failure accounts for approximately 70 percent of ARF cases. Prerenal events result in a decrease in blood flow to the kidney. Examples include congestive heart failure, hypovolemia, sepsis, myocardial infarction, prolonged hypotension, and vascular disorders of the renal artery or vein.

Intrarenal. Approximately 25 percent of ARF cases are caused by intrarenal factors. Any event that damages the kidney tissue, structure, and function is categorized as intrarenal ARF. The damage, which may involve the glomeruli, the tubules, or both, interferes with the ability of the kidneys to carry out their normal functions. The most common cause of intrarenal failure is damage to the tubules. This is called *acute tubular necrosis* (ATN). ATN is caused by severely reduced blood flow leading to prolonged ischemia, or by direct toxic insult to tubular cells. In oliguric ATN, urine flow falls to about 20 ml/hr, and BUN and serum creatinine, phosphate, and potassium levels rise. With nonoliguric ARF, the patient may remain in better fluid balance, but elimination of waste products is impaired. Ischemic injury to the kidneys can occur when the mean arterial blood pressure drops below 60 mm Hg for over 30 minutes. Massive hemorrhage, transfusion reaction, sepsis, cardiovascular collapse, or major trauma can cause ischemic renal injury.

Substances that injure the kidneys are called nephrotoxins. The most common are medications such as antibiotics and nonsteroidal antiinflammatory agents. Other medications, including anesthetics and cancer chemotherapy agents, as well as street drugs, are toxic to the kidney in varying degrees. Radiologic contrast dye used for intravenous pyelography, cardiac catheterization, and computed tomography (CT) is potentially nephrotoxic. Other nephrotoxins include hemoglobin (from hemolysis of red cells), and myoglobin from muscle breakdown (rhabdomyolysis), because of crush injury, heat stroke, or seizure.

Postrenal. Postrenal causes account for approximately 5 percent of ARF cases. Postrenal failure is usually the result of obstruction in the flow of urine anywhere from the kidney to the urinary meatus. The obstruction can be functional or mechanical. Functional causes include diabetic nephropathy, medications such as ganglionic blocking agents that block the autonomic nerve supply to the urinary system, and neurogenic bladder subsequent to spinal cord injury or cerebral vascular accident (CVA). Tumors, stones, prostatic hypertrophy, and urethral strictures are some mechanical causes of postrenal failure.

Does a patient with acute renal failure have urine output?

Some patients with ARF have significant urine output, referred to as nonoliguric renal failure. Most patients progress through several stages from oliguria to anuria to polyuria, depending on the phase of ARF.

Oliguric-anuric phase. Oliguria is defined as urine volume less than 400 ml/24 hours. Anuria is a urine output of less than 50 ml/24 hours. This phase can last from 2 days to 30 days or longer. The longer the oliguria/anuria continues, the prospect of returning to normal urine output worsens. Proper management of fluid volume is essential.

Diuretic phase. This phase begins when the urine output reaches 1 L/24 hours. The renal indices may stabilize, then start to approach normal with gradual return of renal function. A 24-hour urine volume can increase to as much as 4 to 5 L. Accurate evaluation of the patient's status to avoid dehydration leading to hypoperfusion of the kidneys is mandatory. Laboratory values are monitored closely with the expectation that they will return to normal in the late phase of ARF.

Convalescent phase. This period begins with the stabilization of serum chemistries and gradual return of normal kidney function. This phase may last from 3 to 6 months. Return to normal glomerular filtration rate (GFR), if it occurs, may take up to a year.

What are the clinical presentations of acute renal failure?

These include all the symptoms, signs, and findings of rapidly developing uremia (see Chapter 3).

What biochemical changes are present in acute renal failure?

The damaged kidneys are unable to excrete the products of normal body metabolism. There is elevation of the serum urea and creatinine, and altered electrolyte levels. Increased hydrogen ion concentration causes acidosis and a low serum pH. Hyperkalemia or hypokalemia, hypocalcemia, hyperphosphatemia, hypermagnesemia, and a low bicarbonate may be observed.

How is acute renal failure treated?

Many treatment options are available depending on the cause of the renal failure, the severity of symptoms, and the overall condition of the patient. Options include hemodialysis, isolated ultrafiltration, peritoneal dialysis, continuous renal replacement therapy (CRRT), and charcoal hemoperfusion.

What are the indications for treatment?

The most common indications for acute dialysis include the following:

Uremia. Acute dialysis is initiated when a patient becomes symptomatically uremic (see Chapter 3), regardless of BUN or creatinine level. Dialysis may be started prophylactically when the BUN reaches 100 mg/dl, even if the patient has few or no symptoms.

Pulmonary edema. Acute pulmonary edema is a life-threatening complication of ARF that necessitates immediate dialysis. Acute pulmonary edema can result from fluid overload directly attributable to ARF or as the result of an acute myocardial infarction or from overzealous administration of fluid.

Hyperkalemia. Hyperkalemia is a result of the damaged kidney's inability to secrete potassium and the release of intracellular potassium (because of acidosis and tissue breakdown). Hemodialysis is effective in lowering potassium and is initiated when rapid reduction of plasma potassium is indicated. Peritoneal dialysis is an acceptable treatment option, although its effects are slower than that of hemodialysis. Hyperkalemia can be managed in an emergency, while waiting for hemodialysis, by intravenous administration of glucose and insulin in combination with intravenous sodium bicarbonate. These shift extracellular potassium into the cell, where it cannot cause cardiac arrhythmia. Calcium gluconate may be given intravenously to reduce myocardial irritability. Sodium polystyrene sulfonate cation exchange resin (Kayexalate) by mouth or by enema can be administered when slower correction of potassium is acceptable or in the initial management of hyperkalemia.

Acidosis. Metabolic acidosis is caused by inability of the kidneys to excrete hydrogen ion and to reabsorb bicarbonate. Acidosis can be treated temporarily by intravenous sodium bicarbonate. Hemodialysis may be required because of the added sodium, which increases the danger of volume overload.

Neurologic changes. Toxic effects of uremia can result in central nervous system changes. Headache, insomnia, and drowsiness are early symptoms; confusion, convulsions, and coma may occur later. Dialysis is indicated when any of these serious symptoms are seen, and preferably before they occur.

Drug overdoses and poisonings. Dialysis is indicated for the treatment of some drug intoxications. Drugs normally excreted by the kidneys, or water-soluble drugs of low molecular weight, will diffuse rapidly across cellulosic dialysis membranes. Such drugs are readily removed with hemodialysis. Examples include ethanol, lithium, methanol, and salicylates. Water-soluble drugs with high molecular weight such as vancomycin and amphotericin B diffuse across cellulosic membranes much more slowly and are less well removed. If the intoxicant is protein-bound (e.g., digoxin and acetylsalicylic acid) or lipid-soluble (e.g., glutethimide), hemodialysis is not useful. However, both of these intoxicants are removed by hemoperfusion with a charcoal cartridge or with a plasma membrane filter.

What type of vascular access is used for acute dialysis?

The most common access to the circulation for acute dialysis is a double-lumen venous catheter. The catheter may be placed in the subclavian, internal jugular, or femoral vein. Insertion of a catheter into the subclavian or internal jugular vein must be followed by an x-ray examination to determine correct placement, and to rule out pneumothorax or hemothorax before the catheter is used (see Chapter 8).

Can an AV fistula or graft be used for acute dialysis?

Patients with an AV fistula or graft may require acute dialysis, and the fistula or graft can be used after its patency is determined. (See Chapter 8 for additional information.)

How often are patients dialyzed?

Frequency of dialysis is determined by the patient's response to treatment. Patients may be hemodialyzed daily for a few days until the BUN, serum creatinine, potassium level, and acidosis are considered acceptable. Daily dialysis may be necessary for volume overload, or if parenteral nutrition is to be given.

What are complications that may occur with acute renal failure?

Congestive heart failure (CHF) is a common occurrence. It is most often caused by hypertension, volume excess, and/or anemia.

Hypertension. Fluid removal by dialysis may correct the hypertension. Antihypertensive medication may be necessary.

Hypotension. Hypotension may result from blood loss, a strict fluid restriction, sepsis, myocardial infarction or pericarditis. To prevent additional kidney damage, the underlying cause of the hypotension must be corrected to maintain adequate renal perfusion. The use of a vasopressor such as dopamine may be necessary.

Anemia. In acute renal failure the release of erythropoietin is decreased. The usual response to therapy with recombinant erythropoietin or epoetin (EPO) requires 3 to 4 weeks, so it is not of immediate help. Uremic red cells also have a shortened life span. Blood loss from bleeding is often present. See Chapter 14 for additional information about complications.

What is the most serious complication of acute renal failure?

Infection is the leading cause of death in ARF. Uremia causes immune suppression, which predisposes the patient to sepsis. Strict aseptic technique must be used for all invasive procedures, including initiating and discontinuing dialysis, starting an intravenous line, and caring for the bladder catheter.

Are there special considerations when dialyzing a patient for the first time?

An infrequent syndrome known as the "first-use" syndrome results from an allergic-type reaction to new dialyzers and is characterized by itching, hypotension, chest and back pain, and breathing difficulties. In a severe case, cardiopulmonary arrest may occur. Symptoms are usually manifested during the first 15 to 30 minutes of dialysis. Cuprophan dialyzers are most often implicated. Cellulose acetate, modified cellulosic and synthetic membranes (polysulfone, polyamide and polyacrylonitrile) are less likely to cause first-use syndrome.

What is the treatment for "first-use" syndrome?

When the symptoms are severe, the blood must not be returned to the patient, and the dialyzer is discarded. The physician should be notified and an assessment of symptoms, particularly cardiopulmonary status, performed. The use of a more biocompatible membrane may be necessary. When the symptoms are less severe, symptomatic treatment (e.g., nasal O_2 or oral Benadryl) is adequate. In this situation, dialysis can continue because the symptoms usually subside after the first hour.

Are there special precautions when dialyzing someone with acute renal failure?

Patients requiring acute dialysis are generally critically ill with multisystem failure. A thorough and accurate total assessment of the patient is essential before initiating dialysis (see Chapter 9). The nephrology nurse must be highly cognizant of changes, be prudent in assessing and monitoring the patient's vital signs, and respond appropriately.

Controlled anticoagulation with heparin may be necessary to minimize clotting of the dialyzer; however, dialysis can be performed with little or no heparin. Careful monitoring of clotting times may be necessary to prevent complications related to heparinization during hemodialysis. A baseline clotting time must be obtained before the start of dialysis; a normal ACT is 60 to 90 seconds. The Clinical Laboratory Improvement Act (CLIA) now requires quality control checks for ACT machines to meet CLIA requirements. These requirements are resource intensive and may not permit bedside monitoring of ACT levels during dialysis. (See Chapter 10.)

The physician determines the technique of anticoagulation. "Tight" or no heparin may be used for patients at high risk for bleeding. In tight heparinization, clotting times are performed every 30 minutes. The ACT is kept at 1.25 times the baseline with additional heparin, as indicated when the ACT falls below the 1.25 baseline value. With systemic heparinization, generally the ACT values are allowed to range from 2.5 to 3 times the baseline.

"No heparin" dialysis requires a blood flow between 250 and 300 ml/min, or significant dialyzer clotting will occur. The dialyzer is flushed every 20 to 30 minutes with 100 ml of normal saline so that it can be easily examined visually for clotting, and so that proteins and clotting factors will be moved away from the dialyzer membrane surface. Before the start of dialysis this extra volume is calculated into the required fluid loss in order to achieve the planned fluid removal goal. The risk of clotting the dialyzer, resulting in an average blood loss of 150 ml, must be weighed against the risk of administering an anticoagulant to a high-risk patient.

Patients in an intensive care unit are often attached to a cardiac monitor. It is important to watch for arrhythmias during dialysis, since these may relate to the dialysis. However, it is not uncommon to see some aberrant beats or premature ventricular beats during dialysis.

What measures may be taken during acute dialysis to counteract hypotension?

Abnormalities causing hypotension must be identified and corrected as much as possible. These usually involve intravascular volume, cardiac output, and/or vasomotor tone. Although patients are often overhydrated and edematous, some may have hypotension from low intravascular volume and need infusion of normal saline or dextrose and water. Patients who do not respond to normal saline infusion may require colloid or hyperosmolar products such as human plasma protein fraction (Plasmanate) or albumin. These colloids will increase the oncotic pressure and attract fluid from the extracellular space into the vascular space. Hypotension resulting from decreased red cell mass from hemorrhage or other causes may require transfusion of red blood cells. When hypotension is caused by low cardiac output, cardiotonic drugs, particularly inotropic (dopamine) and antiarrhythmic (lidocaine) agents may be helpful. It may be appropriate to reduce the blood flow rate to between 150 and 200 ml/min for an apparent decrease in cardiac output. The physician will need accurate assessment data on duration of dialysis, blood flow rate, ultrafiltration estimate (or weight), BP readings, and all medications administered to determine the most appropriate treatment. NOTE: When the blood flow is lowered, dialysis efficiency is reduced; that is, there is a decrease in urea reduction, Kt/V and creatinine clearance.

If hypotension is caused by poor vasomotor tone, patients may be maintained above their ideal weight to promote vascular filling and normotensive blood pressure.

What measures are appropriate for hypertension?

Most hypertension in acute dialysis patients is related to fluid excess and responds to ultrafiltration. If it is not controlled with fluid removal, the physician may prescribe an antihypertensive medication. Patients on antihypertensive agents may be subject to hypotensive episodes. Administration of antihypertensive agents may need to be deferred prior to hemodialysis if ordered accordingly by the physician.

What is the disequilibrium syndrome?

This is a complex of signs and symptoms ranging from headache, restlessness, and impaired mental concentration to confusion, twitching, jerking, and occasionally culminating in a grand mal seizure. It may occur during or soon after dialysis.

What causes dialysis disequilibrium?

Disequilibrium is believed to be related to cerebral edema. The blood-brain barrier has a selective effect on the transfer of solute and of water between the plasma and the brain. During dialysis, plasma solute concentration is lowered faster than brain solute, and the plasma becomes hypotonic in relation to the brain cell water, causing water to shift from the plasma to the brain.

When should disequilibrium be anticipated?

Disequilibrium is most common in the more severely catabolic patient or in those in whom azotemia is severe (BUN greater than 200 mg/100 ml).

What are ways to prevent or minimize disequilibrium?

Prevention is best. Care must be taken not to lower the urea level too rapidly; it is best to do short (2- to 3-hour) dialysis at 24-hour intervals for the first few treatments. A reduced blood flow rate of 150 to 200 ml/min may lessen the risk of dialysis disequilibrium by slowing the rate of solute shift. Using a small dialyzer with lower clearance properties will help. Configuring the extracorporeal blood circuit with the dialysate flow concurrent—rather than countercurrent—to the blood flow is an easy means of decreasing the rapid removal of urea by lowering clearance throughout the treatment. Decreasing the dialysate flow rate also will lead to decreased removal of urea. The physician may also prescribe a high osmotic solution such as 25% mannitol intravenously at the beginning of treatment. Disequilibrium manifested by seizures and coma is unusual with frequent and less aggressive dialysis. Early detection of the potential for severe neurological changes must be promptly reported to the physician.

PROCEDURES

What is isolated ultrafiltration?

Isolated ultrafiltration is a process by which excess fluid is removed with little or no change in solute concentrations of the blood. Very small amounts of urea and creatinine are removed from the patient's serum passively along with the ultrafiltrate. The rate and amount at which the fluid can be removed depends in part on the amount of excess extracellular fluid present, the patient's intravascular volume, and cardiovascular stability.

What are the indications for using isolated ultrafiltration?

Isolated ultrafiltration is indicated to remove fluid when the removal of solute is not a priority. Isolated ultrafiltration can be performed immediately before, after, or independently of hemodialysis treatment.

What equipment is needed for ultrafiltration?

Isolated ultrafiltration is performed with the same dialyzer and tubing used for hemodialysis. The dialysate flow is turned off, or placed in "by-pass" mode. The dialyzer membrane does not come into contact with the dialysate solution. With conventional equipment, the total of the negative pressure applied to the dialysate side of the membrane plus the venous pressure represents the transmembrane pressure and determines the amount of ultrafiltration. With volumetric equipment, the set value for UFR determines the fluid to be removed. A blood pump, air detector, blood leak detector and pressure monitors are standard equipment to perform the procedure safely.

Are there complications with isolated ultrafiltration?

Rapid removal of fluid can cause hypotension and muscle cramps.

What treatments besides hemodialysis are available to treat acute renal failure?

There are many alternatives to conventional hemodialysis (see Chapter 5). Continuous renal replacement therapy (CRRT) has become the treatment of choice for ARF. CRRT is the umbrella acronym for the five approaches for this treatment: i.e., slow continuous ultrafiltration (SCUF), continuous arteriovenous hemofiltration (CAVH), continuous arteriovenous hemodialysis (CAVHD), continuous venovenous hemofiltration (CVVH), and continuous venovenous hemodialysis (CVVHD). Originally SCUF, CAVH and CAVHD were very popular because they do not require special equipment or the constant attention of nephrology personnel. Now CVVH and CVVHD are being prescribed more. The principles of CRRT are the same, but special equipment is necessary for CVVH or CVVHD. The procedures are limited to the critical care setting for the treatment of ARF. A collaborative approach utilizing the collective expertise of critical care and nephrology personnel is strongly recommended.

What is slow continuous ultrafiltration (SCUF)?

SCUF is a method of gradual fluid removal. As with isolated ultrafiltration, little solute removal takes place; therefore intermittent hemodialysis may be needed to treat azotemia and maintain electrolyte balance. The amount of fluid removed is usually 2 to 6 L in a 24-hour period.

What are the indications for SCUF?

Many patients with ARF have a high rate of protein breakdown and require large volumes of total parenteral nutrition (TPN) fluid. A few hours of hemodialysis may be inadequate to remove such large volumes of fluid, particularly in the patient with hypotension and hemodynamic instability. SCUF allows for the slow continuous removal of fluid, alleviating the large volume administered.

What equipment is used in SCUF?

A highly permeable hemofilter, similar to a dialyzer, is used. SCUF is performed without blood pump assistance, relying on the patient's cardiac output and mean arterial pressure (MAP) to provide adequate blood flow through the filter. The hydrostatic pressure of the blood forces the ultrafiltrate across the membrane, and it is collected in a drainage bag for disposal. The length of tubing from the hemofilter to the fluid collection device creates a negative pressure which supports the UFR.

Do patients require heparin during the procedure?

Usually an initial bolus of 500 to 2000 units of heparin is injected, followed by a continuous drip of 250 to 500 units (U)/hr, or 5 to 10 U/kg/hr. Clotting times are monitored. The procedure can be used without heparin by using normal saline flushes, but the chances of clotting the hemofilter are greatly increased.

What problems are associated with SCUF?

The most common problem is failure to obtain the desired quantity of ultrafiltrate. The reasons are usually clotting of the hemofilter or decrease in blood flow through the circuit. A problem with the patient's access, a kink in the tubing, or a drop in the patient's arterial pressure can also result in a low ultrafiltration rate.

What is continuous arteriovenous hemofiltration (CAVH)?

CAVH is the continuous flow of blood through an extracorporeal circuit to remove excess fluid and solutes over an extended period of time. There are specific hemofilters in different sizes available to perform CAVH. Product specifications, membrane properties, and hemofilter sizes vary considerably.

What are the indications for CAVH?

CAVH is indicated when large volumes of fluid must be removed from hemodynamically unstable patients. Fluid loss is generally 8 to 15 L a day for adult patients. The large amount of fluid loss allows the removal of solutes from the blood. The solutes are removed by convection in proportion to their plasma water concentration. Replacement fluid will hemodilute the concentration of solutes such as urea, creatinine, and other uremic toxins, correct the levels of potassium, calcium, and sodium in the plasma, and allow for a net loss of fluid, which can be tolerated by the patient.

What equipment is used during CAVH?

The extracorporeal circuit is similar to that used in SCUF. CAVH (Fig. 13-1) is also performed without blood pump assistance, and is dependent on the adequacy of the patient's blood pressure to push the blood through the circuit. As with SCUF, the patient's MAP must be maintained at greater than 60 mm Hg, or ideally 70 mm Hg. A drainage bag is attached to a port on the filter to collect the ultrafiltrate.

Fig. 13-1 CAVH schematic.

What monitoring is required during the procedure?

It is essential to keep accurate hourly intake and output records because of the large volume of hourly ultrafiltration. If too much volume is being removed, the ultrafiltration rate can be slowed by raising the level of the collection device up to the hemofilter. Serum chemistries are monitored routinely to avoid electrolyte imbalance and to ensure that replacement fluid is adequate.

How do SCUF and CAVH differ?

The larger amount of fluid removed with CAVH allows for an increased transfer of solute across the membrane and replacement with a balanced electrolyte solution. With SCUF no replacement is needed because the patient's oral and intravenous intake generally are adequate to avoid a significant loss of total body fluid. CAVH is usually sufficient therapy for a patient with low to moderate azotemia and a need for considerable volume removal.

What is continuous arteriovenous hemodialysis (CAVHD)?

CAVHD (Fig. 13-2) is a modification of CAVH, with the addition of dialysate flowing through the filter at a slow rate, for combined removal of fluid and solutes by diffusion (dialysis) and by convection (ultrafiltration).

Fig. 13-2 CAVHD—Continuous arteriovenous hemodialysis. Courtesy Baxter Healthcare, Renal Division, McGraw Park, Illinois.

What are the indications for CAVHD?

When CAVH does not provide adequate waste product removal, CAVHD becomes the preferred treatment option. CAVHD may be more appropriate for patients who are anuric, hyperkalemic, or severely acidotic.

How is the procedure different from CAVH?

The procedures are similar except that dialysate is circulated around the hemofilter membrane in CAVHD for more efficient clearance of urea and creatinine. The dialysate used may be standard peritoneal dialysis solution containing 1.5% to 2.5% dextrose, which is infused into the hemofilter via one of the ultrafiltrate ports at a rate of 15 to 40 ml/min, or 1 to 4 liters/hour. Custom dialysate fluid may be necessary to avoid hyperglycemia and lactic acidosis, or for patients with liver failure. The increased solute removal reduces uremia, acidosis, and potential electrolyte imbalance so that replacement fluid may not be necessary.

What type of access is required for these treatments?

Access to the arterial circulation is necessary because no blood pump is used. Generally, a single-lumen catheter is inserted into the femoral artery, with the blood returning to the femoral vein via another catheter. The subclavian vein can also be used for the return of the blood.

What is continuous venovenous hemofiltration (CVVH)?

CVVH (Fig. 13-3) is a form of continuous therapy, similar to CAVH, but a blood pump is employed to control the blood flow through the hemofilter. The blood pump equipment includes an arterial pressure monitor, a venous pressure monitor and a venous drip chamber with an air alert detector. The use of a blood pump replaces the patient's MAP as the driving force for the extracorporeal system.

What is continuous venovenous hemodialysis (CVVHD)?

CVVHD (Fig. 13-4) is similar to CAVHD in principle, but like CVVH, a blood pump is employed to control the blood flow rate. Unlike CVVH, CVVHD requires the use of dialysate running countercurrent to the blood flow through the extracorporeal circuit. The indications for CVVHD are the same as for CAVHD. Intermittent hemodialysis would be insufficient therapy for these patients, plus they may be too unstable to tolerate aggressive hemodialysis.

Vein

Filtrate

Pump

Fig. 13-3 CVVH—Continuous venovenous hemofiltration. Courtesy Baxter Healthcare, Renal Division, McGraw Park, Illinois.

Fig. 13-4 CVVHD—Continuous venovenous hemodialysis. Courtesy Baxter Healthcare, Renal Division, McGraw Park, Illinois.

What are the primary advantages of CVVH/CVVHD over CAVH/CAVHD?

Arteriovenous extracorporeal circuit require the prolonged cannulation of an artery. This can lead to compromised blood flow to the extremity, infection, and impaired ability to move the patient. Venovenous extracorporeal circuits do not require use of an artery. A single dual lumen catheter can be used. Preferred sites are the subclavian or internal jugular vein. Blood flow through the hemofilter is consistent and controlled by the nurse, generally between 100 to 200 ml/min.

What are the disadvantages of venovenous access?

CVVH and CVVHD require more bedside equipment that must be monitored by the critical care nurse. Inservice education must be provided to assist the critical care nurses to be comfortable with the system.

Is the anticoagulation the same for CAVH/CAVHD and CVVH/CVVHD?

Heparin is the primary anticoagulation used with all approaches of CRRT. Generally a bolus of 500 U to 2000 U is administered into the blood circuit upon initiation of therapy followed by a heparin infusion of 5 to 10 U/kg/hr. If activated clotting times (ACT) are permitted in the institution, an appropriate range for CRRT would be 150 to 200 seconds. An alternative or adjunct therapy is to routinely flush the hemofilter and blood circuit with normal saline. This may prolong the life of the hemofilter. Trisodium citrate anticoagulation has been used successfully, but requires additional monitoring of serum sodium, calcium and bicarbonate to avoid compromising the patient. Venovenous circuits have fewer clotting problems because of the consistent blood flow.

What are the complications associated with CRRT?

Patient complications include hypotension, cardiac dysrhythmias, dehydration, electrolyte imbalance, blood loss, infection, and air embolism. There are technical complications which include blood leak, membrane rupture, clotted hemofilter, disconnection of the arterial or venous tubing, equipment malfunction, position of catheters, kinked tubing and inexperienced personnel.

Who is responsible for CRRT?

The ideal situation is for the critical care and nephrology professionals to work collaboratively. Generally, the nephrologist prescribes the therapy and then shares the monitoring and appropriate interventions with the intensivists. The nephrology nurses set up the system, provide inservice teaching, assist with nursing interventions, such as catheter dressing changes, and remain available on-call for troubleshooting or problem solving. The critical care nurses are responsible for the 24-hour monitoring, documentation of intake and output, replacement fluids, heparinization, and discontinuing a clotted circuit. CRRT offers an approach that focuses on providing the patient with 24-hour renal replacement, rather than attempting to correct a multitude of problems in a 3- or 4-hour hemodialysis treatment. The delineation of clinical responsibilities must be decided upon before initiating a CRRT program for critically ill patients.

What substances can be removed by dialysis or hemoperfusion?

As a general rule, substances completely or almost completely excreted by the normal kidney will be removed by dialysis. Substances metabolized by the liver, or their by-products, may not be removed by hemodialysis. Information about the site of metabolism and excretion of most drugs is often obtainable from the package insert or from pharmacology texts. The *Physician's Desk Reference (PDR)* is another quick resource. A computerized textbook of treatment options for drug overdoses and poisonings, or *Poisindex*, should be available. Information on this system can be very useful because it is updated regularly. Regional poison centers have information on drugs or poisons. The intoxicating substance(s) should be identified and quantified as soon as possible. Often quantitative results may take several hours and are not available when most urgently needed.

What if the substance is not known or cannot be readily verified?

The decision to treat or not, and by what modality, becomes a clinical one, to be made by the physician. If the patient is severely ill and the circumstances suggest one or more of the substances ingested is likely to be removable by hemoperfusion or dialysis, treatment should be started. This is because the duration of coma, morbidity, and mortality may be reduced by early initiation of treatment.

For what toxic agents is dialysis recommended as specific treatment of choice?

Alcohols, such as methyl alcohol and ethylene or propylene glycol (antifreeze), are easily dialyzed. Salicylates (aspirin), lithium carbonate, and aminophylline dialyze well. Certain mushrooms (*Amanita phalloides*) call for immediate hemodialysis therapy. Early removal of toxins may prevent the blindness, liver necrosis, renal failure, or death that can result from such poisons. Accidental therapeutic intravenous drug overdose from such agents as theophylline, antibiotics, or mannitol may require emergent dialysis to decrease the risk of serious complications.

Is there any particular type of dialyzer preferable for poisonings?

In poisoning, the objective is to remove as much of the offending agent as rapidly as possible. Therefore a dialyzer with the largest surface area the patient will tolerate should be used. High–middle molecule clearance devices, i.e., 500 to 20,000 daltons, may be the dialyzer of choice.

What poisonings are best treated by charcoal hemoperfusion?

Sedatives, including barbiturates, ethchlorvynol, and glutethimide and many insecticides and herbicides have better removal by hemoperfusion than by hemodialysis.

What about bloodstream access for dialysis of poisons?

The most appropriate access, if the patient does not already have a permanent vascular access, is a temporary catheter placed in a large vein, such as femoral, subclavian, or internal jugular. The greater the blood flow, the greater the removal of toxins.

Does peritoneal dialysis have any place in the treatment of poisoning?

It is rarely appropriate, and only if hemodialysis is not available or will be delayed. Peritoneal dialysis has low clearance rates and takes longer in removing drugs than hemodialysis and hemoperfusion. However, if preparation for hemodialysis will be delayed, and peritoneal dialysis can be instituted at once, it can be a temporary treatment option.

Should hemodialysis and charcoal hemoperfusion be used together?

Hemoperfusion has a greater affinity and faster clearance for many toxins than does hemodialysis. However, hemoperfusion does not provide the ultrafiltration that may be needed for hypervolemia or pulmonary edema. Perfusion alone does not correct acid-base imbalance or electrolyte abnormalities, which may be very important in the acidosis associated with many intoxications. Sometimes sequential use of hemodialysis and hemoperfusion is recommended. The appropriate treatment is dictated by the properties of the poison or drug that needs to be removed.

What special patient problems may be encountered in dialysis or hemoperfusion of ingested or intravenous poisons or drug overdoses?

Such patients are generally critically ill, possibly with multisystem failure. Most are hemodynamically unstable. Specific problems may include the following:

Hypotension. This responds poorly to volume replacement; infusion of a pressor agent such as dopamine is frequently necessary; however, the pressor agent's effect may be reduced by the dialysis or hemoperfusion.

Respiratory depression or apnea. The patient may have an endotracheal tube or tracheostomy and may require ventilatory assistance equipment.

Severe acid-base imbalance. Patients who have an alkalosis from the drug intoxication may experience worsening of the condition with the dialysis treatment. The amount of bicarbonate in the dialysate may have to be adjusted. Often custom dialysate is required with changes during the treatment.

DIALYSIS IN RELATION TO TRANSPLANT

Many patients receive dialysis as part of the plan for kidney transplant (See Chapter 15). Dialysis may be initiated immediately pretransplant as preparation for surgery, during surgery, or following transplantation as support because of technical complications or complications during rejection episodes. Patients who require dialysis during posttransplant dysfunction or acute rejection require special treatment considerations.

What is posttransplant kidney dysfunction?

This is a form of acute renal failure seen occasionally with living donor kidneys and more often with cadaveric kidneys. It is usually related to the length of the "warm and cold ischemia time." This is the time measured from the kidney removal to its revascularization in the transplanted patient. The mechanism is similar to that of acute tubular necrosis. The kidney usually begins to function in about 10 days, occasionally going as long as 3 to 4 weeks before producing quality urine. (See Chapter 15.)

DIALYSIS OF PATIENTS WITH TRANSPLANT REJECTION

What are special problems in the dialysis of posttransplant patients?

Maintenance of fluid balance is essential to the function of the transplanted kidney. Care must be taken not to be overly aggressive with fluid removal; the resulting hypotension could cause hypoperfusion of the new organ and lead to renal dysfunction. In the early postoperative period, such patients have all the problems of recent major surgery. "No Heparin dialysis" should be used to prevent bleeding at the operative site. Because of steroids, patients may be intensely catabolic, with BUN disproportionately high in relation to serum creatinine. Hypertension may be aggravated by steroid treatment. Wound healing may be slow, and some drainage is common. Patients who have lost a transplant to severe rejection usually have been treated with steroids. Their tissues are often edematous and extremely friable. Patients with infections and rejection are almost always catabolic, edematous, and hypoproteinemic. Their cardiopulmonary and cardiovascular systems are often labile, and hypotension or cardiac dysrhythmias and pulmonary congestion should be anticipated.

Complications of Chronic Dialysis Therapy

Allen R. Nissenson

Chronic dialysis therapy has extended the lives of hundreds of thousands of patients. The treatment, however, can be associated with significant acute and chronic complications. Although the availability of sophisticated dialysis delivery machines has led to a decrease in hypotension, cramps, nausea, and headache for some patients, this has been offset in part by the increasing acuity of the patients treated with chronic dialysis. A slow improvement in patient survival over the past several years has also led to an increased likelihood of chronic complications of dialysis, the most common of which is dialysis-related amyloidosis. A clear understanding of the acute and chronic complications of dialysis will enable the practitioner to better understand, and influence to the extent possible these conditions, and should lead to a better tolerated treatment with improved patient outcomes.

What does maintenance hemodialysis mean?

Maintenance hemodialysis means the repetitive dialysis procedures necessary to keep a person with end-stage renal disease (ESRD) alive and as healthy as possible.

How often is hemodialysis required in ESRD?

Ideally, treatment would be continuous, to more closely approximate normal kidney function. Practically, most patients receive treatment three times each week. The accumulation of metabolic wastes and fluid determines the frequency and duration of dialysis required by a given patient.

Why is frequent dialysis desirable?

Changes in the fluid and biochemical state of the body affect total body function by the *extent* of such changes and by the *rate* of change. A large accumulation of wastes or fluid makes the patient ill. On the other hand, rapid reduction of the accumulation can also make the patient ill because of the shifts between intracellular and extracellular compartments. Frequent hemodialysis reduces the interval for accumulation of metabolic wastes and fluid. Total accumulation is less, and rate of reduction during dialysis is less.

Why not dialyze every day?

Equipment and supplies are expensive. The dialysis procedure takes time, which the patient would prefer to spend elsewhere. The duration and frequency of most dialysis prescriptions are a compromise between what is best for the patient's health and the practical limitations of money and time.

COMPLICATIONS OF ESRD AND DIALYSIS

What adverse reactions are associated with maintenance hemodialysis?

Many complications in patients with ESRD are part of the uremic syndrome and are unrelated to the dialysis treatment itself. Other abnormalities are directly related to the dialysis process. The goal of every dialysis should be to provide a safe, smooth, and comfortable treatment while accomplishing those chemical and fluid changes required for the best long-term care of the patient.

What central nervous system abnormalities occur during dialysis?

Some degree of central nervous system (CNS) abnormality occurs in a significant proportion of patients during or immediately after dialysis. Headache, weakness, fatigue, apathy, or nausea and emesis are common. A few persons become restless or agitated.

These symptoms are probably related to the rate and extent of fluid and chemical shifts between body compartments during the procedure. They represent a form of the disequilibrium syndrome and are caused by brain swelling during dialysis. Better dietary and fluid control between dialyses, reduced ultrafiltration, a change of dialyzer, or longer and slower dialyses may relieve these symptoms. When neurologic symptoms relate to a need to remove a larger volume of fluid, hemofiltration or sequential ultrafiltration and dialysis may be used. These techniques minimize osmolar and volume shifts between the body compartments (see Chapter 2).

Strokes have occurred during or following dialysis. This unfortunate occurrence may be related to hypertension or to subdural or intracerebral bleeding as a result of heparin. Extremes of high or low blood pressure may also play a role.

What causes hypotension as dialysis is begun?

Hypotension at the beginning of dialysis occurs in some patients with a relatively small blood volume (children, small women). This is the result of volume shifts as the dialyzer is filled with the patient's blood. It is much less frequent with small-volume dialyzers than with larger ones. This type of reaction is rarely serious and usually does not last long. It will respond to the infusion of small amounts of saline or albumin. Careful technique in starting the dialysis will minimize the occurrence of these episodes.

What about hypotension occurring later during dialysis?

Later hypotension is usually attributable to removal of fluid from the vascular space (ultrafiltration) in excess of the patient's ability to compensate for this. The hypotension may be asymptomatic until there has been a fall of 40 to 55 mm Hg in systolic pressure. It usually responds to fluid replacement. Most modern dialysis machines remove fluid at a steady rate set by the practitioner. Removing more than 1 percent of a patient's dry body weight as fluid per hour often results in hypotension.

Some patients with gross edema become hypotensive early during a dialysis. Why does this occur?

Patients with gross fluid overload may have heart failure or a low serum albumin. The dialysis removes fluid from the *vascular* compartment, but the low serum protein does not exert sufficient oncotic pressure to mobilize fluid from the interstitial space. There is another group of patients in whom cardiac failure or hypoproteinemia are not obvious causes, who have problems with overhydration, and who have vascular instability during dialysis. These people, during conventional dialysis with ultrafiltration, become symptomatically hypotensive with tachycardia, nausea, and vomiting. The causes are likely to be multifactorial. Changes in serum osmolality, effects of acetate if this is used as the buffer, and norepinephrine depletion have been suggested or demonstrated. Infusion of hypertonic saline, mannitol, or use of a higher than usual sodium in the dialysis fluid may all be beneficial. Sequential ultrafiltration followed by dialysis may also give good results.

What is sequential ultrafiltration and dialysis?

The application of ultrafiltration as a means of fluid removal during dialysis was instituted by Alwall in 1947. The concept of *convective* transport rather than diffusion (see Chapter 4) is currently put to use in the hemofiltration approach. Several dialyzers have membranes or fibers of sufficient permeability and strength to give ultrafiltration of several liters per hour at safe transmembrane pressures.

Application of ultrafiltration alone before conventional dialysis with minimal ultrafiltration is known as sequential ultrafiltration and dialysis. During the ultrafiltration phase blood circulates normally through the dialyzer, but the dialysis fluid does not. The ultrafiltration resulting from the negative pressure gradient across the membrane is collected at the outflow side and measured. Patients tolerate fluid removal by this method at a rate and quantity greater than with conventional dialysis without hypotension or symptoms. Severely hypertensive patients are able to achieve better BP control than would otherwise be obtainable.

What is sodium modeling?

During dialysis small solutes, primarily urea, are removed from the extracellular fluid (ECF) resulting in a fall in ECF osmolality. This fall in ECF osmolality causes a shift of water into cells, aggravating hypotension. One way of preventing this phenomenon is by replacing the lost osmoles (urea) with sodium. This can be done automatically by the dialysis machine and may prevent or minimize hypotension.

Are there complications of sodium modeling?

Some patients experience increased interdialytic thirst, weight gain, and BP when sodium modeling is used. In such patients, adjustment of the dialysate sodium concentration may be required.

What about a fall in blood pressure not related to any of the above?

Occasionally patients have a decrease in BP after dialysis is started but before significant volume loss has been achieved. This fall may be from antihypertensive medication, or sedatives, or other medication. It may be advisable to instruct the patient not to take such medications for 6 to 8 hours before dialysis.

Does hypertension occur during dialysis?

A small minority of patients develop a rise in BP during dialysis. Some have a gradual rise throughout the run, whereas others experience an elevation soon after starting. In some patients the rise in pressure is the result of increased cardiac output as fluid overload is relieved. In other instances there may be an increase in peripheral vascular resistance on a reflex or hormonal basis. Angiotensin-converting enzyme (ACE) inhibitor therapy or bilateral nephrectomy may be indicated in cases in which high renin levels are present, while the hypertension in very young and elderly patients may respond to a lower blood flow rate and the use of a smaller surface area dialyzer.

Is congestive heart failure seen in ESRD patients?

Yes, this may be the result of fluid overload, and ultrafiltration or hemofiltration will relieve it. Often such patients are protein- and calorie-deficient as well as fluid-overloaded. In many patients, however, this is related to left ventricular dysfunction caused by fluid overload, anemia, and hypertension.

A few patients develop a peculiar cardiomyopathy with a greatly dilated, flabby heart. Such patients are prone to arrhythmias, tolerate ultrafiltration poorly, and are very difficult to manage during dialysis. Extreme care and close monitoring of vital signs are essential during their dialyses. Patients with poor dietary control and failure to take phosphorus-binding medication develop a very high calcium-phosphorus product with metastatic myocardial calcification, conduction defects, and heart failure. In addition, aluminum excess (from phosphate-binding gels) may lead to myocardial failure. These abnormalities are largely reversed by renal transplantation.

Are arrhythmias common during dialysis?

As more older patients and persons with complicating diseases enter ESRD programs, arrhythmias become frequent. They are most often caused by underlying heart disease. The physician should make the presence of such problems and their significance known to the dialysis personnel. Evaluation of a new, or different, rhythm developing *during* dialysis requires an electrocardiogram. The patient should be queried as to medications, and a review of recent serum potassium, calcium, and magnesium values should be made. Patients with myocardial damage may develop arrhythmias of various types in response to volume change or a shift in electrolytes, particularly potassium. Patients receiving digitalis may pose particular problems.

What if a patient develops chest pains during dialysis?

Some patients have chest pain that comes on during dialysis. Often these persons have a history of underlying heart disease, and the pain must be presumed to be angina. It may go away if blood flow is slowed or saline is infused. Often a tablet of nitroglycerin or other medication for angina taken just before hookup will prevent the symptoms. Some patients on occasion have a vague chest distress or low back pain. The mechanism is obscure but often seems related to blood volume change or decreased hematocrit. When new or unexpected chest pain occurs in a patient with no known history of cardiac disease, it is always advisable to obtain an electrocardiogram.

Is the dialysis procedure altered for the patient with pericarditis?

Yes, patients who have pericarditis or pericardial effusion should be dialyzed gently and frequently, using no-heparin protocols. Meticulous monitoring is necessary, with special attention to the appearance of pulsus paradoxus, increase in heart rate, or declining BP, which are clues to developing pericardial tamponade. Daily dialysis is usual until the chemistries, weight, and vital signs are stable.

What causes muscle cramping during dialysis?

The cause is probably fluid shift or osmolar change, although pH change may play a role. Use of sodium modeling may be preventative, while rapid infusion of hypertonic saline or a 50 percent dextrose solution usually brings relief once cramps occur. Heat and pressure over the painful area are temporary measures. In patients in whom there may be preexisting small-vessel disease (usually older men), oral administration of quinine before dialysis may reduce or prevent cramping. Many patients respond to 400 U vitamin E taken 30 minutes before dialysis.

Discuss febrile reactions during dialysis.

Chills and fever occur infrequently during dialysis. In the event of a definite chill followed by a temperature elevation, bacteremia should be suspected. Blood cultures should be taken, with a notation to the laboratory to "check for unusual organisms." A frequent site for bacterial contamination is the access puncture site.

A subclavian catheter may be the source for bacterial seeding. Removal of the catheter is necessary, and the catheter, as well as blood specimens, should be sent to the microbiology laboratory with appropriate identification.

Many febrile reactions are unexplained. It is likely that they are pyrogen reactions. Pyrogenic material is usually protein in nature, from breakdown products of blood in reused items or from breakdown of killed bacteria. Any reused item that comes in contact with blood is suspect. Formalin used as a sterilizing agent does not destroy organisms but denatures and fixes any residual proteinaceous material.

Endotoxin produced by bacteria may be able to cross the apparently intact dialysis membrane or adhere to the membrane and trigger a pyrogen reaction. Endotoxin has been demonstrated in the bloodstream of some patients with febrile reactions. Samples of blood and dialysis fluid should be checked for endotoxin in the event of a reaction, to locate the source.

Chemical agents such as formalin may cause febrile reactions when inadvertently introduced into the blood. On a few occasions, 2-chloroethanol, formed by ethylene oxide and water, has been implicated.

Do patients have allergic reactions to dialysis?

Yes. There are several types of such reactions, both of which occur immediately on starting dialysis, or within 30 minutes. The first is a true allergic reaction to ethylene oxide (ETO) gas, used as a sterilant for the dialyzer and tubing. These reactions are characterized by chest pain, shortness of breath, itching, bronchospasm and, if severe, cardiac collapse. They are treated as other forms of anaphylaxis, with antihistamines and sympathomimetics. They occur almost exclusively with hollow fiber dialyzers.

The second reaction is caused by activation of serum complement by contact of blood with the dialysis membrane. This occurs primarily with cellulosic membranes and results in the generation of hormones (lymphokines) that can cause chest pain, shortness of breath, fever, nausea, and vascular collapse. This syndrome is treated acutely like an allergic reaction, and the patient should subsequently be dialyzed with a synthetic membrane dialyzer.

Another reaction is seen in patients dialyzed with high flux synthetic membranes who are also taking ACE inhibitors. As blood pressure falls with ultrafiltration with these membranes, bradykinin, a vasodilator is released. It is normally degraded by an enzyme that is inactivated by ACE inhibitors. If the patient is taking ACE inhibitors, bradykinin is not inactivated and severe hypotension can occur.

What causes itching?

Many uremic patients are troubled by pruritis (itching). The mechanism is not clear. The skin is dry and lacks lubrication. Most patients are improved by dialysis, but an occasional patient develops itching associated with the dialysis procedure. Some of these persons have a high serum phosphorus level and are not taking adequate phosphate-binding medication. Some patients have hyperparathyroidism related to renal osteodystrophy.

Soothing skin creams or lotions may give temporary relief of pruritus. Oral agents such as cyproheptadine (Periactin) or antihistamines occasionally help. Use of Keri-Lotion, Eucerin Cream, or plain baby oil after bathing and at other times will often be helpful.

MEDICAL PROBLEMS ASSOCIATED WITH END-STAGE RENAL DISEASE

Hematologic Problems

The hematocrit for normal men is 46 to 52 percent and for women it is 40 to 45 percent. People with uremia or on maintenance dialysis are anemic and have considerably lower hematocrit values.

What causes the anemia?

Causes include (1) failure of production, or inhibition of action, of erythropoietin, a hormone produced by the kidney that stimulates the bone marrow to produce red blood cells; (2) a shortened life span of the red blood cells; (3) impaired intake of iron; (4) blood loss, including a tendency to bleed from the nose, gums, gastrointestinal tract, uterus, or skin, caused by platelet abnormalities; and (5) blood loss related to the dialysis procedure itself.

How does dialysis influence the anemia?

Incomplete blood recovery after dialysis, dialyzer leaks, and frequent blood sampling contribute to anemia. The patient who is receiving adequate dialysis, is in a good nutritional state, and has adequate iron stores and intake will usually stabilize with a hematocrit between 20 and 30 percent. It is unusual for the hematocrit to go much higher except in persons with polycystic kidney disease, in whom there may be greater than normal production of erythropoietin.

To minimize blood loss related to dialysis, particular care must be taken to (1) pretest dialyzers to prevent leaks, (2) monitor heparinization to prevent clotting, (3) return blood as completely as possible, (4) prevent damage to blood cells from incorrect pump occlusion or equipment malfunction, and (5) minimize the volume and number of blood samples drawn.

Does the anemia produce symptoms?

In chronic renal failure the anemia has usually been present for many weeks or months, and the patient has become adjusted to it. As the hematocrit improves on dialysis, he or she begins to feel better. These people still have considerably fewer red blood cells than normal and become dyspneic and tire easily. Other symptoms attributable to anemia include poor exercise tolerance, weakness, sexual dysfunction, anorexia, and inability to think clearly.

When should EPO be given?

Recombinant human EPO is now available for ESRD patients. In appropriate doses it will raise the hematocrit to normal levels. Any ESRD patient with a hematocrit less than 30 percent should receive EPO. The target hematocrit should be 32 percent to 36 percent, depending on patient symptoms.

How is EPO given?

EPO is given either intravenously or subcutaneously, usually three times per week at the end of a regular dialysis treatment.

What are the complications of EPO?

The major complication of EPO is an elevation in BP. This usually occurs during the initial 12 weeks of therapy, while the hematocrit is rising, and is treated with antihypertensive medications and fluid removal with dialysis.

As the hematocrit rises, the efficiency of dialysis falls somewhat since the red blood cells do not release their toxins (e.g., creatinine, potassium) very readily as they pass through the dialyzer. Close attention to blood chemistries is essential in EPO patients, and some adjustment of the dialysis prescription may be necessary.

When should transfusions be given?

The routine administration of blood at a certain hematocrit value is not done. If the patient suffers a large blood loss from a dialyzer leak or from hemorrhage, the blood should be replaced. If the patient becomes short of breath or excessively fatigued or has angina, a transfusion will often relieve the symptoms. In general, increasing the dose of EPO to improve the anemia is more desirable than transfusion.

What are some of the complications of transfusions?

The most common complications include the following:

*   *Incompatibility reactions* caused by major or minor blood group incompatibility may occur. Chest or back pain, chills, and fever occur soon after blood is started. If this occurs, the transfusion should be stopped immediately. A blood specimen should be drawn from the patient for evidence of hemolysis and for recheck of type and crossmatch. Chills or fever should be treated symptomatically. Intravenous steroids may be used if symptoms are severe.
*   *Allergic reactions* to leukocytes, platelets, or protein of the donor blood may occur. Manifestations include chilling, fever, or skin eruption developing about 30 to 60 minutes after the start of the transfusion. These are treated by slowing the rate of infusion. An antihistamine, such as diphenhydramine (Benadryl), 20 to 50 mg, or steroids should be given intravenously if symptoms are severe.
*   *Infections*—whether caused by HB, HA, or hepatitis C, CMV, EBV or human immunodeficiency (HIV) viruses—may be transmitted by blood. The onset is from 1 to 4 months after the transfusion.
*   *Preformed antibodies* may result from minor incompatibility or allergic reactions. These are particularly important to the patient awaiting a renal transplant. Some dialysis units with transplantation affiliation give a limited number of transfusions on a regular basis. This has an enhancing effect on graft survival.

What can be done to minimize the anemia?

A good dietary intake of protein is important. Adequate iron intake is essential if the patient's iron stores are depleted prior to starting EPO. Maintenance iron therapy will be needed in most patients to ensure adequate iron stores and an optimal response to EPO. Oral iron supplements are rarely adequate. They often cause gastrointestinal upset, nausea, gas, vomiting, or anorexia. Intravenous iron, such as the saccharated iron dextran, can be given in 100-mg doses, usually for a total course of 1 g, depending on the adequacy of iron stores. In patients on EPO, iron deficiency is almost inevitable, since iron is used rapidly under EPO stimulation of red blood cell (RBC) production and is continually lost from the patient. Patients on EPO may benefit from regular administration of small doses of parenteral iron. Folic acid and vitamin B_{12}, both of which are important in red blood cell formation, are water soluble and theoretically could be depleted by dialysis. Although there is little evidence that these vitamins are seriously deficient, it is the usual practice to give a supplement, particularly of the former.

Abnormalities of Calcium and Phosphorus Metabolism: Renal Osteodystrophy

Disturbances of calcium and phosphorus metabolism are common in persons who develop renal insufficiency gradually and are often apparent even before dialysis is required. During the progression of renal failure there is loss of ability to excrete phosphate. Phosphate ions accumulate in the body fluids and lead to a reciprocal decrease of serum calcium. The parathyroid glands seek to maintain a normal concentration of calcium in body fluid and respond by increased production of PTH. This causes calcium to be resorbed from the bones, resulting in loss of bone density and strength. In addition, the active form of vitamin D, needed for normal bone metabolism, is manufactured in the kidney and is deficient in ESRD patients. Dialysis does not fully correct the disordered calcium-phosphorus metabolism, and progressive osteodystrophy (the term for several bony manifestations) is a serious problem for many ESRD patients.

Are there other factors involved in the bone disorder?

The absorption of dietary calcium from the intestinal tract is decreased in end-stage renal failure. There is resistance to the action of PTH, which normally enhances the resorption of calcium from bone. Chronic acidosis enhances calcium reabsorption from bone, further contributing to loss of bone density. In addition, the aluminum-containing phosphate binding gels cause a form of renal bone disease. The aluminum in these gels is absorbed and deposited in bone, leading to a form of osteomalacia.

What are the bony changes seen in osteodystrophy?

These include adynamic bone, osteomalacia, osteitis fibrosa, osteoporosis, osteosclerosis, and growth retardation (in children); in addition, metastatic calcification also occurs. Adynamic bone is bone with little or no metabolic activity; osteomalacia is deficient calcification of bone; osteitis fibrosa is excessive destruction of bone by osteoclasts, with replacement by fibrous tissue; osteoporosis is deficiency of both bone matrix and calcification; and osteosclerosis is abnormally dense bone. The term *renal osteodystrophy* spans the totality of these various bone diseases in the uremic patient.

Metastatic calcification results when the product of serum calcium times phosphorus (measured in milligrams per deciliter) is 75 or greater. One should therefore keep this calcium and phosphorus product below 70.

What symptoms does osteodystrophy cause?

Many patients complain of sore, painful feet or back pain. Fractures, when they occur, are painful and heal poorly. Metastatic calcification causes precipitates in soft tissue around joints. Less apparent, but more dangerous, are diffuse

deposits of calcium in the heart muscle and in the lung. Itching may be intensi-
fied in the presence of a high calcium-phosphorus ratio. Skin ulcerations and
gangrene of the tips of toes and fingers have occurred. Aggravation of hypertension is frequent.

How is osteodystrophy treated?

A priority system is necessary in the management of uremic osteodystrophy.
The first objective is to maintain a low serum phosphorus to prevent metastatic
calcification and hyperparathyroidism. The serum phosphorus level depends on
intake, removal by dialysis, and binding of phosphate within the gastrointestinal
tract. Restriction of dietary protein intake also limits phosphate intake. A variety
of agents are available to bind phosphate to prevent absorption from the gastrointestinal tract. Those containing aluminum should be avoided and calcium-
containing compounds should be used instead. Their activity depends on the
surface area available for binding. The problem is to find the dose of phosphate
binder that provides sufficient surface area throughout the day and is palatable
enough for patient compliance. A change in medication periodically may make
it more acceptable. Failure to bind phosphate adequately usually represents failure of the patient to take the phosphate binder.

Once serum phosphate is lowered to about 4 mg/dl, elevation of serum calcium above 10 mg/dl reduces the parathyroid stimulation of osteoclasts that
causes osteitis fibrosa. One must be cautious, however, not to reduce the PTH
too much. Adynamic bone disease will occur if the PTH is decreased to normal.
The goal should be a PTH between 1.5 and 3 times the upper limit of normal.
Elevation of serum calcium can be achieved in several ways. The usual concentration of diffusible calcium in dialysis fluid is well above that of the serum, so
each dialysis provides a surge of calcium. The administration of 1 to 2 g of calcium orally will often lead to an improved serum calcium level even in the
absence of normal quantities of potent vitamin D compounds. If the desired
level of serum calcium does not result from these efforts, 1,25 DHC may be
administered either orally or intravenously. Vitamin D may also be helpful in
maintaining bone formation, apart from its role in the gastrointestinal absorption
of calcium. Finally, one must not forget that alleviation of chronic acidosis of
uremia is another objective of treatment. Some patients will develop hypercalcemia on this regimen and will require a lower calcium in the dialysis bath.

Even if the treatment is successful in maintaining a low serum phosphorus
and a high serum calcium, some patients may persist with the problems of renal
osteodystrophy. Those with bone pain are likely to have a component of adynamic bone or osteomalacia. Those with fractures and a high alkaline phosphatase may suffer to a large extent from osteitis fibrosa. Persistence of renal
osteodystrophy, with x-ray film changes consistent with hyperparathyroidism,
high PTH levels, and a high alkaline phosphatase, may warrant a parathyroidec-

tomy: either a four-gland removal or a subtotal parathyroidectomy. A bone biopsy is advisable before parathyroidectomy.

Joint Disorders

Uric acid is frequently elevated in ESRD patients. The hyperuricemia may be associated with a goutlike involvement of one or more joints. Occasionally there is a true gouty attack, but most episodes are of pseudogout. Dialysis amyloidosis may also be seen in long-term dialysis patients.

What is pseudogout?

Pseudogout is an acute inflammation, usually involving a single area at or near a joint. The back of the hand or wrist, finger joints, and shoulders are common locations. Pain comes on abruptly, followed rapidly by tenderness, swelling, and limitation of motion. This lasts 3 to 5 days or longer unless treated.

How can it be treated?

Colchicine or one of the nonsteroidal antiinflammatory agents often relieves distress in 24 to 36 hours.

Are there residual effects of pseudogout?

Soft tissue swelling may persist for several weeks. Areas of metastatic calcification at the site sometimes are seen on an x-ray examination.

Is there any preventive treatment?

Frequent dialyses usually keep the uric acid below serious levels. If a very high level of uric acid persists, use of allopurinol may be considered.

What is dialysis amyloidosis (DA)?

Amyloid is a peculiar form of protein that precipitates in various body tissues. There are many different kinds of amyloid, including amyloid composed of β_2-microglobulin that is unique to dialysis patients. This protein is normally excreted by the kidneys, but is poorly dialyzed and therefore accumulates in the blood of patients with ESRD. This protein then deposits in joints and periarticular structures of the shoulders, hands, wrist, neck, and elsewhere, causing pain and limitation of motion. If progressive, this can be extremely debilitating.

Who gets dialysis amyloidosis?

Patients on dialysis for long periods of time (> 3 years) are prone to this complication. Of patients on dialysis over 10 years, the majority will have DA. Patients dialyzed with high flux, synthetic membranes are less likely to get this complication.

What is carpal tunnel syndrome (CTS)?

CTS in dialysis patients is compression of the median nerve at the wrist by the carpal tunnel sheath, which has been thickened by deposition of amyloid. CTS causes pain, numbness, and tingling of the thumb and first two digits.

Can DA be treated?

Pain medications, nonsteroidal antiinflammatory drugs (NSAIDs), and deep therapeutic ultrasound may ease joint symptoms. Renal transplantation usually causes a rapid disappearance of symptoms.

Gastrointestinal Problems

Is peptic ulcer disease common in dialysis patients?

Some reports cite an increased incidence of peptic ulcer disease in dialysis patients, others do not. There are reports of higher than normal gastric acidity related to high blood levels of gastrin, which may relate to parathyroid overactivity. Other studies indicate low gastric acidity related to increased urea and ammonia content of gastric juice. Our own experience suggests that the incidence of ulcer disease is about the same as for the nonuremic general population.

Why is prevention of constipation important?

Because of a restricted diet, limited fluid intake, and regular ingestion of phosphate binders, ESRD patients tend to become constipated or to develop fecal impactions. As older patients are taken into dialysis programs, there is more functional constipation. Such persons have a high incidence of diverticula of the colon. In addition, diverticulitis or perforation is not rare. Hematomas of the bowel and perforation caused by injudicious enemas have occurred. Cathartics and laxatives should be avoided. Stool softeners seem to work well, although they are often required in larger than usual doses. Patients should be encouraged to eat a high fiber diet, to adhere to a program of regular exercise, and to plan a regularly scheduled time for bowel movements to reduce the problems of constipation. Severe constipation may also cause hyperkalemia, since stool potassium losses account for up to 40 percent of total body potassium losses per day in dialysis patients. (See Chapter 12.)

Does ascites occur in ESRD patients?

Ascites (a massive fluid collection in the peritoneal cavity) is an infrequent problem that is very troublesome. Most cases are related to repeated fluid over-load, poor nutrition, and cardiomyopathy. Although some patients overcome ascites, deterioration and death are frequent outcomes.

Hepatitis

What is hepatitis?

Hepatitis means inflammation of the liver (Greek, *hepar:* liver) without regard to etiology.

Are there different kinds of hepatitis?

There are many varieties of hepatitis: bacterial; parasitic; toxic, caused by chemicals or medications; and viral.

Which kinds of hepatitis occur in dialysis patients?

The most common is viral hepatitis. Liver involvement from medications occurs sufficiently often to make its differential diagnosis difficult.

What are some features of viral hepatitis?

There are several distinct and identifiable viruses including A, B, C, D, F, and G. Hepatitis C was until recently called "non-A, non-B" hepatitis.

It is thought that about 50 percent of all clinical cases of acute hepatitis in the United States are caused by type B virus, and types A and C account for the other 50 percent. Type C accounts for most of the morbidity and mortality in dialysis patients.

Hepatitis A infection has an incubation period of 15 to 30 days, and the incubation period of hepatitis B virus is 50 to 160 days; the incubation period for hepatitis C infection appears to overlap with both hepatitis A and hepatitis B. The viruses of all three types can be transmitted parenterally.

What are the differences between the hepatitis viruses?

Hepatitis A virus particles are similar to the viruses of intestinal influenza and respiratory tract infections. The hepatitis B virus particle is larger than and has a central core similar in size to the hepatitis A virus particle, with an outer shell that contains the surface antigen. Hepatitis C virus is a small RNA virus, and has a number of variants.

What are the symptoms and findings of acute hepatitis?

Jaundice (icterus) is the classic finding of hepatitis. However, cases of active hepatitis *without* jaundice (anicteric) greatly outnumber those with jaundice among dialysis patients. Most cases are recognized by a sudden rise in liver enzymes ("transaminitis")

Other symptoms include malaise, poor appetite, and nausea, with migratory joint pains and skin eruptions in about 30 percent of infections with hepatitis B or hepatitis C virus. There is often tenderness over the liver.

Serum bilirubin may be minimally elevated in anicteric patients. Liver enzymes and other function tests usually correlate with the extent of parenchymal involvement.

What is the risk of hepatitis in dialysis units?

In the United States' general population the reported incidence of all types of hepatitis is 2 to 3 per 1000, or 0.2 to 0.3 percent.

In the 1970s the prevalence of hepatitis B surface antigen (HB_sAg) positivity in ESRD patients receiving dialysis reached or exceeded 50 percent in some areas of Europe and the United States. However, this incidence has been greatly reduced in most programs by the practice of screening new patients, by hepatitis testing of staff and patients, by hepatitis vaccination, and by the use of rigid techniques to prevent cross contamination (see Chapter 18). Recent data suggest a prevalence of 1.4 percent among patients and of 0.3 percent among staff. The incidence of antibodies to hepatitis C varies from 0 to 51 percent in North American dialysis facilities (average 8 percent).

Why is hepatitis such a problem in dialysis units?

There are a number of explanations.
- First, the uremic individual has a diminished immune response and may have hepatitis without symptoms and with minimal laboratory findings other than HB_sAg positivity or slightly elevated enzymes. Only 30 percent of patients develop jaundice. Patients who become HB_sAg positive may remain so without developing HB_s antibody for prolonged periods and are chronic carriers.
- The dialysis environment is unique in its potential for virus spread. Limited space, frequent blood and fluid spillage, and innumerable uses of needles provide ideal conditions for spread of the virus once introduced.
- Emergency dialysis may bring unscreened patients (who may be carriers) into the unit.
- Before EPO was available, blood transfusions were frequently given and these at times transmitted hepatitis.

- Longer survival on dialysis increases the liklihood of hepatitis C infection.
- Transmission of hepatitis C may occur within dialysis facilities.
- Patients returning to dialysis after a failed transplant have an increased incidence of hepatitis C.

How can hepatitis spread be minimized?

The entire dialysis area must be regarded as continually contaminated with blood and body fluids. Personnel as well as patients are subject to intense exposure once hepatitis virus has been introduced. Personnel are at particular risk because of the chances for accidental needle sticking, cuts, or abrasions, leading to parenteral introduction.

Hand-to-mouth contact is very important. Forty percent of personnel infections in the United States study did not involve tissue penetration. Eating or drinking by personnel in the unit should *not* be permitted. New gloves should be worn at each patient contact. Thorough handwashing before and after each patient contact and on leaving the working environment is mandatory.

Isolation of hepatitis C patients or their machines in the dialysis unit is not currently recommended.

Does patient-to-patient transmission of hepatitis virus occur?

Several sources of cross contamination are possible. With central delivery systems (rarely used now, except for bicarbonate mixing), once virus gets into the plumbing it may be passed on if the disinfection process is not adequate to kill the virus. In central supply systems this applies to the individual station units. It applies also to individual proportioning systems used by more than one patient.

Monitoring devices attached to the blood lines by "disposable" lines may be a factor in patient-to-patient transmission. Virus-contaminated fluid can reach the pressure bellows or transducer surface of monitors, areas that may not be routinely disinfected. Hydrophobic (change of color upon fluid contact) 0.22 μmm filters should be used in the monitoring lines. Such filters will *not* be a barrier to the virus, but they will stop the fluid carrying it and will identify the contamination. Contamination in the reprocessing room may be another source of within-unit transmission. It is recommended that the barriers be changed between patients.

What about immunization for hepatitis?

A purified and inactivated hepatitis B vaccine became available in 1982. The Public Health Service Advisory Committee on Immunization Practices recommends vaccination for all dialysis personnel and for patients who are not known to have *antibody* to HB_sAg already. According to package labeling (since dosages from different manufacturers vary), a series of three or four doses of vaccine resulted in seroconversion with demonstrable anti-HB_s antibodies in 95 percent of staff and 60 percent of patients. After the initial vaccine injection, administration of booster inoculation at 1 and 6 months appears to extend protection for 3 to 5 years.

The vaccine does not afford protection against hepatitis A or C. A hepatitis A vaccine is now available. In addition, high-titer immune serum globulin (ISG) provides effective, though transient, passive protection against hepatitis A infection, and probably against hepatitis C as well.

Neuropathy

What is uremic neuropathy?

Neuropathy indicates deterioration of nerve function. It may develop gradually as renal failure progresses, or it may appear suddenly after an intercurrent infection or an episode of fluid overload.

What are the symptoms?

A frequent early symptom is the "restless legs" syndrome; the person cannot sit or lie still but moves the legs in a restless manner. There may be a complaint of tingling or painful burning of the feet. As the disorder worsens, there may be loss of reflexes, then loss of sensation, and finally loss of muscle strength, or paralysis. Changes usually begin at the toes and progress upward. The upper extremities may be involved, but less often than the lower ones.

How does neuropathy develop?

Neuropathy may come on slowly so that the patient is unaware of it or is unable to recall the onset. Occasionally, it develops explosively after a bout of infection or heart failure. Often the patient is malnourished.

Is neuropathy common?

Neuropathy, in subclinical or clinical form, has been reported in up to 80 percent of persons with ESRD. It is often seen at the time dialysis begins, possibly because that is when a careful search is done. Clinically significant neuropathy is less common with earlier institution of dialysis.

Can neuropathy be detected before symptoms appear?

Nerve conduction velocity measurements are used to detect and to quantitate progression or improvement of neuropathy. Most patients with moderately advanced azotemia have some delay in nerve conduction, often long before symptoms appear.

The test, while not difficult, is subject to many variables that make its reproducibility questionable and small changes difficult to evaluate.

Is neuropathy relieved by dialysis?

If dialysis is begun early, when only prolongation of conduction time is demonstrable, frequent dialysis may prevent worsening. More severe nerve damage responds very slowly to dialysis. If the amount and frequency of dialysis are not adequate, neuropathy may develop or, if already present, will worsen.

How does the dialysis prescription relate to neuropathy?

When adequate dialysis is prescribed and delivered (Kt/V_{urea} greater than or equal to 1.2 with PCR 1 g/kg/day), neuropathy is rarely seen. If it does develop, it strongly suggests that underdialysis and urea kinetic modeling should be performed to assess this. Even if the modeling parameters fall within an acceptable range, worsening neuropathy requires intensification of the dialysis procedure (larger dialyzer, more time, higher blood flow).

What is the cause of neuropathy?

This is not known. The pathologic changes in the nerves are similar to those seen in some cases of diabetes mellitus, in certain vitamin deficiency states, and in chronic alcoholism. A number of authorities believe it results from accumulated middle- to large-sized toxic metabolites in the body. However, specific toxic agents have not been identified.

Is there involvement of other than the peripheral nerves?

A few patients develop deafness, for which no other cause can be demonstrated. Other patients on dialysis have developed gastric atony or bowel dysfunction resembling the autonomic disturbances seen in some diabetic individuals. Impotence *may* also be related to uremic toxin accumulation.

Reproduction Problems

Does chronic dialysis contribute to menstrual dysfunction?

Women commonly have cessation of menstruation as a part of the uremic syndrome. A few pregnancies in women on maintenance dialysis have been reported. Other reports suggest that fewer than 20 percent of such women of childbearing age ovulate at all. Most are amenorrheic or have oligomenorrhea of an anovulatory nature. A significant proportion are troubled by galactorrhea.

Endocrine studies suggest a defect at the hypothalamic-pituitary level, such that the hormonal feedback mechanisms do not function normally.

To prevent unnecessary (undesirable) blood loss, patients should be instructed to report any abnormal or excessive menstrual flow. Early detection of the problem may eliminate the need for surgical intervention.

What about infertility?

Infertility, both male and female, is very common. Research studies indicate poor sperm formation in most men. The exact mechanism is less clear in women but, as indicated before, is presumed to be endocrine in nature.

What other sexual problems have been associated with chronic dialysis?

Sexual dysfunction is a very real problem for the majority of maintenance dialysis patients. Reduction of libido and impotence in men are common as uremia develops. Various sociologic and psychologic studies, largely depending on questionnaire responses, have suggested that total or partial impotence is a problem in 60 percent of men receiving maintenance dialysis. However, another study suggests that 50 to 70 percent of the impotence of male dialysis patients has an organic basis—whether neuropathic, endocrine, or vascular is unknown. In addition, medication (particularly antihypertensive agents) must always be considered a potential cause of impotence.

The reproductive problems described above are often relieved after correction of anemia with EPO. The mechanism for this is unclear, but several successful pregnancies in women receiving EPO have now been reported.

Insomnia

Describe the potential for insomnia in this patient population.

Inability to sleep or fitful sleeping during the usual hours of rest is a common problem in ESRD patients. Often the patient sleeps throughout the dialysis procedure, and it may be that the need for sleep at other times is reduced. Other patients seem to have a pathologic inability to rest soundly.

Response to sedatives and tranquilizers is usually poor and the risk of dependency is considerable. We have seen no adverse effects from the lack of sleep and suspect the problem is most often one of fitful or interrupted sleep, which is interpreted as "no sleep." Sleep apnea is more common in ESRD patients than in the general population. The reason for this is unclear, but formal sleep studies may be useful in selected patients.

Dialysis in the Elderly

Can elderly patients be dialyzed?

Yes, and very successfully. Both hemodialysis and peritoneal dialysis have been used in this group. Careful attention to hemodynamic stability is necessary if hemodialysis is used, but an excellent result and quality of life can be achieved. (See Chapter 21.)

Why is so much attention being given to dialysis in the elderly?

In 1987 nearly 47 percent of all ESRD patients were over the age of 65. By 1996, this had grown to nearly 60 percent. The over 65 age group is the only one projected by Health Care Financing Administration (HCFA) to continue to increase in number into the next century.

Are there special medical concerns related to elderly ESRD patients?

These patients present complex challenges related to their underlying physiologic state. Of concern is the propensity in the elderly for diminished cardiovascular reserve, immunodeficiency, bone disease, and malnutrition.

What is the outcome for the elderly on dialysis?

Mortality on dialysis increases with increasing age. Hospitalizations are more common and longer in older compared with younger dialysis patients. In spite of these concerns, many elderly dialysis patients lead satisfying, high-quality lives.

Exercise

Is exercise beneficial in dialysis patients?

Exercise is very important in dialysis patients. It is useful to maintain good muscle tone and strength and thus promote normal activities. In addition, exercise can lead to important physiologic changes including a rise in hematocrit, a fall in BP, and an improvement in lipid abnormalities. A carefully monitored thrice-weekly program, 30 minutes each session, can achieve these results.

Is exercise safe in dialysis patients?

Exercise can be carried out safely in dialysis patients. The muscle exertion involved can lead to a slight rise in serum potassium during or following exercise, and this needs to be watched for. It is probably best to minimize exercise in the period immediately before a dialysis treatment.

Diabetes Mellitus

Is diabetic nephropathy a common cause of ESRD?

Over 40 percent of new ESRD patients in the United States have diabetic nephropathy as a primary etiology. This number is even higher in some ethnic groups, particularly Hispanics and Native Americans.

Are there special problems with dialysis in patients with diabetes?

Yes. These patients have many problems with hemodialysis. Repeated heparinization may exacerbate retinopathy; BP and blood sugar are often difficult to control; orthostatic hypotension may limit fluid removal with dialysis; accelerated atherosclerosis may lead to limb amputations; vascular access may be difficult to maintain. (See Chapter 17.)

What is dialysis dementia?

This is a rare syndrome, first described in 1972. It may appear after a few months or several years in patients who are seemingly well dialyzed and doing well. There is a peculiar complex of garbled speech (dyspraxia), asymmetrical muscle jerking, mental deterioration, and seizures, along with characteristic electroencephalographic (EEG) changes. A number of studies have implicated aluminum accumulation as a cause, primarily from administered aluminum hydroxide. With the use of calcium-containing phosphate binders in place of aluminum hydroxide, this syndrome has largely disappeared.

Do children on dialysis grow normally?

Growth is markedly impaired in children with chronic renal failure. Neither hemodialysis nor peritoneal dialysis significantly alters this abnormality. Recently, recombinant growth hormone has been shown to lead to catch-up growth in some patients and may prove to be a breakthrough in this regard.

What are the psychological consequences of long-term dialysis?

Dialysis may have a major impact on a patient's psychosocial status. Some patients have a gradual decline in quality of life, particularly as medical complications become more severe. This can lead to depression and an increased risk of suicide. Other patients experience an excellent quality of life and are highly rehabilitated and productive. What distinguishes these two patient groups remains uncertain. Close attention to psychosocial adaptation, with psychiatric intervention and counseling when needed, can help patients optimize the quality of their lives while on dialysis.

Transplantation

Gwen E. McNatt

Nephrology nurses who primarily care for patients undergoing dialysis treatment have several roles involving transplantation. They educate and counsel patients regarding the option of transplantation, and they may assist patients undergoing the pre-transplant evaluation. They may also need to provide dialysis treatments for transplant recipients experiencing temporary loss of renal function from acute tubular necrosis (ATN) or a rejection episode and patients with permanent loss of a transplanted kidney. Nephrology nurses and technicians may also provide dialysis for recipients of transplanted non-renal organs (such as liver or heart), who are experiencing acute or chronic renal failure.

What are the advantages of renal transplantation?

The most important advantage of renal transplantation is improved quality of life. Patients with a successful kidney transplant report a higher quality of life compared to patients receiving other forms of renal replacement therapy. With no need for dialysis treatment and more complete resolution of uremic symptoms, successful transplant recipients can experience a more "normal" lifestyle including family, social, and vocational activities. Another benefit is cost. Although the initial year of transplantation is more costly than dialysis treatment, the subsequent years' costs are significantly less. Finally, although the long-term survival rate for patients undergoing dialytic therapies has vastly improved, transplantation may offer patients an opportunity for a longer survival. Since the introduction of cyclosporine, survival rates for transplant recipients are longer than for dialysis patients. This difference is most pronounced in individuals with diabetes mellitus.

What are the disadvantages to renal transplantation?

The disadvantages of transplantation stem from the need for lifelong immunosuppression to prevent the body from rejecting the organ. The necessity for daily medication compliance is a minor nuisance for some patients and an insurmountable hurdle for others. Especially in the initial post-operative period, family support can be crucial in ensuring adherence to what is often a daunting medication regimen.

Probably a more important disadvantage to transplantation is the vast potential complications of immunosuppression. Direct consequences of suppressing the immune system are increased risk of infection and of some malignancies. The medications also carry the potential for some non-immunological complications such as bone disease, cataracts, diabetes mellitus, hyperlipidemia, hypertension, and gastrointestinal complications such as ulcers, hyperuricemia, and hyperkalemia. Obesity as well as more cosmetic side effects such as hirsutism and gingival hyperplasia may also occur.

Another major hurdle for many patients is the difficulty paying for the costly immunosuppressive medications. While Medicare will provide 80 percent coverage for the first 36 months after transplantation, many patients do not have other insurance coverage. Nephrology nurses practicing in transplantation, along with social workers, assist transplant recipients in finding solutions to this problem.

The process of transplantation—from evaluation and waiting for a donor organ to the surgical hospitalization and threatened or actual rejection—places a great deal of stress on both the patient and family members. Again, strong social support is a crucial component of successfully coping with the stress of transplantation. Table 15-1 summarizes the risks and benefits of transplantation.

Table 15-1   The Transplant Trade-Off

Improved quality of life vs	Lifelong Immunosuppression
Freedom from dialysis	Necessity for daily medication
More normal lifestyle	Increased risk of infection
Longer survival rate	Increased risk of malignancy
Increased ability to pursue normal activities—work, home, school	Loss of sick role
More complete resolution of *uremic symptoms:* •normal calcium/phos. •improved cardiac function •improved appetite •less restrictive diet •improved sexual function •increased feeling of wellness •increased mental acuity	Potential medication side effects: •steroid bone disease •hypertension •ulcers/dyspepsia/other GI effects •hyperkalemia, hyperlipidemia, obesity •body image changes: hirsutism, gingival hyperplasia •diabetes mellitus, gout, cataracts, tremor •psychological stress
Less costly than dialysis (after first year)	Difficulty paying for costly medications

What are the risks and benefits of combined kidney-pancreas transplantation?

Dialysis patients who also suffer from diabetes mellitus may want to consider a combined kidney-pancreas transplant. The major benefits of this procedure are:

- Euglycemia, which may halt or slow the progression of diabetic sequelae.
- Freedom from frequent insulin injections and fingersticks for glucose measurement.
- For those individuals with hypoglycemic unawareness, the combined procedure is a lifesaver.

The combined kidney-pancreas transplant procedure is more complicated and involves more risks than kidney transplantation alone. These risks are associated with:

- Longer surgery
- Exocrine drainage of the pancreas. Many transplant surgeons choose to drain amylase, a digestive enzyme made by the pancreas, to the urinary bladder using a piece of donor duodenum as a conduit. Although this procedure allows for monitoring of pancreatic function by measuring urinary amylase, the amylase may cause acute or chronic cystitis or urethritis. In addition, the patients lose a great deal of bicarbonate and fluid and thus have a tendency to develop acidosis and dehydration.
- Increased immunosuppression-associated risks. The transplanted pancreas is much more prone to stimulate the body's immune system than is a transplanted kidney, thus greater amounts of immunosuppression are required.

Who should be considered as a transplant candidate?

In general, all patients should be offered the option of consultation with a transplant team to determine his or her eligibility. The following box summarizes absolute and relative contraindications to transplantation.

Absolute and Relative Contraindications to Transplantation

Absolute Contraindications
 Active infection
 Active malignancy
 Active substance abuse
 Inability to comply with medication regimen

Relative Contraindications
 Age: Very young or over 65
 Severe comorbidities
 Lack of family support
 Mental/psychological problems

What is the immunologic basis of transplantation?

The immune system protects the body from foreign invasion by identifying the invaders and then destroying them. Anything that produces this response is called an *antigen*. The basis of immunology in transplantation is to identify how the body recognizes foreign antigens. Transplant immunologists have identified two main antigen systems that affect the acceptance or rejection of a transplanted organ or tissue. These two systems are blood groups and the human leukocyte antigen (HLA). Blood groups are the first determinant of compatibility for solid organ transplantation. In general, an organ must be ABO compatible with the recipient to be transplanted. For this reason, transplant recipient waiting lists are arranged by ABO group. The rhesus (Rh) factor is not applicable to solid organ transplantation.

The HLA system is comprised of a group of genes found on the sixth chromosome. Three main sites or loci on this chromosome—A, B, and DR have been identified as influencing the recognition of foreign tissue. As each individual has two of each chromosome, one donated by each parent, six loci are identified for each person. When tissue is introduced to the body with different HLA genes, the immune system is triggered and the rejection process begins.

The components of the immune system that are most important in transplantation are the T cell and B cell lymphocytes. T cell lymphocytes recognize the foreign tissue and initiate the rejection process. B cell lymphocytes recognize the foreign antigen and produce antibodies to destroy the invader. Once presented, both T and B cells will remember a foreign antigen and attack it more quickly in subsequent presentations. Humans develop immunological memory to HLA antigens through exposure via blood transfusions, pregnancy, and transplantation.

What is meant by tissue typing?

Tissue typing refers to blood tests designed to identify the HLA genetic markers. Although HLA matching is used to distribute organs objectively, modern immunosuppressive medications have made HLA matching increasingly less important in successful outcomes. Many centers transplant organs with no HLA similarities (0 matched organs), as long as the crossmatch is negative, with excellent results. When the body recognizes and forms immunity to one HLA antigen, it often forms immunity to other related antigens, even though these antigens were not presented to the body. This crossover immunity has been recognized by the development of cross-reactive antigen groups (CREG) tests. CREG matching may improve outcomes in minority groups. The United Network for Organ Sharing (UNOS) began pilot studies with CREG matching in 1997.

What is crossmatching?

Monthly serum samples from potential recipients are used to perform cross-matching tests. Crossmatching tests are blood tests that determine whether a recipient has acquired immunity to a given donor organ tissue. The tests are performed when a donor organ becomes available. Serum from all eligible recipients is tested with donor lymph cells. A positive crossmatch means that the recipient has memory or acquired immunity to the donor and therefore cannot receive the organ. The routine test is the Amos and antiglobulin test, which takes about six hours to complete, although more sophisticated and time-consuming tests, such as flow cytometry crossmatches, may sometimes be performed. In living donor transplantation, an additional test called a mixed leukocyte reaction (MLR) may be ordered, although this takes several days to complete and has not proven to be of great value.

What is meant by PRA levels?

Another important crossmatching test is called panel reactive antibody (PRA). The potential recipient's serum is tested against a panel of random donors. The number of positive reactions to donor panel is expressed as a percentage. This percentage represents the risk of a positive crossmatch and thus incompatibility with any random donor. Therefore, the higher a potential recipient's PRA, the less likely that any given organ will be compatible. For this reason, patients with high PRAs are given preference in the distribution of cadaver organs.

What is the purpose of the monthly serum samples? Why send them in every month?

The numbers of sensitized lymphocytes that constitute pre-formed immunity to any particular antigen may wax and wane over time. Sometimes the number may be so low that the PRA may fall. Because of this phenomenon, sometimes a specific crossmatch using current serum will be negative even though the crossmatch using older or historic serum is positive. Because immunosuppression will be applied to block the memory response, a current negative crossmatch may indicate a window of opportunity for a potential recipient. On the other hand, immunity provoked by a blood transfusion after the most current serum sample was obtained could give a falsely negative crossmatch. The variability of immune status necessitates monthly serum samples for potential recipients.

What does the recipient workup entail?

The evaluation process before a kidney or other organ transplant begins with referral to the transplant center. The potential recipient and family meet members of the transplant team. This team usually consists of transplant nurse coordinators, transplant surgeons, transplant nephrologists, and social workers. Once the team has determined the initial eligibility of a candidate, the transplant nurse coordinator works with the patient, dialysis health care team, and primary health care provider to facilitate the evaluation. Although the evaluation may find that transplantation is not a viable option for some potential recipients, the ultimate goal of the pre-transplant workup is to find out as much about the patient as possible in order to perform a successful transplant.

The evaluation generally consists of blood, urine and other diagnostic tests such as chest radiograph and electrocardiogram, as well as careful review of the patient's records. Special attention is given to the following areas:

- Cardiovascular assessment, which may include cardiac arteriogram, echocardiogram, and stress testing.
- Infection surveillance, which usually includes a dental examination
- Malignancy detection
- Genitourinary tract assessment
- Psychosocial evaluation, which may include screening for illicit drugs.

What are the possible sources for organs?

Two main sources of kidneys for transplantation are: living donors or cadaveric donors. Living donors can be related to the recipient by blood, such as a parent or sibling, or related to the recipient emotionally such as a spouse, close friend or adopted child. The key requirements for living donation are completely voluntary, informed consent and a completely healthy donor.

Cadaveric donors are individuals who have died from irreversible brain death. The bodies of these individuals are kept functioning by artificial ventilation and medications. With the consent of next of kin, the organs and tissues are procured by the organ recovery team and distributed by the regional organ and tissue bank in accordance with national guidelines. There is no expense to the donor family and usual funeral arrangements are not affected by organ and tissue donation. There is currently a shortage of cadaveric organs in the United States.

What happens after a patient is placed on the cadaver donor waiting list?

After a candidate is considered eligible for transplantation and no living donors are available, the transplant center places the candidate's name on the cadaver waiting list. Kidneys are distributed by a point system. Points are given for length of time on the waiting list and degree of HLA match. Because of the difficulty in finding suitable kidneys for these patients, additional points are given to patients with high PRAs. In general, cadaveric kidneys from donors in one blood group are only offered to recipients in that same blood group; therefore, the waiting list is divided by blood group. When cadaveric kidneys are procured, the organ bank offers them to transplant centers *in this order*:

1. Any potential recipient anywhere in the country that matches with the donor at all six HLA loci.
2. Locally according to the point system.
3. Regionally and then nationally according to the point system.

Most kidneys are used locally. Other organs are also distributed in an equitable, objective manner, locally first, with medical need as the main determinant.

What is the responsibility of the dialysis team while the patient waits for a kidney?

Many patients wait one to two years before receiving their organ. It is important for the dialysis health care team to keep the transplant center informed regarding the health status of potential recipients and make certain that no recipient misses his or her chance at an organ because of missing serum samples.

Where are transplant kidneys placed? How long is the surgery?

The transplanted kidney is usually placed extraperitoneally in the right or left iliac fossa of the recipient. The incision extends from above the iliac crest and to just above the symphysis pubis. Although the right iliac fossa is generally preferred for primary transplantation, either side may be used. If the recipient has had a previous transplant, the transplant surgeon will generally select the side not previously used. The donor renal artery is anastomosed end-to-end with the recipient internal iliac (hypogastric) artery or end-to-side with the external iliac artery. The venous anastomosis is generally end-to-side to the recipient's external iliac vein. The donor ureter is attached to the recipient's bladder or rarely, the recipient's ureter (see Fig. 15-1). If a pancreas is also being transplanted, it will be placed in the opposite iliac fossa (see Fig. 15-2). The kidney transplantation procedure generally lasts 2 ½ to 4 hours.

The iliac fossae are preferred placement sites even when the patient has had two or more transplants. Occasionally, adhesions and scarring from multiple transplantation or other surgical procedures or severe atherosclerotic disease precludes the use of these sites. In these extremely rare cases, the surgeon may place the kidney intraperitoneally and use other vasculature including the abdominal aorta.

How long do patients stay in the hospital after transplantation?

Transplant recipients are usually discharged at 3 to 5 days after the transplantation procedure. Of course, surgical or medical complications may delay discharge, but the hospital stay may also be prolonged if the transplant team has concerns about the patient's or the patient's family's ability to provide adequate post-operative care.

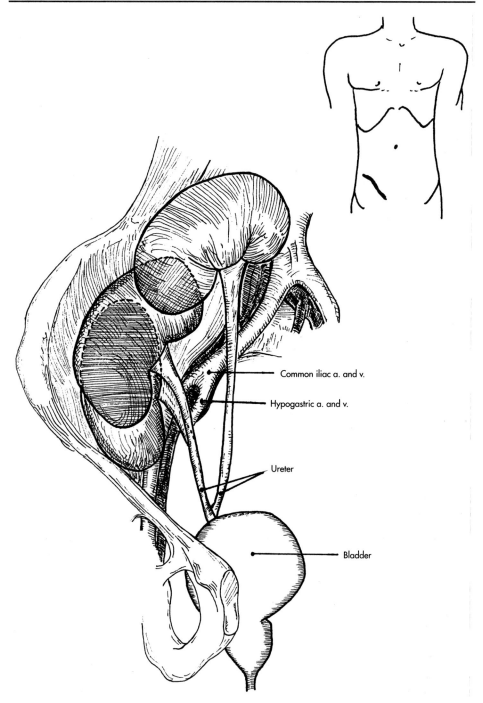

Common iliac a. and v.

Hypogastric a. and v.

Ureter

Bladder

Fig. 15-1   Various positions of the kidney allograft using either the common iliac or hypogastric vessels in the iliac fossa. Adapted from Starzl TE et al.: Technique of Renal Hemotransplantation, *Archives of Surgery* 89:96, 1964.

Figure 15-2 Technique of combined kidney-pancreas transplantation with the duodenal segment bladder drainage technique. (From Sollinger HW, Stratta RJ, D'Alessandro AM, et al.: *Ann Surg* 208(4):475-483, 1988.)

Why do some transplant recipients require dialysis?

Like other individuals, organ transplant recipients may require dialysis treatment for fluid removal, electrolyte imbalance, uremia, or a combination of these reasons. Renal—as well as extra-renal (such as liver and heart)—transplant recipients often need hemofiltration after surgery because of the vast amounts of fluids used to maintain cardiovascular stability during the procedure. The patient's new kidney may be slow to respond to this fluid load. Kidney transplant recipients with acute tubular necrosis (ATN) or an acute rejection attempt may require temporary dialysis. Recipients of extra-renal organs often have concomitant renal disease or acute renal failure. Uremia and/or electrolyte imbalances may occur in these patients as well. Fluid and solute removal via traditional hemodialysis, peritoneal dialysis, or methods such as slow, continuous ultrafiltration (SCUF) or continuous arterio-venous hemofiltration (CAVH) may be employed.

What is ATN?

Acute tubular necrosis (ATN) occurs in up to 45 percent of all cadaveric donor kidney transplantations and rarely in living donor transplantations. ATN is characterized by oliguria (although high urine output ATN is occasionally seen) and failure of the serum creatinine to fall after a technically successful transplantation procedure. Its etiology is not well described, but it is probably due to a combination of factors including preservation injury, prolonged cold storage time, vascular instability of the donor or recipient during the harvest or transplant procedure or reperfusion injury. Cyclosporine may exacerbate or prolong ATN and thus the initiation of cyclosporine therapy may be delayed in recipients with ATN. These individuals may require dialysis until the kidney begins to function, which is generally in several days to two weeks. ATN can last for several months with a good eventual outcome; however, oliguria and uremia that extend beyond two weeks may also be caused from rejection or drug-induced nephrotoxicity. A percutaneous biopsy of the kidney is usually performed to establish a diagnosis. Patients with ATN need reassurance and support from their caregivers. It is helpful to allow them to ventilate their feelings about still requiring dialysis and to inform them that most transplanted kidneys with ATN eventually function well.

What special precautions should be taken when dialyzing a transplant recipient?

The following precautions are most notable:
- During the initial 24 hours after surgery, internal bleeding is a concern, so hypotension should be carefully monitored and brought to the attention of the physician.
- Because of the susceptibility of the transplanted kidney to ischemia, avoid hypotension, even at the cost of decreased fluid removal.
- The integrity of the surgical incision must be maintained.
- Anticoagulation is also a concern in transplant recipients. Heparin-free or minimal anticoagulation is preferred, especially in the immediate post-operative period or if they have undergone a diagnostic percutaneous renal biopsy.
- Electrolyte imbalances are common after transplantation. The most common is hyperkalemia. Hyperkalemia is common in patients with impaired graft function but is also caused by medications such as cyclosporine and tacrolimus. Other electrolyte abnormalities are outlined in Table 15-2.

Table 15-2   Electrolyte Abnormalities After Transplantation

Abnormality	Predisposing Factors	Treatment
hyperkalemia	ATN cyclosporine tacrolimus trimethoprim-sulfa blood transfusions	dialysis IV 50% dextrose/insulin Kayexalate diuretics diet
hypokalemia	rapid post-tx diuresis diuretics	K+ supplements diet
hypocalcemia (often w/ hyper- phosphatemia)	parathyroidectomy hyperparathyroidism + ATN	calcium supplements increased calcium dialysate Rocaltrol phosphorus binders

hypercalcemia
(often w/ hypo-
phosphatemia)
	hyperparathyroidism
	  + functioning kidney
		diet
		phosphorus supplement
		Rocaltrol to suppress PTH
		  (if calcium < 11.0)

hypomagnesemia	diuresis cyclosporine	magnesium supplement
acidosis	ATN rejection cyclosporine pancreas transplant w/ bladder drainage	sodium bicarbonate dialysis sodium citrate

Is there an increased risk of infection after transplantation?

Increased risk of infection is an inevitable consequence of immunosuppression. In the immediate postoperative period, bacterial infections in sites such as the wound, urinary tract and lungs are more common, while viral infections such as cytomegalovirus (CMV), herpes simplex, and herpes zoster are more prevalent after the first several weeks following transplantation. CMV is a major cause of morbidity and mortality in transplant recipients. Many centers employ prophylactic medications such as ganciclovir or hyperimmune gamma globulin to prevent CMV infection or reactivation. Strict adherence to universal precautions should reduce the number of infectious complications in these patients. Isolation is rarely required and transplant recipients pose no special risk to other patients or staff.

Does any one immunosuppressive medication place the transplant recipient at higher risk for malignancy?

Transplant recipients have demonstrated a higher risk for lymphoma, Kaposi's sarcoma, cervical cancer, vulva and perineal cancer, hepatobiliary cancers, sarcomas, and lip cancers than the general population. No one immunosuppressant has been found to increase the risk; rather, the risk increases as the total amount of immunosuppression increases. When detected early, many of these cancers respond well to treatment.

What are the most commonly used immunosuppressive medications?

Immunosuppressive medications can be classified into five groups: steroids, calcineurin inhibitors, antimetabolites, antilymphocyte agents, and chimeric monoclonal antibodies. Table 15-3 outlines the major immunosuppressive medications used in organ transplantation. Most centers employ triple drug maintenance immunosuppressant therapy consisting of steroids, a calcineurin inhibitor, and an antimetabolite. Antilymphocyte preparations are used for a short time as rejection prophylaxis or treatment. All immunosuppressive medications carry the risk of infection and malignancy.

Steroids

Oral prednisone and intravenous methylprednisolone sodium (Solumedrol) are the most commonly used steroids. Steroids are used to both prevent and treat rejection. Steroids, while easy to use and inexpensive, have the potential for a vast number of side effects. These side effects can be minimized by using the lowest possible dose.

Calcineurin inhibitors

Cyclosporine (Sandimmune, Neoral) and tacrolimus (FK 506, Prograf) are both immunosuppressant drugs derived from fungi. These drugs block T cell action by blocking the chemical signal calcineurin. Cyclosporine and tacrolimus have similar side effect profiles. Nephrotoxicity is a major problem with both medications, complicating the diagnosis of rejection. Tacrolimus offers the advantage of not sharing the cyclosporine effects of hirsutism, or gingival hyperplasia, and may not have as deleterious an effect on serum lipids as does cyclosporine, but is more likely than cyclosporine to cause diabetes and gastrointestinal symptoms. Tacrolimus is a more powerful immunosuppressant than cyclosporine, and thus the doses used are much smaller. The doses of both medications are based on blood levels obtained 12 hours after the last dose of medication. In most cases, these drugs are not used in combination but used interchangeably. A change of medication is usually precipitated by a severe rejection episode or intolerable side effects while receiving one of these medications. Cyclosporine—either as Sandimmune or Neoral, the more readily absorbed microemulsion form—is the primary drug used in kidney and heart transplantation. At many centers, tacrolimus is the primary agent employed in pancreas, liver, and small bowel transplantation.

Antimetabolites

Azathioprine (Imuran) and mycophenolate mofetil (Cellcept) are both antimetabolites. Mycophenolate mofetil is rapidly replacing azathioprine in transplantation as it appears to have an improved immunosuppressive effect, including action against B cells. This B cell blocking action makes mycophenolate mofetil the only immunosuppressant that may treat chronic rejection.

Antilymphocyte Preparations

ATGAM and OKt3 (Orthoclone) are the primary antilymphocyte agents used as prophylaxis against or to treat rejection. These powerful immunosuppressants are made by immunizing an animal with human lymphocytes and using the resultant antibodies. These antibodies block the function of T cells in the recipient. ATGAM is a polyclonal preparation, which means it has antibodies against a host of human blood cells, including platelets and red blood cells. It is administered in a manner similar to that used for other serum products, using a central vein catheter. OKt3 is a product of genetic engineering; the only specific antibodies present are those that block the function of certain T cells known as CD3 cells. This monoclonal preparation is given as an intravenous push medication via a peripheral vein. The most serious side effects from OKt3 occur after the first one or two doses and thus special precautions, including avoiding fluid overload, are observed.

Chimeric monoclonal antibodies

Several new monoclonal antibodies have been developed for use in transplantation. Basiliximab (Simulect) and daclizumab (Zenapax) are similar drugs developed to prevent transplant rejection. They are both humanized or chimeric antibodies: that is, the majority of the antibody is partial human immunoglobulin with only a small portion being murine antibody. This humanization means that the body is less likely to recognize it as a foreign protein, and thus first-dose side effects are minimized, and the drug enjoys a prolonged half life. Both drugs prevent rejection by interfering with interleukin-2 binding of lymphocytes. They are given intravenously in the first weeks after transplant. Baciliximab is given in 2 doses (2 hours before transplant and on post-operative day 4), while the recommended course of daclizumab is 5 doses beginning immediately before surgery and then every other week. Both drugs appear to be similar in efficacy and safety.

Table 15-3   Immunosuppressant Medications

Medication	Action	Side Effects	Dia
Steroids (prednisone, Solumedrol)	Blocks interleukin-1	Cushingoid appearance, glucose intolerance, hyperlipidemia, bone disease, muscle wasting, cataracts, gastric ulcers, sodium retention, increased appetite, night sweats, skin thinning, delayed healing, psychosis, pancreatitis	HD-Y PD-U
Cyclosporine (Sandimmune, Neoral	Blocks interleukin-2	Nephrotoxicity, hypertension, hyperlipidemia, tremors, numbness or burning in hands and feet, headaches, nervousness, gingival hyperplasia, hirsutism, hyperuricemia	HD-N PD-N
Tacrolimus (Prograf)	Blocks interleukin-2	Nephrotoxicity, headaches, tremor, gastric distress, glucose intolerance, neurotoxicity	HD-N PD-U
Azathioprine (Imuran)	Prevents lymphocyte proliferation	Myelotoxicity: leukopenia, thrombocytopenia, anemia; hepatotoxicity	HD-Y PD-NA
Mycophenolate mofetil (Cellcept)	Prevents lymphocyte proliferation	Gastrointestinal distress, gastric ulcers including perforation and hemorrhage, constipation, leukopenia, anemia, albuminuria	HD-N PD-N
ATGAM	Blocks action of T cells	Thrombocytopenia, neutropenia, anemia, anaphylactic reaction	HD-U PD-U
Daclizumab (Zenapax)	Blocks interleukin-2 receptors of T and B cells	Uncommon—nausea, vomiting, other gastrointestinal effects; headache, fever, hypotension, hypertension	HD-U PD-U
Basiliximab (Simulect)	Blocks interleukin-2 receptors of activated T cells	Uncommon—nausea, vomiting, other gastrointestinal effects; headache, fever, hypotension, hypertension	HD-U PD-U

(continued)

Table 15-3 (cont'd)

| Muromonab-CD3 (OKt3, Orthoclone) | Blocks action of CD3 T cells | First dose: pulmonary edema, fever, chills Note: Prevented by premedication and avoiding fluid overload Subsequent doses: flu-like symptoms: fever, chills, headache, arthralgias, myalgias; aseptic meningitis | HD-U PD-U |

Key: DIA = Dialysis of drug
HD = Hemodialysis PD = Peritoneal dialysis
Y = yes N = no U = unlikely NA = data not available

What is meant by rejection?

When the body's immune system recognizes the transplanted organ as foreign, it will attempt to destroy it. This phenomenon is called rejection. Rejection is carried out in two ways: cellular rejection or humoral rejection. Cellular rejection is initiated by T cells, while humoral rejection refers to destruction of the transplanted organ by specific antibodies.

What are the different kinds of transplant rejections?

There are basically three types of rejection processes: hyperacute rejection, acute rejection, and chronic rejection. Rejection episodes represent a great amount of stress to the recipient and his or her family.

Hyperacute rejection

Hyperacute rejection is a humoral rejection process primarily caused by preformed antibodies to the transplanted tissue HLA or ABO antigens. This type of rejection occurs within minutes to hours of the transplantation procedure. The onslaught of specific antibodies causes massive intravascular coagulation and cell death. There is no treatment for hyperacute rejection. It is prevented by careful crossmatching.

Acute rejection

When helper T cells recognize tissue cells as foreign, they initiate the cascade of events known as acute rejection. Acute rejection usually occurs weeks to months after transplantation. This form of cellular rejection generally occurs the initial time the immune system is presented with a specific foreign tissue cell or antigen. The majority of immunosuppression is directed at preventing and treating acute rejection.

Chronic rejection

In humoral rejection, B cells, stimulated by non-self antigens produce antibodies to destroy the transplanted organ. Chronic rejection is a slow humoral rejection process that occurs months to years after transplantation. The hallmark of chronic rejection is slow gradual loss of function caused by fibrosis in the organ's blood vessels. Chronic rejection of the kidney may be difficult to distinguish from chronic cyclosporine toxicity.

How is rejection diagnosed and treated?

Increased serum creatinine, in the absence of other causes, is most commonly used as the diagnostic indicator of rejection. A percutaneous biopsy may be used to confirm the diagnosis.

Hyperacute rejection

Hyperacute rejection is often diagnosed as soon as the vascular anastomoses are completed and the clamps released. The kidney will rapidly turn black and fail to produce urine, or the recipient may suffer severe symptoms of oliguria, fever, and pain soon after the transplant procedure. There is no treatment; the organ must be surgically removed.

Acute rejection

Oliguria, fever, edema, weight gain, and graft tenderness are the cardinal physical symptoms of acute renal transplant rejection. However, modern immunosuppression blocks these symptoms, causing transplant clinicians to rely on biochemical markers. A rapid rise in the serum creatinine over several days with or without physical symptoms may indicate acute rejection. Nephrotoxicity is also a possible diagnosis, especially if drug levels are high.

Many rejection attempts can be treated by increased steroids. The steroids are delivered by intravenous boluses or "pulses" of methylprednisolone and/or increased oral prednisone that is rapidly tapered over several days back to baseline dose. If the rejection is severe or does not respond to steroids, antilymphocyte preparations (ATGAM, OKT3) are used. Most acute cellular rejections are successfully treated.

Chronic rejection

Patients with chronic rejection often do not experience symptoms until the rejection has progressed to serious renal compromise. The serum creatinine slowly increases over months to years until the kidney ceases to function. Definitive diagnosis is made by biopsy. Traditionally, there has been no treatment for chronic rejection; however, mycophenolate mofetil (Cellcept), which has action against antibody-inducing B cells, has demonstrated some success in treatment. Because it probably begins as very mild acute rejection, chronic rejection is best prevented by adequate immunosuppression and regular laboratory follow-up.

Who should provide long-term care/health maintenance after transplant?

A variety of health care providers are qualified to provide long-term care to successful transplant recipients. These care providers include transplant physicians, nephrologists, internists, family practice physicians, and nurse practitioners. The goal of long-term care is to assist the patient in achieving his/her maximum health potential. This goal is achieved by routine health maintenance, as well as a focus on the prevention, early detection and treatment of the consequences of immunosuppression. As cardiovascular disease remains the number one cause of death in the first decade after successful renal transplantation, particular attention is paid to this area. Cancer and infection surveillance are also focus areas. The degree of rehabilitation to career, family, and social life is assessed and interventions implemented if necessary.

What happens when the transplanted kidney irreversibly fails?

When the transplant team has determined that the transplanted kidney has irreversibly failed and that further treatment would be unsuccessful or detrimental, the patient returns to maintenance dialysis treatment. Except in the cases of hyperacute rejection, early vascular catastrophe, or untreated acute rejection, the transplanted kidney usually slowly scars and shrinks as function ceases, thus surgical removal is not necessary. Failed transplanted kidneys are removed for severe hematuria, infection, or malignant hypertension. Immunosuppression is discontinued gradually to prevent superimposed acute rejection and to allow the adrenal glands to regain function.

These individuals require special nursing care. In addition to the effects of immunosuppression, which may remain for several months, the failed transplant represents a crisis for the patient and family. The loss of the transplanted kidney may provoke depression, feelings of hopelessness, anger, and worthlessness. Individuals may experience the grieving process similar to the process described for those experiencing death and dying. Emotional support is essential for these patients. The dialysis staff should encourage the individual to seek another transplant, if appropriate.

Peritoneal Dialysis and Home Dialysis Therapies

Margaret S. Holloway, Christopher R. Blagg, and Sandra Smolka-Hill

Peritoneal Dialysis

Peritoneal dialysis (PD) is an alternative dialytic modality for the patient with ESRD. There is great worldwide variation in the usage of PD from a low of 3% in Poland to a high of 46% in the United Kingdom. Approximately 35% of the ESRD population of the United States is currently on PD. PD is primarily a home dialysis therapy for chronic renal failure, but it can also be a treatment option for the patient with acute renal failure in the hospital setting.

What is peritoneal dialysis and how does it work?

PD is a process during which the peritoneal cavity acts as the reservoir for the dialysate and the peritoneum serves as the semipermeable membrane across which excess body fluid and solutes, including uremic toxins, are removed (ultrafiltrate). The peritoneal membrane surface area is approximately equal to the body surface area (1.73 m^2). The peritoneum consists of the lining of the inner surface of the abdominal and pelvic walls, including the diaphragm (parietal peritoneum) as well as the covering of the abdominal organs (visceral peritoneum). In males the peritoneum is a closed cavity, but in females the fallopian tubes and ovaries open into the peritoneal cavity.

The peritoneal membrane is in contact with the rich blood supply to the abdominal organs. Dialysate is infused into the peritoneal cavity via a catheter, allowed to dwell for a predetermined amount of time and then drained (effluent). This process is called an exchange. Dextrose is used in the dialysate to create an osmotic gradient that causes water to be moved into the peritoneal cavity. The excess fluid is removed when the effluent is drained. Electrolytes and uremic toxins are removed by diffusion from an area of higher concentration (bloodstream) to an area of lower concentration (peritoneal cavity). Solute removal is further enhanced by "solute drag," created when hypertonic dialysate is used, which increases ultrafiltration (UF) and causes additional low molecular weight solutes to be "dragged" along with the UF by convective transport.

What solutions are used for peritoneal dialysis?

Commercially available solutions approximate the composition of extracellular body water except for potassium because many patients tend to be hyperkalemic. Potassium may be added (2 to 4 mEq/L) if necessary to correct hypokalemia. Dextrose provides the osmotic gradient between the plasma and the dialysate that leads to fluid and solute removal. The more hypertonic the dialysate, i.e., 2.5% and 4.25% dextrose, the greater the UF. After a 2 L exchange has been dwelling for 4 hours, an average of 200 ml of ultrafiltrate will be obtained with a 1.5% exchange and 600 to 1000 ml with a 4.25% exchange. Table 16-1 highlights some commercially available solutions.

Are there different ways to perform peritoneal dialysis?

PD can be done either manually or automatically with a cycler. The manual form of PD is called Continuous Ambulatory Peritoneal Dialysis (CAPD). In CAPD, four or more exchanges are performed each day. The patient connects to a tubing system, drains the effluent, and infuses new dialysate to dwell for a prescribed amount of time. Most patients do "bagless" CAPD; they disconnect from the tubing system at the end of the exchange, leaving a short transfer set or

Table 16-1   Commercially Available Peritoneal Dialysis Solutions

Solution	Vol (ml)	% Dextrose	Na	Cl	Ca (mEq/L)	Mg	Lactate
Dianeal PD-2 (Baxter Healthcare, Inc.)	250,500,750, 1000, 1500, 2000, 2500, 3000, 5000, 6000	1.5 2.5 4.25	132	96	3.5	0.5	40
Dianeal PD-1 (Baxter Healthcare, Inc.)	2000, 5000	1.5 2.5 4.25	132	102	3.5	1.5	35
Dianeal Low Ca (Baxter Health-care, Inc.)	1500, 2000, 2500, 3000, 5000, 6000	1.5 2.5 4.25	132	95	2.5	0.5	40
Delflex (Fresenius USA)	1000, 1500, 2000, 3000, 5000	1.5 2.5 4.25	132 132	102 96	3.5 or 3.5	1.5 0.5	40 40
Delflex (Fresenius USA)	1500, 2000, 2500, 3000, 5000	1.5 2.5 4.25	132	95	2.5	0.5	40

the capped catheter. Most CAPD tubing systems involve a Y configuration that enables the patient to "flush" any contaminants that might have been introduced while connecting to the system or spiking the bag into the drain bag before infusing fresh dialysate.

What is automated peritoneal dialysis?

Automated peritoneal dialysis (APD) is performed with a cycler, usually at night while the patient sleeps. Cyclers perform the following functions: (1) measure the volume of dialysate to be infused; (2) warm the dialysate to body temperature before infusion; (3) time the frequency of exchanges; (4) count the number of exchanges and; (5) measure UF. Cyclers can be programmed for volumes from 50 cc to 3000 cc per exchange, have a last bag option to accommodate a unique diurnal (day) dwell (volume, percentage, additives), and the ability to program one or more exchanges during the daytime hours. All machines can be programmed to perform tidal PD. APD enables the patient to mix dextrose concentrations to achieve the desired UF, e.g., 2.5% mixed with 4.25% to get 3.3%.

What are the different forms of APD?

Continuous cycling peritoneal dialysis (CCPD). Several exchanges are performed nightly with a full diurnal dwell. The diurnal dwell improves the clearance of middle molecules.

Nocturnal intermittent peritoneal dialysis (NIPD). Several exchanges are performed nightly, but there is a minimal or no diurnal dwell. NIPD is indicated in patients who are unable to tolerate a diurnal dwell, e.g., those with hyperpermeability of the peritoneum to dextrose, resulting in absorption of diurnal dwell; those with problems exacerbated by increased intraabdominal pressure, including hernias, low back pain, cardiopulmonary compromise, etc.

Intermittent peritoneal dialysis (IPD). Several frequent exchanges are performed three to four times a week, and the peritoneum is left "dry" between treatments. IPD is appropriate for patients with residual renal function or institutionalized patients. Also, it is used in economically underdeveloped countries because of the financial constraints imposed by daily peritoneal dialysis.

Tidal peritoneal dialysis (TPD). An initial volume of dialysate is infused, followed by partial drainage of effluent at the end of each exchange (leaving a constant reserve volume); finally a "tidal" volume of fresh dialysate is infused. TPD is intended to enhance clearance by maintaining continuous contact of dialysate with the peritoneum and maintenance of the dialysate/plasma gradient. TPD may improve clearances by 20% but increases costs because of the need for additional dialysate.

What kinds of catheters are used for peritoneal dialysis?

Catheters for both acute and chronic PD must transport fluid into and out of the peritoneal cavity as rapidly as possible as well as be biocompatible (maintain normal structure and function of the tissues near the catheter tract). Catheters manufactured for both acute and chronic PD come in sizes to accommodate neonates to adults.

Catheters for acute PD are usually placed at the patient's bedside and include rigid catheters or soft silicone catheters. The patient should have an empty bladder and the rectum should be free of stool at the time of insertion to minimize the risk of organ perforation. Placement may be by direct insertion with a trocar or guide wire or by use of a peritoneoscope. Dialysis may be initiated immediately after insertion. Risks with the rigid catheter include bowel or organ perforation, dialysate leaks, peritonitis, discomfort, and inadvertent catheter loss. Silicone catheters, used for acute dialysis, are more comfortable and may be used for chronic dialysis if necessary.

Catheters used for chronic PD are usually placed surgically during a laparotomy or laparoscopically. The exit site should be directed in a downward or lateral direction and located in the right or left midquadrant area avoiding the belt line, scars and skin folds. Catheters are made of silicone or polyurethane with a radiopaque stripe for x-ray visualization. Catheters may be straight or coiled and have one or two cuffs. Coiled catheters are believed to minimize catheter migration out of the pelvis and have fewer outflow problems than straight catheters. Cuffs are made of Dacron polyester or velour and provide for tissue ingrowth to stabilize the catheter. Cuffs are also intended to prevent migration of bacteria along the subcutaneous tunnel into the peritoneum. When placing double-cuffed catheters, the internal cuff is placed in the rectus muscle, and the external cuff is placed in the subcutaneous tissue proximal to the exit site. Implanted catheters (Fig. 16-1) consist of the following: an intraperitoneal segment containing side holes and an open tip for fluid flow; a subcutaneous segment that passes through the peritoneal membrane, muscles, and subcutaneous tissues; and an external segment that extends from the external cuff out to the exit site. There are several versions of chronic catheters including the Tenckhoff, column disc, Toronto Western, swan neck, Cruz, and Moncrief catheters. All include features intended to improve dialysate flow and decrease catheter complications.

What is meant by catheter break-in?

Catheter break-in is the period after the chronic catheter is placed, during which there is healing and tissue ingrowth into the cuff(s). The goals are to promote healing and prevent complications such as dialysate leaks, infections, or catheter obstruction. Healing may take up to six weeks and includes scab formation, granulation of tissue at the exit site, and epitheliazation of the sinus tract. Full-volume dialysis, especially CAPD, should be avoided for at least 10 to 14

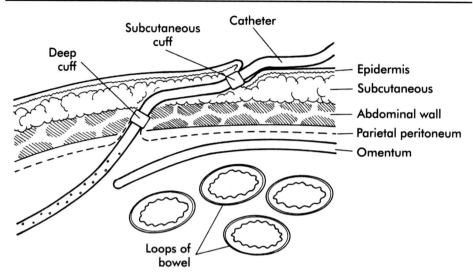

Fig. 16-1 Placement of a double-cuffed Tenckhoff catheter. (From Ash SR, Carr DJ, and Diaz-Buxo JA: Peritoneal access devices. In Nissenson AR, Fine RN, and Gentile DE, eds: *Clinical dialysis*, ed 2, Norwalk, CT, 1990, Appleton & Lange.)

days to allow healing to occur. This healing period may necessitate the placement of a temporary hemodialysis access if the patient is severely uremic, or is fluid-overloaded and in need of immediate dialysis. Postoperatively, the patient should remain supine when possible and avoid activities that increase intraabdominal pressure such as straining to defecate, excessive coughing, crying, and lifting. Treatment options during the postoperative period include:

- Infusion of heparinized saline solution (1-10 units heparin/ml saline), 25 to 100 ml every 4 to 8 hours for 1 to 3 days postoperatively. This protocol will not detect catheter malposition or outflow problems.
- Low volume in and out exchanges with heparinized saline or dialysate done several times a day until the effluent is no longer bloody, then daily for 1 to 2 weeks and weekly thereafter until the patient is on PD. A small volume of heparinized solution should remain in the peritoneum to inhibit the formation of fibrin (whitish protein formed in response to bleeding, inflammation, or infection) and prevent the development of adhesions. There is no systemic anticoagulation from the administration of low-dose intraperitoneal heparin.
- Low-volume dialysis in the patient who needs immediate dialysis but who is unable to undergo hemodialysis. Frequent, low-volume exchanges (500 to 1000 ml) are performed using a cycler with the patient in the supine position. The volume is gradually increased to eliminate the signs and symptoms of uremia.

How is exit site care performed?

The goals in the immediate postoperative period are to stabilize the catheter, promote healing, and prevent infection. The exit site dressing should not be changed for 5 to 7 days postoperatively unless there is excessive drainage under the dressing (blood, exudate, dialysate). The first dressing change should be performed by trained dialysis personnel and may then be taught to the patient. It is recommended that masks be worn during dressing changes to avoid contamination with oral or nasal flora. The skin around the exit site may be pink, similar to a healing scar, or it may have a brownish or purplish discoloration. During dressing changes, the exit site should be assessed for signs of infection (erythema, exudate, induration, tenderness); the subcutaneous tunnel should be palpated for tenderness; and the catheter and connections should be inspected for integrity. The exit site should be cleansed with an antibacterial soap and water and covered with a sterile nonocclusive dressing such as gauze and tape or an air-permeable adhesive sheet. Cytotoxic agents such as 1% povidone-iodine, 3% hydrogen peroxide and 0.5% sodium hypochlorite may interfere with wound epitheliazation during the postoperative period. The catheter should be secured to the patient's skin with tape or an immobilization device to avoid tension on the catheter and trauma to the exit site.

The goal of chronic exit site care is the prevention of infection. Exit site care is usually performed in the shower and consists of daily cleansing with an antibacterial soap with careful rinsing and drying. An antibacterial solution (1% povidone-iodine, 3% hydrogen peroxide, 0.5% sodium hypochlorite, etc.) is then applied in a circular motion to the skin around the exit site. The exit site should not be submerged in bath water. Many programs allow swimming in chlorinated pools and the ocean. After the healing period (4 to 6 weeks), a dressing may or may not be worn, according to patient or unit preference. It is extremely important to secure the catheter to the skin with tape or an immobilizing device to avoid trauma and infection should the catheter be accidentally tugged.

How is the adequacy of peritoneal dialysis determined?

The clinical condition of the patient should be paramount when evaluating the adequacy of PD. Important elements of the evaluation include careful attention to both overt signs of uremia—laboratory values, fluid overload—and covert signs, such as sleep and concentration disturbances, anorexia, and nutritional indices. Because PD is primarily a home therapy, patient compliance with the prescribed regimen must also be assessed in the evaluation of dialysis adequacy.

The efficiency of PD depends on the ability of the peritoneal membrane to ultrafiltrate fluid and solutes. Peritoneal clearance of solutes is determined by diffusion, which is driven by the concentration gradient between dialysate and plasma and by the "solute drag" created by hypertonic dialysate. Solutes and fluid may move from the intravascular compartment to the peritoneal cavity or from the peritoneal cavity to the intravascular compartment. Other substances lost in the effluent include protein (8.8 to 12.9 g/day), amino acids, water-soluble vitamins, trace minerals, and certain hormones.

UF and solute clearance in PD are influenced by: (1) permeability of the peritoneal membrane, (2) volume of the exchange, (3) dialysate glucose concentration, (4) dwell time, and (5) molecular size of the solute. Clearance of solutes is expressed as the dialysate/plasma ratio (D/P) at a given point in time during the exchange. Equilibration is achieved when the D/P ratio approaches one. Small solutes such as urea (molecular weight = 60 daltons) are highly diffusible and approach equilibration at 4 hours. Creatinine (molecular weight = 113 daltons) moves more slowly toward equilibration, never reaching it during the typical 4-hour CAPD exchange. Table 16-2 demonstrates solute clearances that can be achieved with different types of peritoneal dialysis.

The peritoneal equilibration test (PET) is a standardized test of peritoneal membrane permeability used to determine solute transport characteristics, glucose absorption, and net UF. The PET assists in prescribing therapy and in making changes based on the current transport characteristics of the peritoneum. The PET involves giving the patient an exchange of 2.5% dialysate and obtaining a serum sample at hour 2 and dialysate samples at hours 0, 2, and 4. Samples are analyzed for urea, creatinine, and glucose. Urea and creatinine are also analyzed from the long dwell (12 hours) obtained when the patient arrives for the PET.

Table 16-2   Solute Clearances with Various PD Modalities

| Modality | Clearance (L/Day) | | Schedule | | |
	Urea	Creatinine	*n* exchanges	Volume	Duration (hr)
Acute PD	24	16	24	2	24
CAPD	8.1	6.2	4	2	24
CCPD	8.0	6.0	Nocturnal 4	2	10
			Diurnal 1	2	14
NPD	7.7	5.3	12	2	8
TPD	10.4	6.3	—	TV[a] 1.5	8
				RV[b] 1.5	
				Total[c] 27	

From Diaz-Buxo JA: Clinical use of peritoneal dialysis. In Nissenson AR, Fine RN, and Gentile DE, eds: *Clinical dialysis*, ed 2, Norwalk, CT, 1990, Appleton & Lange.
[a]*TV*, Tidal volume
[b]*RV*, Residual volume
[c]*Total*, Total dialysis volume/8 hr.

The D/P ratios are calculated and plotted on the graphs below (Fig. 16-2). Decisions are made as to the best dialytic therapy according to Table 16-3, based on the solute transport characteristics of the patient.

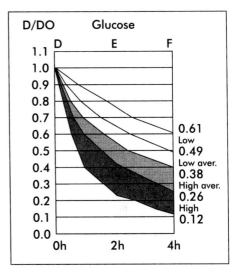

Calculate D/P and D/DO as follows:

$$D/P \; = \; \frac{\text{dialysate concentration of corrected creatinine}}{\text{serum concentration of corrected creatinine}}$$

at 0, 2 and 4 hours

$$D/DO \; = \; \frac{\text{dialysate concentration of glucose at 2 and 4 hours}}{\text{dialysate concentration of glucose at 0 hrs}}$$

Fig. 16-2 Plotting graphs for PET. (Redrawn from Twardowski ZJ, Nolph KD, Khanna R, et al.: *PD Bull* 7:138, 1987.)

While the PET will help determine the transport characteristics of the peritoneum, a 24-hour collection of urine (residual renal function) and effluent (dialysis clearance) must be obtained at regular intervals to determine whether adequacy targets are being met. These collections are analyzed for urea and creatinine and the weekly Kt/V and creatinine clearance are determined. The current adequacy targets recommended by the Dialysis Outcomes Quality Initiative (DOQI) of the National Kidney Foundation are summarized in Table 16-4.

Table 16-3   Baseline PET Prognostic Value

Solute Transport	Predicted Response to CAPD		Preferred Dialysis Prescription
	UF	Dialysis	
High	Poor	Adequate	NIPD, DAPD[b]
High average	Adequate	Adequate	Standard dose PD[a]
Low average	Good	Adequate	Standard dose PD[a]
		Inadequate[c]	High-dose PD[d]
Low	Excellent	Inadequate[c]	High-dose PD[d] or hemodialysis[e]

From Twardowski ZJ: Blood purification, vol 7, Berlin, New York, 1989, S. Karger.

[a]Standard-dose PD, Standard-dose CAPD with 7.5–9.0 L of dialysis solution used per 24 hours or Standard-dose CCPD, 6–8 L of dialysis solution used overnight and 2 L daytime.

[b]NIPD, IPD performed every night for 8 to 12 hours using 10–20 liters of dialysis solution. DAPD, Ambulatory peritoneal dialysis performed only during daytime using 3 to 4 exchanges.

[c]Inadequate dialysis likely in patients with body surface area > 2.00 m^2.

[d]High-dose PD. CAPD with > 9.0 L of dialysis solution used per 24 hours or CCPD with > 8 L of dialysis solution used overnight or > 2 L daytime.

[e]Hemodialysis may be needed in patients with body surface area > 2.00 m^2.

Table 16-4   DOQI Peritoneal Dialysis Adequacy Targets

	Kt/V	Creatinine Clearance (1/week/1.73m^2)
CAPD	2.0	60
CCPD	2.1	63
NIPD	2.2	66

From Clinical Practice Guidelines for Peritoneal Dialysis Adequacy. DOQI. Medical Education Institute, Madison, WI, 1997.

What complications are encountered in peritoneal dialysis?

Table 16-5 summarizes the common complications encountered in PD, including the causes, signs, symptoms, and interventions.

Table 16-5   Complications of Peritoneal Dialysis

Complication	Cause	Signs/Symptoms	Interventions
Peritonitis Infections of the peritoneal cavity	Invasion of peritoneal cavity with microorganisms, usually due to break in closed system; may also enter along outer surface of catheter and through bowel wall	Cloudy effluent; abdominal pain; nausea/vomiting; peritoneal fluid cell count with greater than 100 WBC and greater than 50% neutrophils; Culture results: gram + gram – multiple organisms FUNGI other no growth no culture done	Prompt diagnosis & treatment; flushes with 1.5% dialysate; intraperitoneal antibiotics are as effective as IV; coverage for gram + and gram – until organism identified; heparin added (.5–1 unit/ml dialysate) to combat fibrin and adhesions *PERITONITIS TREATMENT DECISION TREE* (Fig. 16-3)
Exit Site Infection Purulent drainage and erythema of the skin at catheter exit point through the skin	Microorganisms in epidermal area; may be related to trauma, *S. aureus* nasal carriage Causative organisms: *Staph, epidermidis, S. aureus, Pseudomonas*	Erythema; purulent drainage; positive culture; induration; pain	Oral/IV/IP antibiotics; exit site care increased to BID; duration of therapy unknown; may lead to peritonitis; catheter removal may be necessary for recurrent or resistant infections *S. Aureus* nasal carriages mupirocin ointment intranasally bid x 5 dqn or Rifampin 300 mg bid x 5d q 3 mo

Table 16-5   Complications of Peritoneal Dialysis—cont'd

Complication	Cause	Signs/Symptoms	Interventions
Tunnel Infection Inflammation along the subcutaneous tunnel-catheter tract	Migration of microorganisms along the tunnel	Erythema or thickening along the tunnel—"sausage" appearance; pain; may or may not be exit site drainage	IV/IP antibiotics; often leads to peritonitis; often results in catheter removal
Fibrin Formation	Formed in response to inflammation due to decreased fibrinolysis of fibrinogen; increased during peritonitis	Whitish strands/clots seen in effluent or catheter; may lead to catheter obstruction if untreated	Heparin added to dialysate to prevent fibrin production and adhesion formation (500–1000 units/L)
Hemoperitoneum	Menstruating women (retrograde menstruation); trauma; ovarian cysts; ovulation; peritonitis; post colonoscopy or enema	Blood effluent; 2 ml blood/L will result in blood-tinged effluent; effluent hematocrit greater than 5%, indicative of major bleeding; usually resolves spontaneously	In-and-out flushes with room temperature dialysate (vasoconstriction); addition of heparin to prevent obstruction
Inflow/Outflow Problems	Obstruction of catheter with fibrin, blood, omentum; catheter migration out of pelvis; loculation of fluid in abdominal cavity due to adhesions; constipation	Dialysate will not inflow or outflow; resistance when catheter irrigated	Relief of constipation; x-ray for internal kink, catheter position; inspect catheter for external kinks; irrigation of catheter with heparinized saline; irrigation with urokinase (70,000 units for adults); reposition/replace catheter; peritoneogram with contrast medium to identify loculation

Table 16-5 Complications of Peritoneal Dialysis—cont'd

Complication	Cause	Signs/Symptoms	Interventions
Air in Peritoneum	Air entering peritoneal cavity due to air in system/loose connections	Shoulder pain; peritoneal eosinophilia	Drain pt. in knee-chest position or Trendelenburg; may need to resolve over time; tighten connections
Dialysate Leak Around exit site or into subcutaneous tissue	Increased intraabdominal pressure; delayed healing after catheter placement	Clear fluid from exit site; abdominal, penile, scrotal edema	Dextrostick to document glucose; resuture exit site of acute catheter; stop PD for 2 or more weeks to allow healing; decrease volume with APD in supine position if unable to stop PD; stabilize catheter; catheter replacement
Hernias	Increased intraabdominal pressure caused by presence of dialysate in peritoneum, seen in pts. with congenital or acquired defects or previous abdominal surgeries	Swelling in inguinal, ventral incisional, umbilical area, nonpainful, reducible	APD with minimal or no diurnal dwell; decreased exchange volume; surgical repair
Pain on Inflow	Migration of catheter; catheter resting against pelvic wall; rapid infusion of dialysate; hyperosmolarity of dialysate; acidity of dialysate	Pain when dialysate is entering peritoneum	Slower infusion of dialysate; addition of $NaHCO_3$ to increase pH; local anesthetic (2% lidocaine, 3–5 ml/L dialysate IP); surgical revision/replacement of catheter

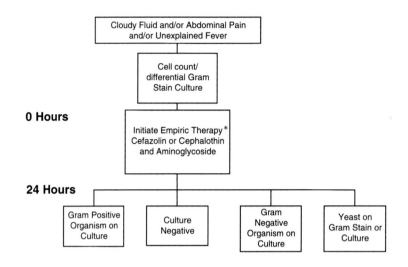

0 Hours

24 Hours

* Empiric Therapy

Agent	Continuous Dose	Intermittant Dose (in 1 exchange/day)	
		Residual urine output (mL/day)	
		Anuria (< 500)	Non-anuria (> 500)
cefazolin or cephalothin	500 mg/L load, then 125 mg/L in each exchange	500 mg/L (or 15 mg/kg)	Increase dose by 25%
gentamicin netilmicin tobramycin	8 mg/L load, then 4 mg/L in each exchange	0.6 mg/kg body weight	1.5 mg/kg initial loading dose. See footnote for maintenance dose recommendations
amikacin	25 mg/L load, then 12 mg/L in each exchange	2 mg/kg body weight	5 mg/kg initial loading dose. See footnote for maintenance dose recommendations

Fig. 16-3   Peritonitis treatment tree. Keane, Alexander, et al.: Peritoneal dialysis-related peritonitis treatment recommendation: 1996 update, *Peritoneal Dialysis International* 16(6):557–573, 1996.

24–48 Hours

96 Hours

Duration of Therapy

24–48 Hours

96 Hours

120 Hours

Duration of Therapy

*If methicillin-resistant *S. aureus* is cultured and the patient is not responding clinically, clindamycin or vancomycin should be used.

Fig. 16-3 continued

24–48 Hours

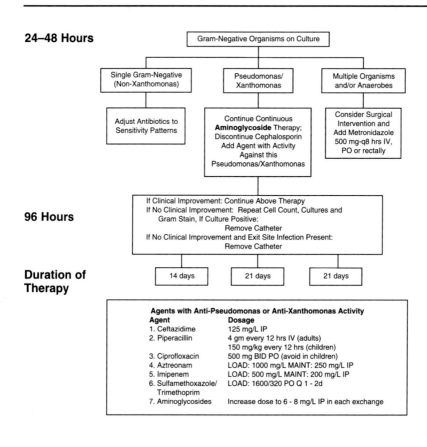

96 Hours

Duration of Therapy

24–48 Hours

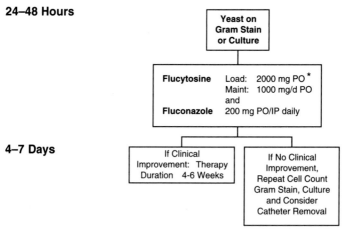

4–7 Days

*Pediatric doses: Flucytosine 50–100 mg/kg load PO, 25–50 mg/kg maintenance PO; fluconazole 1–3 mg/kg IP every 2 days.

Fig. 16-3 continued

Can diabetics be treated with peritoneal dialysis?

PD offers many advantages to the diabetic patient. In PD, there is a steady physiologic state without the drastic biochemical or fluid fluctuations seen with hemodialysis in the diabetic patient with cardiovascular instability or autonomic neuropathy. There is no need for a vascular access. Blood sugar is well controlled with intraperitoneal administration of regular insulin because the peritoneal cavity containing insulin provides a steady, gradual, and prolonged appearance of insulin in the peripheral circulation. The total daily intraperitoneal (IP) dose of insulin may need to be much higher than the previous subcutaneous dose because of any or all of the following factors: its slow absorption from the peritoneal cavity; the effect of dilution in the dialysate on insulin absorption; extra insulin needed because of the dextrose in dialysate; binding of insulin to the plastic bags and tubing (10%); and hepatic degradation of insulin. Although IP insulin requires the daily addition of medication to the dialysis bags, the incidence of peritonitis is no higher than in other PD patients. There are numerous protocols for the IP administration of insulin.

Home Dialysis Therapy: Peritoneal

How are patients selected for peritoneal dialysis as a home dialysis therapy?

Before a person is selected as a home peritoneal dialysis patient, there must be a thorough evaluation by the interdisciplinary dialysis team. The following areas need to be assessed:

1. Relative medical contraindications for peritoneal dialysis such as:
    * Abdominal adhesions
    * Concurrent abdominal disease such as neoplasms
    * History of ruptured diverticulum
    * History of recurrent hernias
    * Documented inability of peritoneal membrane to ultrafiltrate or diffuse solutes (PET results)
    * Opening between the peritoneal and pleural cavities
    * Patients weighing > 70 kg without residual renal function

2. Psychosocial evaluation including:
    * Patient motivation for self-care
    * Life-style (job, school)
    * Educational background
    * Health beliefs
    * Support system within the family/community
    * Patient's decision-making abilities
    * History of compliance with medical treatment
    * Distance from a dialysis center

- Characteristics of the home (cleanliness; availability of water, electricity, and telephone; space for storage of supplies, etc.)
- Availability of alternate caregiver (spouse, sibling, parent, friend, etc.)

3. Physical characteristics/limitations of the patient including:
   - Vision
   - Strength
   - Dexterity
   - Fine motor coordination

Peritoneal dialysis may be medically indicated in the patient with cardiovascular difficulties.

Home peritoneal dialysis is particularly well suited to the pediatric patient as it allows for the "normalization" of the child's and the family's life (normal school attendance, fewer dietary restrictions than hemodialysis, fewer needle sticks, steady state of body fluid and electrolyte status, independence, etc.).

How is a patient trained for home peritoneal dialysis?

If possible, training is delayed for at least 2 weeks after the catheter is inserted to allow time for healing to occur and for the patient to recover physically and psychologically from surgery. Another family member should train with the patient for support and backup. It is important that the patient be trained by a primary nurse who establishes a trusting relationship with the patient and family and subsequently acts as the liaison between the patient and the dialysis team. Training is performed primarily on an outpatient basis. Medicare will fund 15 outpatient training sessions and up to 18 sessions with written medical justification.

Content and method of presentation must be individualized to the patient's learning abilities. Content of training includes normal kidney function and the effects renal failure has on body homeostasis; mechanism of peritoneal dialysis; performance of aseptic technique; catheter and exit site care; monitoring of weight and BP; dialysis record keeping with weight, BP, and dialysis treatments performed; CAPD exchange procedure; use of cycler if on APD; decision-making regarding dialysate to be used to maintain dry weight and normalize BP; recognition of the signs and symptoms of infections (exit site, tunnel, peritonitis); importance of adequate PD, treatment of peritonitis; medications; dietary counseling by the dietitian; ordering dialysis supplies; and management of complications. There must be ample time for return demonstration of dialysis techniques and attainment of all training objectives before the patient is allowed to perform peritoneal dialysis independently at home. At the completion of training, a home visit may be made by the primary nurse. Additional support is provided by having a peritoneal dialysis nurse on call to assist the patient with problems encountered during the off hours.

How is quality of care monitored in peritoneal dialysis?

Quality assurance programs are mandated by the JCAHO and by the HCFA, whose mandates are administered by the regional ESRD Networks (see Chapter 22). The focus of quality assurance should be continuous improvement in the quality of care patients receive.

The following are examples of quality assurance indicators:

- Incidence of infections such as peritonitis, exit site/tunnel infections
- Incidence of catheter complications such as pericatheter leaks, migration, obstruction necessitating catheter replacement, holes/cracks in the catheter, etc.
- Patient morbidity (number of hospital days/year and causes for hospitalization) and mortality
- Attainment of adequacy targets
- Revision of policies and procedures to improve patient care

PD is a viable dialytic modality for both the acute or chronic patient with ESRD. Acute PD is appropriate in the patient who cannot tolerate hemodialysis. Care must be taken in the selection of patients for chronic home PD to optimize the chances for success. Ongoing evaluation of patient satisfaction and compliance with the treatment, incidence of complications, and adequacy of PD in removing uremic toxins and excess fluid must be undertaken and adjustments made to ensure quality patient care.

Are there drawbacks to peritoneal dialysis?

Recently, concern has grown about the frequency of malnutrition and of inadequate dialysis in peritoneal dialysis patients. Protein malnutrition is frequent as a result of the loss of amino acids and protein in the dialysate, and because of appetite suppression resulting from inadequate dialysis and the glucose load absorbed from the dialysate. The latter often causes hypertriglyceridemia, and the increased calorie intake results in weight gain, especially in patients already overweight when they started on peritoneal dialysis. The other major concern is adequacy of dialysis. In the past, most CAPD patients used four exchanges of 2 to 2.5 liters daily, but it has now become clear that many peritoneal dialysis patients are getting inadequate dialysis once they lose their residual renal function.

The hospitalization rate for peritoneal dialysis patients is 14 percent higher than for in-center hemodialysis patients, even after adjusting for comorbid conditions. Similarly, the adjusted relative risk of death in peritoneal dialysis patients is also higher, particularly in older patients and diabetics, and deaths from infection, cardiac disease, cerebrovascular disease and withdrawal from dialysis are more frequent, compared with those of hemodialysis patients.

The *Clinical Practice Guidelines For Peritoneal Dialysis Adequacy,* recently developed by the National Kidney Foundation-Dialysis Outcomes

Quality Initiative, state that adequate dialysis with CAPD requires a Kt/V of at least 2.0 per week and a creatinine clearance of at least 60 liters/1.73m^2 per week. (See page 333 for additional information on NKF-DOQI.) Corresponding figures for CCPD are a Kt/V of 2.1 and a weekly creatinine clearance of 63 liters/m^2. For patients who are malnourished, even more dialysis is recommended. As a result, more CAPD patients are now using five exchanges daily, often with larger volumes of up to 3 liters, and/or supplementing this with cycler dialysis overnight. This may increase the patient time required for carrying out the procedure, as well as increased discomfort.

What are the implications of these findings?

One implication of these findings is that the use of peritoneal dialysis in the United States may have peaked. Continuous ambulatory peritoneal dialysis and cycler dialysis are good initial treatments for many patients, allowing them to experience the advantages of home dialysis after only a few days of training. However, as their residual renal function declines, many patients will become inadequately dialyzed on peritoneal dialysis. They will then need to change to hemodialysis, and unfortunately at present, home hemodialysis is not likely to be available to many of them.

A significant proportion of peritoneal dialysis patients have always transferred to hemodialysis each year. There are many reasons for this, including inadequate dialysis or inadequate ultrafiltration once residual renal function has been lost, repeated episodes of peritonitis, and inability to do the dialysis. Some patients put on hemodialysis while treating a catheter infection or peritonitis may elect to stay on this treatment permanently. The USRDS reports that, of those patients on CAPD or CCPD 90 days after starting treatment in 1990–1992, only 40.7 percent were still on these treatments after 2 years; 14.1 percent were on outpatient hemodialysis, and 12.8 percent were transplanted. This compares with 55.1 percent of the patients on outpatient hemodialysis at 90 days who were still being treated with this modality at 2 years.

Home Dialysis Therapy: Hemodialysis

Home hemodialysis is an excellent but under-utilized alternative to dialysis in a center for many patients with end stage renal disease (ESRD). This section briefly recounts the history of home dialysis in the United States, describes the use of home hemodialysis today, and discusses its advantages in comparison with peritoneal dialysis.

What is the history of home hemodialysis?

Dialysis for the treatment of ESRD became possible with development of the Teflon arteriovenous shunt by Belding Scribner and coworkers at the University of Washington in 1960. For the first time, it was possible to get repeated access to the bloodstream for long-term hemodialysis. Clyde Shields, the first patient so treated, lived for some eleven years, latterly on home hemodialysis, and died from a myocardial infarction.

In 1963, home hemodialysis programs were started in Boston, London and Seattle, the prime reason for this being financial. At that time, there was no funding for long-term dialysis from insurance or from government sources other than research funds, and so this expensive treatment was paid for by patients themselves or from public donations. It soon became obvious that suitably trained and supported patients could do hemodialysis safely themselves at home for a fraction of the cost of staff-assisted dialysis in a hospital or dialysis unit. Furthermore, these patients were better rehabilitated and had a better quality of life than those treated as outpatients in a dialysis center. For the next ten years, until introduction of the Medicare ESRD Program in 1973, funds for dialysis in the United States remained in very short supply. In consequence, in 1973 some 42 percent of the 10,000 or so dialysis patients in the United States were on home dialysis, almost all of these on home hemodialysis for 6 to 8 hours 3 times weekly.

Intermittent peritoneal dialysis (IPD) for the treatment of ESRD patients also was developed in the 1960s and early 1970s. This was usually done at home, overnight for 12 hours, 3 nights weekly, using sterile dialysate from plastic bags or bottles or prepared by a machine. However, this was a time-consuming and inconvenient treatment and, because survival was not as good as with hemodialysis, it did not become widely used.

What was the impact of the Medicare ESRD program on home dialysis?

The Medicare ESRD Program in 1973 provided almost universal entitlement to dialysis and transplantation for ESRD patients, and as a result the picture changed radically. Funding was now readily available for outpatient hemodialysis, resulting in rapid proliferation of dialysis units across the United States. Many of these were for-profit units that were often reluctant to present home hemodialysis as a treatment option, and most were directed by nephrologists lacking personal experience with a home hemodialysis program. At the same time, the patient population treated changed rapidly to include many more diabetics, minorities, and elderly patients. As a result, the use of home hemodialysis declined rapidly. By 1995, fewer than 1 percent of all dialysis patients in the United States were treated by home hemodialysis, although a few programs still persist in providing this. In contrast, in 1995 in Australia, 14 percent of patients were on home hemodialysis.

The next home dialysis innovation occurred in the late 1970s with development of continuous ambulatory peritoneal dialysis (CAPD) by Moncrieff and Popovich. This simple technique, coming at a time when access to home hemodialysis training programs was declining rapidly, gave the opportunity for more patients to experience the benefits of self-care dialysis at home. Following the success of CAPD, other varieties of peritoneal dialysis were developed, and two of these now account for about 15 percent of peritoneal dialysis patients in the United States. Continuous cycling peritoneal dialysis (CCPD) uses a cycler for treatment overnight with one or more exchanges during the day, and nocturnal intermittent peritoneal dialysis (NIPD) uses a cycler for nightly overnight peritoneal dialysis. In the United States in 1995, about 28,000 patients (14.5 percent of all dialysis patients) used some form of peritoneal dialysis, and this remains the principle mode of home dialysis.

Recently, interest in home hemodialysis has revived. New dialysis machines are being developed, designed specifically to allow patients to dialyze themselves at home without the need for an assistant. At the same time, there have been reports from Toronto and elsewhere of very impressive results with nightly home hemodialysis. Perhaps equally important, with the emphasis on providing adequate dialysis, peritoneal dialysis is becoming less attractive as a long-term treatment for many patients once their residual renal function is lost.

How does home hemodialysis compare with in-center hemodialysis?

Home hemodialysis does not differ essentially from outpatient hemodialysis in a facility, except that it is done by the patient, aided by a family member or other helper. Currently there are fewer than 2000 home hemodialysis patients in the United States. Nevertheless, this is an important treatment because of its advantages for patients. Also, with the promise of new technology and growing concern about the long-term adequacy of peritoneal dialysis, home hemodialysis could be poised for a comeback in the not-too-distant future.

What is the patient selection process for home hemodialysis?

Suitably trained and supported patients of all ages, including children and the old, can do hemodialysis at home. Contraindications include serious cardiovascular or other problems during dialysis, lack of good blood access, documented noncompliance, lack of an assistant, lack of a suitable home, inability to learn, excessive anxiety on the part of patient or family, and lack of patient motivation and willingness to undertake treatment at home. All other patients should be regarded as potential candidates for self-care and should be given information on the advantages of home dialysis, both home hemodialysis and peritoneal dialysis, when they are selecting a modality of treatment. A multidisciplinary team, working with the patient and family and the patient's nephrologist, should assess the patient's suitability for home hemodialysis, looking at medical, psychosocial and vocational factors that might affect choice of treatment modality.

Inspection of the home itself is important. There must be suitable plumbing, water and electricity, and space to store the equipment and supplies. Many homes and apartments will require only minor modifications to allow for home hemodialysis.

How would you train a home hemodialysis patient?

Home hemodialysis training is best done in a separate area using specialized staff, and, because of its specialized nature, consideration should be given to establishing regional training units. Training should begin as soon as possible once a patient has made the decision to be treated at home and is well enough to absorb information. The most difficult task for most patients is learning to do needle insertion, but this is something patients do best for themselves. From the beginning, they must be reassured that home hemodialysis is a relatively simple and safe procedure, and that when any problems occur at home, support and advice are always available from the training staff by telephone. In addition to the technique of dialysis, the patient must learn about diet, the disease and its complications, and the medical regimen. He or she should meet with a social worker, a financial counselor, a nutritionist, and an exercise coach and, where appropriate, a vocational counselor.

Training usually takes between 3 and 8 weeks once the patient becomes proficient with fistula puncture, and progress should be assessed at regular intervals. The training schedule should be arranged to allow the patient maximum opportunity to continue to work or to have access to vocational and other rehabilitation services as required.

What are the qualifications of home hemodialysis training staff?

Selection of home hemodialysis training staff is most important. They should be experienced in dialysis, have good teaching skills, be committed to encouraging independence and self-care, and be willing to allow patients to learn by making mistakes. Written materials, videotapes, films, posters, models and other educational aids can facilitate training.

What patient support services are required?

Provision of support services for home hemodialysis patients is most important. These should include follow-up visits to the physician's office at least once a month, monthly routine laboratory testing, review of dialysis records, provision of supplies, equipment maintenance and repair, availability of on-call advice from a training nurse at all times, regular follow-up visits to the home by a training nurse, and access to social, nutritional and other services as required.

Patients can take their own blood samples for laboratory tests and mail these to the laboratory. The results of these are shared with the nephrologist, the patient, and the home dialysis training program.

Back-up dialysis in a facility must be available for when a patient develops medical, technical or social problems that make dialysis at home difficult. Patients are able to take vacations, either by arranging to dialyze at a center elsewhere, or by using portable equipment. Back-up dialysis should also be available to give the opportunity for the family member or other helper to have a vacation.

What are the advantages of home hemodialysis?

Although home dialysis was first introduced for financial reasons, its other advantages for the patients soon became obvious. These included the increased patient independence, a feeling of accomplishment, opportunity to schedule dialysis into daily life, better quality of life, greater opportunity for rehabilitation, and a reduced risk of exposure to hepatitis and other infections. In contrast, patients treated in a dialysis unit have a fixed schedule and very easily become dependent on nursing and technical staff. Interestingly, very similar advantages have been reported with other treatment technologies that have been moved into the home. As Scribner pointed out thirty years ago, with any chronic disease, the more a patient understands about the illness, and the more responsibility and control taken for their own care, the greater the opportunity for adjustment and rehabilitation. A major aim in treating ESRD patients should be to maximize quality of life and encourage rehabilitation to the greatest extent possible. Studies have shown that the quality of life of home hemodialysis patients is better than that of CAPD patients, and in turn, that the quality of life of CAPD patients is better than that of patients dialyzing at a center.

Patient survival with home hemodialysis is also better than with other forms of dialysis. A recent national study using data from the United States Renal Data System (USRDS) has shown this to be the case, even with adjustment for demographic factors, diabetes and comorbid conditions. Many patients have lived very successfully for ten or even twenty years on home hemodialysis, and most of the patients active politically over the years have also been on home hemodialysis.

Recently revived interest in more frequent hemodialysis also has implications for home hemodialysis as it is much easier for patients to treat themselves six times weekly at home than to have to come to a center. Reports from Toronto, Italy, and elsewhere have shown that with such a regimen, much more dialysis can be provided. This results in remarkable improvements in blood chemistry, patient well being, quality of life and rehabilitation. As a result, knowledgeable patients are likely to be demanding home dialysis in the future.

In summary, CAPD and CCPD are relatively short-term but very effective initial treatments for many ESRD patients. When treatment becomes inadequate, these patients usually transfer to outpatient hemodialysis because they do not have access to home hemodialysis. Fortunately, attention is again being paid to improving home hemodialysis, and with the advent of safe, effective, and easily used equipment, patients will have the opportunity for better and more frequent dialysis and improved quality of life. Those patients, physicians and nurses with experience of home hemodialysis continue to believe that this provides, by far, the greatest benefits for patients who can undertake it. Consequently, now is the time to pursue home hemodialysis again as a readily available treatment option for all ESRD patients.

Diabetes and Hemodialysis

Lesley C. Dinwiddie and Beverly W. Storck

Over 16 million people in the United States of America have diabetes mellitus (DM). The majority of these are Caucasian, but blacks have double the incidence; Hispanics are two and a half times, and Native Americans are five times as likely to have DM as Caucasians.

Diabetes mellitus is the leading cause of end-stage renal disease (ESRD) in the United States. The most recent data show that in 1996 Medicare was providing renal replacement therapy (RRT) for 30,933 diabetic patients, 42 percent of the ESRD patient population of 73,091 (USRDS, 1998). Fifty-seven percent of these patients were age 60 or older. For most Caucasians, Asians, and Native Americans, DM is the dominant cause of ESRD. Hypertension is the leading cause of ESRD for African Americans (30 percent of new cases).

What is diabetes mellitus?

Diabetes mellitus is a disease process that prevents proper metabolism of glucose because of insufficient production or inefficient use of the hormone insulin. Insulin is produced by the beta cells of the pancreas. The function of insulin is to regulate blood sugar (blood glucose). Glucose is "food" for the cells of the body, and insulin facilitates the diffusion of glucose from the bloodstream to the cells. If there is a deficiency of insulin, or if the insulin cannot effect transport of glucose into the cells, the cells will "starve."

What are the 2 types of diabetes?

Type 1, formerly called juvenile diabetes or insulin-dependent diabetes mellitus (IDDM), is due to the destruction of the beta cells of the pancreas. The susceptibility to the disease is inherited, but the actual onset of the disease is due to some environmental trigger such as a virus or allergen. An autoimmune response occurs that leads to beta cell dysfunction.

Type 2, previously known as adult-onset diabetes or non–insulin-dependent diabetes mellitus (NIDDM), accounts for over 90 percent of diabetes in the United States. This number is increasing because of the growth in the more susceptible minority populations. In this condition, insulin requirements are greater than the supply, or the patient's cells are insulin resistant and require help using insulin. Dietary control, exercise, and weight loss are important factors in lowering insulin requirements and increasing insulin utilization. Family history, obesity, hypertension, and smoking are major risk factors for this type of DM.

How is diabetes treated?

Diabetes is best managed with a multidisciplinary approach, in which the physician, nurse, and dietitian plan and implement a comprehensive plan of care. Often these professionals specialize in diabetic care and work with the primary care physician. The diabetologist (physician) determines the severity of the disease and assesses its effects. Other specialists such as nephrologists and ophthalmologists are consulted periodically for assessment of organ damage and for treatment. Annual visits to the ophthalmologist are necessary for all diabetics. A podiatrist should be consulted early to treat existing foot problems, assess risk of future problems, and recommend appropriate footwear. The medical goal is to arrest tissue and organ damage by normalizing the blood sugar. In the Type 1 patient, glycemic control is achieved through diet, exercise, and insulin administration via subcutaneous injection or insulin pump. For the Type 2 patient, the treatment varies and can be diet and exercise alone, or with the addition of an oral hypoglycemic agent and/or insulin injections. Monitoring of blood glucose values dictates the need for medication or dosage adjustments. (See Table 17-1.) The dietitian creates a meal plan based on the American Diabetes Association guidelines and the individual's lifestyle preferences. In addition, the dietitian teaches and counsels the patient about the vital role that diet and exercise play in the patient's long-term outcomes. The nurse coordinates care, educates the patient and family about all aspects of care, and makes follow-up assessments of all parameters of the patient's health, including psychosocial adjustments, response to medication, diet and exercise, foot care, etc.

How is blood sugar measured and what is normal?

There are four blood sugar tests used for diagnosing and monitoring diabetes.
- A *fasting blood glucose* is measured after an 8-hour fast. For a non-diabetic patient, the range is 60–115 mg/dl. A value greater than 126 mg/dl on repeated studies may indicate diabetes.
- A *random blood glucose* greater than or equal to 200 mg/dl is diagnostic if accompanied by classic signs and symptoms.
- The *glucose tolerance test* measures both the blood and urine glucose after the patient drinks a 75 g glucose solution. Normal blood values are less than 200 mg/dl after 2 hours.
- A *finger stick blood sugar* is used by nurses to teach patients or family to perform for ongoing monitoring and evaluation. It is not used to diagnose diabetes. As implied by the name of the test, blood is obtained from a finger stick, and the amount of glucose is measured by a hand-held device called a glucometer.

Table 17-1   Medication Monitoring in Diabetes Mellitus

Drug	Action and Duration of Drug	Dialyzability	Dosing in Renal Failure
Insulin agents	Direct glucose metabolism		As per blood glucose and hemoglobin Alc
Humulin (Human insulin)	Short and long acting	No	Reduced
Humalog (Lispro)	Rapid acting	No	Reduced
Iletin (Beef/pork insulin)	Short and long acting	No	Reduced
Oral Hypoglycemics			
Sulfonylureas	Increased insulin secretion and utilization		
Acetahexamide (Dymelor)	Moderate to long acting	Unlikely	No change
Chlorpropamide (Diabenese)	Long acting	Yes	Avoid
Glipizide (Glucotrol)	Moderate to long acting	Unlikely	No change
Glyburide (Diabeta, Micronase)	Moderate to long acting	No	Avoid
Glimepiride (Amaryl)	Long acting	Unknown	Unknown
Biguanides			
Metformin (Glucophage)	Reduces insulin resistance	Yes	Strictly avoid
Other			
Acarbose (Precose)	Blocks GI glucose absorption	Unknown	Unknown
Troglidazone (Rezulin)	Helps insulin efficiency	Unknown	100%

What is hyperglycemia?

Hyperglycemia means high blood glucose. Signs and symptoms include frequent urination, excessive thirst, nausea and vomiting, weakness, confusion, and dehydration. If hyperglycemia is confirmed by a finger stick test, the episode is treated with insulin and fluids (if dehydrated).

What is hypoglycemia?

Hypoglycemia means low blood sugar. Signs and symptoms include anxiety, confusion, tachycardia, diaphoresis, and tremors. The blood sugar will usually be less than 70 mg/dl, although some patients become symptomatic at higher values. The treatment is to return the blood sugar value to normal by giving glucose-containing liquids either orally or by IV.

Both hyper- and hypoglycemia can lead to coma, a life-threatening emergency. Prior to becoming comatose the patient may appear to be very drunk.

Is there a cure for diabetes?

Not at this time. Prevention of diabetes is being studied by identifying people at risk and instituting treatments designed to delay or prevent damage to the pancreas in Type 1 or the insulin receptors on the patients' cells in Type 2. A successful pancreas transplant can restore normal insulin production, but as with any organ transplant, the patient is immunosuppressed and at risk for adverse effects of those medicines.

What is diabetic nephropathy?

Diabetic nephropathy is kidney disease caused by diabetes. The pathology seen is glomerulosclerosis, a fibrotic thickening of the glomeruli. It is thought to be caused by hyperfiltration and accumulation of glycosolated or "caramelized" proteins. As the disease progresses, the glomeruli lose their ability to filter blood effectively, resulting in the accumulation of waste products such as urea and creatinine in the body.

Diabetic nephropathy occurs in five stages:

- *Stage 1.* Increased blood flow through the kidney (hyperfiltration) results in enlarged kidneys (renal hypertrophy).
- *Stage 2.* This hyperfiltration of the glomeruli damages the membrane, causing it to leak larger molecules that would normally not pass across. The leak of albumin from the blood into the urine in known as microalbuminuria. As the loss of this and other proteins increase, the clearance of waste products such as urea and creatinine decreases.
- *Stage 3.* Microalbuminuria exceeds 200 micrograms per minute.
- *Stage 4.* Glomerular filtration rate has dropped to 75 ml/min or below, proteinuria is significantly increased, and the patient has become hypertensive. This stage is called *advanced clinical nephropathy.*
- *Stage 5.* End-stage renal disease.

Can diabetic nephropathy and progression to ESRD be prevented?

Diabetic nephropathy does not occur in all diabetics and is more likely in Type 1 than in Type 2. Studies show that tight glycemic control can significantly reduce the development and rate of progression of diabetic nephropathy. With an intensive regimen of blood glucose monitoring, insulin and/or oral hypoglycemic agent administration, and adherence to a program of diet and exercise, the majority of patients can maintain normal blood glucose levels.

Three recent studies have demonstrated this conclusion. The Diabetes and Complications Trial (DCT) was a 10-year study from 1983 to 1993. The research showed a 50 percent decrease in the development and progression of diabetic nephropathy in Type 1 patients who maintained their average blood sugar levels at 150 mg/dl, which was 80 mg/dl lower than conventionally managed controls. A comparable trial in Japan with Type 2 patients had similar results. The Minnesota Medical School trial involved the examination of the transplanted kidney tissue of diabetics. Those who had maintained tight glycemic control 5 years post transplant had fewer glomerular lesions than those who had not.

Progression of diabetic nephropathy can be delayed by the use of an angiotensin-converting enzyme (ACE) inhibitor medication. This class of drugs is usually prescribed to control hypertension but is useful for both purposes in the patient with diabetic nephropathy. It is given in Stage 1 to control hyperfiltration.

What determines when a diabetic patient who has nephropathy should start dialysis?

Initiation of dialysis depends on the individual needs and condition of the patient, but a clear indicator is a low creatinine clearance combined with symptomatic edema. Patients with diabetes suffer symptoms of uremia earlier than their non-diabetic counterparts. For this reason, it is usual to begin dialysis when the creatinine clearance is between 10–15 ml/min, but it may be started with a clearance of up to 20 ml/min. Hypertension is very difficult to manage in patients with a clearance below 10–15 ml/min. Blood pressure control is important in the management of diabetic retinopathy, as well as cardiovascular and peripheral vascular disease.

Is hemodialysis better for a patient with diabetes than peritoneal dialysis?

There are advantages and disadvantages to both modalities of treatment. The health care team and the patient must choose the treatment that best suits his/her lifestyle, taking into consideration comorbidities and medical history.

Advantages for the in-center hemodialysis include frequent medical surveillance and smaller loss of protein into the dialysate. Disadvantages are a higher risk of vascular access complications, risk of predialysis hyperkalemia, and an increased incidence of hypotension during dialysis.

Peritoneal dialysis may offer better glycemic control, especially if intraperitoneal insulin is used; it also offers better cardiovascular tolerance and potassium control and does not require vascular access. Contraindications are all the usual problems of peritoneal dialysis magnified. Examples include more episodes of peritonitis due to reduced immune response to infection, protein loss, and increased intra-abdominal pressure complications, such as gastroparesis.

Finally, inability to do peritoneal dialysis because of poor eyesight or fine motor control requires the patient to be dialyzed in-center if he/she does not have an assistant at home.

Can a patient with diabetes receive a transplant?

Yes. Living related donor transplantation is the treatment of choice for these patients because it offers a higher rate of survival than dialysis. Many younger patients with Type 1 diabetes receive combined kidney-pancreas transplants that offer the additional benefit of normal insulin production. However, many are not considered transplant candidates because of advanced age and/or atherosclerosis. A thorough evaluation is required and cardiac surgery is often necessary prior to listing the patient for a cadaveric donor transplant. A higher percentage of transplanted patients with diabetes undergo limb amputation than their dialysis counterparts. Infection and peripheral vascular disease are exacerbated by steroids. However, the increased length of survival post-transplant probably accounts for the development of these complications in this patient population.

Why do diabetics need more dialysis than non-diabetics?

Diabetes affects every cell, tissue, and organ of the body, as does uremia. Patients with diabetes who also have ESRD offer a unique challenge. According to current mortality data, only one in five of such patients who begin dialysis will be alive in five years. In order to have better survival prospects, patients with diabetes need to achieve higher urea clearance rates than other patients. Some sources say they need a Kt/V of 1.4 or greater. But with multisystem organ involvement this may be difficult to achieve. Patients with diabetes and with autonomic neuropathy are at risk for underdialysis because of hypotension in the first hour of dialysis. A diseased cardiovascular and autonomic nervous system cannot adequately respond to intravascular volume changes that occur with ultrafiltration. Dialysis blood flow is frequently lowered to treat this hypotension along with administration of extra saline. Symptomatic hypotension sometimes leads to early termination of treatment, affecting the adequacy of dialysis and leaving the patient fluid-overloaded, thus further stressing the cardiovascular system. Peripheral vascular disease contributes to vascular access problems with subsequent inadequacy of dialysis. Because of steal syndrome and previous graft failures, many patients with diabetes can only dialyze with catheter access.

Why do some dialysis patients say that they are "no longer diabetic" since they started dialysis?

Kidney failure due to diabetes has the paradoxical outcome of making the insulin that is available last longer because it cannot be broken down and excreted as efficiently. Patients with uremia frequently eat a lot less, and so need less insulin. Patients with Type 1 diabetes will always need some insulin injected unless they have a successful pancreas transplant. Type 2 patients, however, frequently no longer need additional insulin or oral medication. If they lose weight, their own insulin will be better utilized. Oral hypoglycemics, especially the long-acting ones, can cause severe hypoglycemia in the hemodialysis patient. These drugs are excreted by healthy kidneys and are not dialyzable.

How does hemodialysis affect the patient with diabetes?

The chemical composition of the dialysate is designed to be compatible with normal blood values. For all patients it has been determined that a dextrose level of 200 mg/dl is optimal. For those with diabetes, this level prevents hypoglycemia and improves hyperglycemia.

Should the diabetic patient with retinopathy get standard-dose heparin?

No. Definitive evidence has been presented to show that heparinization during dialysis puts the diabetic patient at increased risk for progression of retinopathy. On the other hand, heparin requirements should be carefully monitored and dosages adjusted accordingly.

Are insulin or the oral hypoglycemic agents dialyzable?

Insulin is the most common hypoglycemic agent for patients with diabetes on hemodialysis. Insulin and most oral agents are not dialyzable. Exceptions are metformin (Glucophage) and chlorpropamide (Diabenese). These drugs are contraindicated for use in the ESRD patient.

How is hypoglycemia managed during hemodialysis?

Hypoglycemia must be verified with a glucometer. The signs and symptoms of hypoglycemia can be confused with hypotension. Some patients require a snack or some apple juice. However, blood volume diverted to the gut for digestion may increase patients' risk for hypotension. Profound hypoglycemia may require a physician's order for an IV dextrose infusion.

How is hyperglycemia managed during hemodialysis?

If hyperglycemia is verified with a glucometer, the physician may order some regular insulin. Hyperglycemia can be a sign of infection, and the patient must be assessed and treated if an infection is present. Heparin doses may need to be increased if unusual incidences of clotting occur associated with hyperglycemia.

Are diabetic patients more difficult to keep healthy than non-diabetic hemodialysis patients?

Yes. Statistics show a higher mortality rate for patients with diabetes on dialysis. Cardiovascular disease is the leading cause of death, followed by sepsis and voluntary withdrawal from dialysis. The progression of atherosclerosis is accelerated in diabetic patients on hemodialysis, making them more prone to cardiovascular complications such as hypertension, angina, gangrene, and myocardial infarction. Hyperglycemia coupled with uremia delays wound healing and compromises immunity. Gastrointestinal neuropathy resulting in constipation as well as sudden, uncontrollable diarrhea can be a source of great distress to the patient with diabetes. Gastroparesis may cause regurgitation and aspiration.

What is gastroparesis?

Gastroparesis occurs as a consequence of autonomic neuropathy. Delay of gastric emptying is evidenced by difficulty swallowing, heartburn, nausea and vomiting, abdominal pain, and erratic blood glucose values. Treatment includes small, low-fat, and low-fiber meals; the use of drugs to improve gastric motility, such as metoclopramide (Reglan) and cisapride (Propulsid); and improved glycemic control.

Do individuals with diabetes have more vascular access problems than non-diabetic patients?

Along with atherosclerotic peripheral vascular disease, calcification of the vascular tree further limits the quantity and quality of blood vessels normally used to create access. Diabetic patients on dialysis do not experience more episodes of sepsis with their vascular access, but do require more hospitalization and have a poor prognosis. These patients do have a higher rate of graft thrombosis.

How should diabetics modify their diets once they are on hemodialysis?

Patients with diabetes already know about diet modification necessitated by errors of glucose metabolism. Now they must further modify their diets to accommodate renal failure and hemodialysis. Some patients hear about restrictions in the renal diet and feel there is nothing left to eat. Not so! While they must make new adjustments to avoid the dangers of hyperkalemia and bone disease, it is imperative that they eat well to keep up with the demands of hemodialysis, which increases the risk for malnutrition. Hemodialysis removes nutrients by depleting amino acids at the rate of 1 to 2 g/hr during treatment. Blood loss in the dialyzer and lines also contributes to protein loss. Dietary protein replacement should be at a minimum of 1.2 g/kg/day. A caloric intake of 35 kcal/kg is required to prevent the body burning protein stores for energy. Generally, protein should make up about 20 percent of the diet with 30 percent fat (preferably monounsaturated), and 50 percent carbohydrate. Diets should be tailored to patient preferences and customs. The dietary goal is to make eating pleasurable while meeting nutritional needs. Highly refined carbohydrates such as candy, cake, and pie can be incorporated into the diabetic renal diet as long as they are factored into the overall dietary plan. High-calorie, low-nutrient foods must be limited, but are not forbidden. The goal is to maintain good glycemic control.

If diabetic patients on dialysis no longer need medication for blood sugar control, should their blood sugar still be checked?

Yes. Daily checks are important to confirm good glycemic control with more frequent checks if the patient is not feeling well. An elevated blood sugar may indicate the presence of infection.

What is glycosylated hemoglobin?

A glycosylated hemoglobin value is the measurement of glucose bound to the hemoglobin of the red blood cells. Elevated blood sugar levels cause the hemoglobin to become saturated with glucose in the form of glycohemoglobin. Glycohemoglobin is present for the 120-day life span of the red blood cell. An average of the measurement of the glycolated part of the hemoglobin is called hemoglobin A1. It can be measured as subunits designated as hemoglobin A1a, hemoglobin A1b, and hemoglobin A1c. In most laboratories, only hemoglobin A1c is measured because it is the most prevalent form. Other laboratories measure the total glycohemoglobin as A1. Glycohemoglobin A1 values are 2 to 4 percent higher than hemoglobin A1c values, so it is imperative to know which standard of measurement is being used by the laboratories serving the hemodialysis facility. This test is a good indicator of compliance with the prescribed diet and medication regimen because it measures long-term glycemic control. However, studies have not been done to demonstrate that Hgb A1c values are a reliable measurement for evaluating diabetic patients with uremia. The values and interpretations for both tests in the general population, as presented in Table 17-2, allow health care professionals to recommend changes in the patient's diet and medications and to educate the patient on the importance of compliance.

Table 17-2   Values for Hemoglobin A1c and Glycosolated Hemoglobin

Values for hemoglobin A1c		Values for glycosolated hemoglobin
2.2%–4.8%	nondiabetic adult	
1.8%–4.0%	nondiabetic child	
2.5%–5.9%	good glycemic control	<7.6%
6.0%–8.0%	fair glycemic control	7.6%–8.9%
>8.0%	poor glycemic control	≥9.0%

What assessments of diabetic patients on dialysis are critically important?

Though diabetic patients make up only 5 percent of the United States population, 50 percent of all lower limb amputations are performed on this population. Frequent and careful assessment of the feet and legs of diabetic patients on dialysis should be done to identify potential problems of skin breakdown or infection. Early detection and prompt treatment may prevent serious complications.

Can diabetic foot problems be prevented?

Absolutely! Regular foot inspections should be done by the nephrology nurse with referrals to the podiatrist for attention to potential problem areas such as toenails, corns, bunions, etc. Patients should never cut their own corns or calluses and should be warned never to use heating pads, hot water bottles, or unsupervised hot water soaks. Patients and caregivers must be educated in the basics of good foot hygiene. Prosthetic footwear to protect insensitive feet from trauma are a necessity. Medicare now reimburses for prescribed shoes.

Infection Control and Universal Precautions

Georgina Randolph and Eileen Peacock

Infection control is used in the dialysis setting to prevent patients and staff from acquiring infections specific to the dialysis unit. Infection control incorporates policies and procedures that include surveillance and monitoring activities for water treatment, dialyzer reuse, bacterial contamination, and transmission of blood-borne and other infectious diseases.

The Centers for Disease Control (CDC) have issued and updated blood-borne infection control strategies and precautions (including universal precautions) over the years for dialysis centers as well as for other health care agencies. The Occupational Safety and Health Administration (OSHA) has issued regulations that enforce the use of universal precautions and other infection control strategies for all healthcare agencies. The OSHA blood-borne pathogen regulations provide specific measures that healthcare workers and their employers can do together to substantially reduce the risk of healthcare workers contracting a blood-borne disease while on the job. The CDC has also issued recommendations for preventing the spread of drug-resistant organisms and other potentially infectious diseases such as tuberculosis.

This chapter will review information personnel are required to know to help prevent the spread of infectious diseases in dialysis facilities. The chapter also includes a review of blood-borne diseases, universal precautions, as published by the CDC, as well as strategies to prevent the spread of methicillin-resistant staphylococcus aureus (MRSA), vancomycin-resistant enterococcus (VRE), and tuberculosis (TB) will be discussed. Questions commonly asked by dialysis personnel regarding water treatment, bacterial contamination, dialyzer reuse, and infection control issues are addressed in the specific chapters dealing with those subjects.

What are universal precautions?

A recommendation that blood and body fluid precautions be used consistently for all patients, regardless of their blood-borne infection status, is the basic tenet of universal precautions. Blood-borne pathogens, such as the human immunodeficiency virus (HIV) and hepatitis B virus (HBV) infect people of all ages, socioeconomic classes, and from all geographic areas. Healthcare workers may not be able to identify patients who harbor a virus or who may transmit infection. The application of "universal precautions" assumes all patients are infectious.

Reducing exposure to and transmission of blood-borne pathogens through the use of universal precautions involves appropriate work practices such as the use of barrier precautions.

Appropriate barrier precautions are to be used to prevent skin and mucous membrane exposure in contact with blood or any other body fluid of any patient. Barrier precautions also known as personal protective equipment (PPE) include the use of:

- Gloves
- Face shields/masks/protective eyewear
- Gowns

Gloves are to be worn for touching blood and body fluids, mucous membranes, or non-intact skin of *all* patients; for handling items or surfaces soiled with blood or body fluids; and for performing vascular access procedures where blood spill is likely. *Gloves* are to be changed and hands washed after contact with each patient, whenever the gloves are blood stained, and after handling infectious waste containers.

Masks and protective eyewear or face shields shall be worn during any procedure likely to generate droplets, blood splashes, or body fluids near the face. Initiating and terminating dialysis and trouble shooting the vascular access are examples of procedures that may increase a healthcare worker's risk of exposure to blood-borne pathogens if barrier precautions, such as gloves, face shield and impervious gowns/aprons are not used.

Impervious gowns or aprons are to be worn during procedures likely to generate droplets, blood splashes, or body fluids near the body. Before leaving the work area, all personal protective equipment should be removed and placed in a designated area or container for washing, decontamination, or disposal. Hands should be thoroughly washed after the removal of PPE and before leaving the work area. In addition to barrier precautions, employee work practices, such as diligent handwashing, are essential in order to reduce risk of exposure to and transmission of blood-borne pathogens.

Handwashing reduces the risk of transferring contamination from hands to other individuals, to other areas of the body or the other surfaces the healthcare worker may later contact. Hands should be washed when entering or leaving patient care areas, before gloving and after gloves are removed, and after touching an environmental surface such as the dialysis machine, without having gloved first.

Employee work practices include precautions that healthcare workers should take to prevent injuries caused by needles, scalpels and other sharp instruments that may be responsible for the transmission of blood-borne diseases.

Precautions should be taken in the following situations: when cleaning used instruments; during disposal of used needles; and when handling sharp instruments after procedures. Needles should not be recapped, purposely bent, or broken by hand, removed from disposable syringes, or otherwise manipulated by hand. After use, disposable syringes and needles, scalpel blades, and other sharp items must be placed in puncture-resistant containers located as close as practical to the use area.

Sharps containers should not be mounted too high, but should be easily accessible. They also should not be allowed to overfill.

To minimize the need for emergency mouth-to-mouth resuscitation, mouth pieces, resuscitation bags, or other ventilation devices should be available for use in areas in which the need for resuscitation is predictable.

Healthcare workers with exudative lesions or weeping dermatitis should refrain from direct patient care and from handling patient equipment until the condition resolves. All skin defects (cuts, abrasions, ulcers, etc.) must be covered with an occlusive bandage.

Pregnant healthcare workers are not known to be at greater risk of contracting HBV or HIV infection than healthcare workers who are not pregnant; however, if a healthcare worker develops HBV or HIV infection during pregnancy, the infant is at risk of infection resulting from perinatal transmission. Therefore, pregnant healthcare workers should be especially familiar with and strictly adhere to precautions to minimize the risk of HBV or HIV transmission.

What are specific examples of universal precautions in a dialysis unit?

Universal precautions in a dialysis unit can be summarized into four main categories:
- Barrier precautions/personal protective equipment such as gloves, face shield masks, protective eyewear, gowns, aprons.
- Protection against penetration caused by sharps.
- Good personal hygiene.
- Good environmental control/avoidance of environmental contamination.

During initiation and termination of dialysis, or any other time there is a risk of exposure to blood-borne pathogens, a mask, protective eyewear (glasses or face shield), and gloves *must* be worn. An impervious gown or plastic apron should be worn if there is likely to be blood splashed. A sharps container should be positioned within reach of the patient caregiver so that the needle can be disposed of immediately without having to be placed down and picked up a second time. Hands must be washed after removing gloves and before touching any environmental surfaces such as machine knobs, charts, phones, or other equipment. Eating, smoking, applying cosmetics or handling contact lenses in the treatment room must be prohibited. Good environmental controls include maintaining separate areas for clean and soiled areas, as well as adequately cleaning and disinfecting the treatment area and equipment in contact with the patient, such as chair and blood pressure cuff.

What are the most significant blood-borne pathogens?

A blood-borne pathogen simply means a microorganism (usually a virus) transmitted in the blood or body fluids. The two most significant blood-borne pathogens are hepatitis B virus (HBV) and HIV. Other blood-borne pathogens include non-A, non-B (NANB) hepatitis, delta hepatitis, hepatitis C, syphilis, malaria, and cytomegalovirus (CMV). Efficiency of transmission varies among the viruses due to the number of viruses present in the blood.

What is hepatitis?

Hepatitis is an inflammation of the liver caused by infectious agents, medications, or toxins. There are several types of infectious hepatitis (A, B, C, non-A, non-B, and delta), but hepatitis B presents the greatest risk to dialysis personnel. Hepatitis B infects approximately 8700 healthcare workers a year, resulting in more than 400 hospitalizations and 200 deaths a year.

How infectious is HBV?

Hepatitis B is a highly transmissible virus due to the high concentration of the virus in the blood of infected people (1 ml of HB_sAg-positive blood may contain 100 million infectious doses of virus) and the ability of the virus to survive for several days on environmental surfaces at room temperature.

How is hepatitis B transmitted?

In the dialysis unit exposure to blood with the possibility of HBV transmission can be either direct or indirect. Direct exposure consists primarily of penetration of the skin (percutaneous) by sharp objects such as needles, scalpels, and broken capillary tubes, or blood on broken skin and on mucous membranes of the eyes, mouth, or nose.

Indirect exposure involves transmission from environmental surfaces such as clamps, control knobs on dialysis machines and door knobs.

The most common ways hepatitis B is spread in dialysis units are by penetration of the skin by sharps and by contact of blood with broken skin or mucous membranes.

Are there additional precautions necessary to safely dialyze an HB_sAg-positive patient in the dialysis unit?

Patients who are HB_sAg positive should be dialyzed in a separate room designated only for HB_sAg-positive patients. If this is impossible, the positive patient should be separated from hepatitis B seronegative patients in a separate area removed from the mainstream of activity and should be dialyzed on a dedicated machine. The same hemodialysis equipment should not be used for both

HB_sAg-positive and seronegative patients. HB_sAg-positive patients should not participate in a dialyzer reuse program. Ideally, dialysis staff members should not care for both HB_sAg-positive and seronegative patients during the same shift, but can care for HB_sAg-positive and anti-HB_s-positive patients during the same shift. Staff members who are HB_sAg positive may be assigned preferentially to care for HB_sAg-positive patients. If, for some reason, staff members must care for both HB_sAg-positive and seronegative patients during the same shift, they must change gowns between patients, wash hands, and change gloves to prevent cross-contamination.

What are the CDC recommendations for hepatitis B serologic screening?

Patients and staff should be screened for HB_sAg and hepatitis B surface antibody (HB_sAb) to determine their serologic status before they first enter the dialysis unit. Patients and staff are each identified as one of the following: infected-HB_sAg-positive; immune-HB_sAb-positive; or susceptible-HB_sAg-negative and HB_sAb-negative. The CDC (see Table 18-1) recommends periodic screening for each of the above categories of serologic status.

Table 18-1   Recommendations for Hepatitis B Serologic Surveillance in Chronic Hemodialysis Centers

Vaccination and Serologic Status	Frequency of HB_sAg Screening		Frequency of anti-HB_s Screening	
	Patients	Staff	Patients	Staff
Unvaccinated				
Susceptible	Monthly	Semiannually	Semiannually	Semiannually
HB_sAg Carrier	Annually	Annually	None	None
Anti-HB_s-positive*	None	None	Annually	None
Vaccinees				
Anti-HB_s-positive*	None	None	Annually	None
Low Level or no anti-HB_s	Monthly	Semiannually	Semiannually	Semiannually

HB_sAg = hepatitis B surface antigen; anti-HB_s = antibody to HB_sAg.
* At least 10 miU/ml (milli international units)
                    or
  At least 10 SRUs by RIA or positive by EIA.

What about the hepatitis B vaccine?

The CDC strongly recommends the administration of hepatitis B vaccine to susceptible patients and staff as an additional means of preventing HBV in the hemodialysis unit. (See Table 18-2). In addition, if a healthcare worker has the potential to be exposed to HBV on the job, the employer is required by law to make the hepatitis B vaccination available at no cost.

Today's vaccines are safe and effective. Hepatitis B vaccines now used in the United States. are made from yeast and cannot be infected with HIV or bloodborne pathogens. Over 2 million U.S. healthcare workers have already been vaccinated. The complete series of HBV vaccinations is 85 to 97 percent effective at protecting someone from getting the disease or becoming a carrier.

What if I lose antibody protection after a couple of years?

The Public Health Service Advisory Committee on Immunization Practices states that: "Individuals who have initially responded to the hepatitis B vaccine with protective levels of anti-HBs, is and then loose detectable antibodies, do not need to receive booster shots. They are protected and will not develop clinical hepatitis." However, dialysis patients may have less complete vaccine-induced protection that may persist only as long as the antibodies remain at a certain level. Dialysis patients may need a booster dose and should have antibody testing done annually.

Table 18-2 Recommended Doses and Schedules of Currently Licensed Hepatitis B Vaccines for Adults

	Vaccine	
Group	Recombivax HB[a]	Engerix-B[a,b]
Dialysis patients	40 µg (1ml)[c]	40 µg (2ml)[d]
Healthy adults older than 19 yrs	10 µg (1 ml)	20 µg (1 ml)

[a]Usual schedule; three doses at 0, 1 and 6 months.
[b]Alternative schedule; four doses at 0, 1, 2, and 12 months.
[c]Special formulation for dialysis patients.
[d]Two 1.0 ml doses given at one site, in a four dose schedule at 0, 1, 2, and 6 months.

Source: Centers for Disease Control and Prevention: Hepatitis B virus: a comprehensive strategy, *MMWR* 40(RR-13) 1-19, 1991. Adapted from Table 1.

What do I do if I am stuck with a patient's needle or have a blood exposure to non intact skin or mucus membranes?

If you are exposed, report the incident immediately to your supervisor. If you consent, your employer is required by law to provide you with a confidential medical evaluation, necessary blood test, and any post-exposure preventive treatment and follow-up counseling. Depending on your HBV antibody status and the status of the source person (person to who's blood you have been exposed) a booster dose of the hepatitis B vaccine may be indicated. The hepatitis B immune globulin or HBIG may also be indicated.

Table 18-3 reviews a suggested approach for hepatitis B prophylaxis following percutaneous or permucosal exposure.

Table 18-3　Post-Exposure Prophylaxis: Recommendations for Hepatitis B Prophylaxis Following Percutaneous or Permucosal Exposure

Exposed person	Treatment when source is found to be:		
	HB$_s$AG-positive	HB$_s$AG-negative	Source not tested or unknown
Unvaccinated	HBIG x 1[*] and initiate HB vaccine	Initiate HB vaccine	Initiate HB vaccine
Previously vaccinated known responder	Test exposed for anti-HB$_s$ 1. If adequate,[†] no treatment 2. If inadequate, HB vaccine booster dose	No treatment	No treatment
Known nonresponder	HBIG x 2 or HBIG x 1 + 1 dose HB vaccine	No treatment	If known high-risk source, may treat as if source were HB$_s$AG-positive
Response unknown	Test exposed for anti-HB$_s$ 1. If inadequate,[†] HBIG x 1 + HB vaccine booster dose 2. If adequate, no treatment	No treatment	Test exposed for anti-HB$_s$ 1. If inadequate,[†] HB vaccine booster dose 2. If adequate, no treatment

[*]HBIG dose 0.06 ml/kg IM
[†]Adequate anti-HB$_s$ is ≥ 10 SRU by RIA or positive by EIA

What is HIV?

HIV is the human immunodeficiency virus which attacks the body's immune system, causing the disease known as AIDS, or Acquired Immune Deficiency Syndrome. Currently, there is no vaccine to prevent infection.

How infectious is HIV?

The efficiency of HIV transmission in the dialysis setting is much less than HBV due to the lower concentration of HIV in blood when compared to HBV. The concentration of HIV in blood is approximately 10 to 10,000 infectious viruses/ml.

How is HIV transmitted?

Like other bloodborne pathogens, the AIDS virus is present in the blood of infected individuals. HIV is transmitted primarily through sexual contact, but may also be transmitted through contact with blood and body fluids. The virus can also be passed to a newborn infant from an infected mother. Transmission through contact with contaminated environmental surfaces has not been documented. The virus is very sensitive to chemical disinfection and is completely inactivated by a 10% solution of 0.5% sodium hypochlorite (bleach) within 1 minute of exposure.

No airborne transmission of HBV or HIV has been documented. However, splashing, splattering, centrifuge accidents or removal of stoppers from tubes can produce droplet transfer into the mouth, or eyes, or onto defects in the skin surface.

What HIV precautions are necessary in a dialysis unit?

Universal precautions are the only thing necessary to protect patients and staff from HIV infection in the dialysis setting. Patient isolation is not necessary due to the lack of an environmental route for transmission of the virus and the low number of viruses in the blood. It is not necessary to cohort or group together HIV-positive patients. HIV testing is not recommended as a part of infection control in a dialysis unit. Also, it should not be used as a prerequisite for admission to a dialysis unit, but it may be helpful for optimal medical management and counseling. HIV testing should be part of a transplant work-up, as a transplant would be contraindicated in someone who is already immunosuppressed because of the HIV virus. If HIV antibody testing is performed, informed consent, appropriate confirmation testing, appropriate professional counseling and confidentiality of test results must be provided.

How about reuse of dialyzers for known HIV patients?

Although the CDC believes that dialyzer reuse poses no specific threat if done correctly, there are dialysis units that do not reuse dialyzers of known HIV-positive patients.

What if I am exposed to blood of someone known to be positive or test positive for HIV?

As with any blood exposure, you should immediately notify your supervisor. The source patient should be tested for evidence of HIV infection after a consent is obtained. The CDC recommends that workers with occupational exposures to HIV should receive follow-up counseling and medical evaluation, including HIV-antibody tests at baseline and periodically for at least 6 months postexposure (e.g., 6 weeks, 12 weeks, and 6 months), and should observe precautions to prevent possible secondary transmission.

In 1996 Public Health Service published source material and provisional recommendations for chemoprophylaxis (preventive drug therapy) after occupational exposure to HIV, by type of exposure. Though these recommendations are provisional, because they are based on limited data, chemoprophylaxis should be recommended to exposed workers after occupational exposures associated with the highest risk for HIV transmission. For exposure with a lower, but non-negligible risk, postexposure prophylaxis (PEP) should be offered, balancing the lower risk against the use of drugs having uncertain efficacy and toxicity. For exposures with negligible risk, PEP is not justified. If exposed, you should consult your physician regarding chemoprophylaxis.

What is hepatitis C?

Hepatitis C is the most common form of non-A, non-B (NANB) hepatitis worldwide and accounts for 90 percent of post-transfusion hepatitis in the United States. Currently, there is no vaccine to prevent infection.

How infectious is hepatitis C?

Hepatitis C is less concentrated in blood than hepatitis B and does not survive long on environmental surfaces. Concentration of infectious virus is thought to be less than 1000 per ml. However, outbreaks have occurred in dialysis units and are thought to be due to poor infection control practices. Persons at increased risk of acquiring hepatitis C include IV drug users, healthcare workers with occupational exposure to blood, hemodialysis patients and transfusion recipients.

How is hepatitis C transmitted?

Like hepatitis B and other bloodborne pathogens, hepatitis C is transmitted through percutaneous exposure to infected blood.

Are there additional precautions necessary to safely dialyze a hepatitis C-positive patient in the dialysis unit?

Patients who are positive for hepatitis C antibody or who have a diagnosis of NANB hepatitis *do not* have to be isolated or dialyzed separately on dedicated machines. They may participate in dialyzer reuse programs if liver enzyme values are acceptable.

What are the CDC recommendations for hepatitis C serologic screening?

Routine screening of patients or staff for hepatitis C antibody is *not* necessary for purposes of infection control. However, dialysis centers may wish to conduct serologic surveys of their patient populations to determine the prevalence of the virus in their center, and to determine medical management for patients or staff with a diagnosis of hepatitis C.

Although this test has a sensitivity of about 90 percent, it does not distinguish between acute and chronic infection. In addition, the test does not distinguish between people who are infectious and those who have completely recovered and cannot pass the disease on to someone else. While the CDC does not recommend routine screening for hepatitis C, regular monitoring of liver enzymes is recommended for the detection of all types of NANB hepatitis, including hepatitis C.

All patients should be monitored monthly for liver enzymes, alanine aminotransferase (ALT) and aspartate aminotransferase (AST), to detect any type of NANB hepatitis, including hepatitis C. Elevations in liver enzymes are currently more sensitive indicators of acute hepatitis C infection than is detection of hepatitis C antibody.

What is tuberculosis (TB)?

Tuberculosis is an infectious disease caused by the bacterium *Mycobacterium tuberculosis*.

How is tuberculosis transmitted?

The bacterium is carried in airborne particles (droplet nuclei) that are generated when persons with pulmonary or laryngeal tuberculosis, who are not on effective antituberculosis medication, cough or sneeze. The small droplets can remain suspended in the air for prolonged periods. While airborne on normal room current, these droplet nuclei can infect individuals as soon as the inhaled droplets containing the bacilli become established in the alveoli of the lung.

Two to ten weeks after initial infection, the healthy immune system usually limits further multiplication, and the person does not become ill. A positive TB skin test is usually the only evidence of infection.

Approximately 10 percent of these healthy individuals with latent TB will develop active TB months or years later. However, for persons infected with HIV, the risk of progression to active infectious disease is markedly increased. The CDC estimates that approximately 10–15 million persons in the United States are infected with the *Mycobacterium tuberculosis*.

What is the difference between TB infection and active TB?

Persons who progress to active contagious TB are capable of transmitting the disease. Persons infected, but who have *not* progressed on to active TB will have no symptoms, will not be contagious, and will not know they are infected unless they have a positive Mantoux skin test. It may take months or years before the person progresses into active TB, or the person may never develop active TB at all. Symptoms of active TB include prolonged coughing for 3 weeks or more, fatigue, fever, weight loss and night sweats. Medication and therapy are available.

Is tuberculosis a problem in dialysis units?

The number of cases of tuberculosis has increased in the overall U.S. population. Outbreaks have been reported in correctional facilities, hospitals, and some dialysis units. The level of risk for transmission varies by the type of healthcare facility. For example, the risk of acquiring TB may be greater in emergency rooms, where patients are provided care before screening and diagnosis take place.

Can a patient with active contagious TB be safely dialyzed in the outpatient facility?

Patients with active TB disease should not be dialyzed in ambulatory settings while infectious. These patients must be referred to hospitals with appropriate isolation accommodations (separate room, negative pressure, etc.) as prescribed by CDC Guidelines. ESRD Program regulations require freestanding dialysis units to have back-up agreements with a hospital. This may provide the mechanism for referring active TB patients for dialysis treatment until no longer infectious.

What are the CDC recommendations for tuberculosis screening?

Staff should be screened at the onset of employment. TB screening is often done at least annually. Frequency of TB screening is based on an institution's risk assessment including the community TB profile. If you live and work in an area with a high incidence of TB, the frequency of screening may be more often.

Patients should be screened on or before their first dialysis encounter. New dialysis patients may arrive after a hospitalization and/or extensive work-up. If a recent (within past year) chest x-ray or PPD was included, initial screening may not be necessary, unless risk factors are present.

CDC recommends that the two-step Mantoux be used for baseline screening. The Mantoux technique involves intradermal injection of 0.1 ml of PPD tuberculin containing 5 tuberculin units. The two-step procedure (if initial PPD is negative, PPD is repeated 1-3 weeks later) is used for baseline testing in persons who periodically receive TB skin tests to reduce the likelihood of mistaking a booster reaction for a new infection.

Nonroutine screening of patients and staff should be conducted as needed in response to clinical symptoms or documented exposure (active case identified among patients or staff).

What are drug-resistant organisms?

Drug-resistant organisms are bacteria that have mutated to defend themselves against commonly used antibiotics. Resistant strains develop quickly and crossbreed, transferring their resistance to other bacteria. Vancomycin-resistant enterococcus (VRE) and methicillin-resistant staphylococcus aureus (MRSA) are two bacteria known to be resistant to antibiotic therapy. Both VRE and MRSA have become significant nosocomial pathogens in United States hospitals and healthcare facilities. MRSA and VRE may cause infections in patients who are immunosuppressed, including ESRD patients, cancer and HIV patients, the elderly, newborns, and those being treated with multiple antibiotics. Patients at increased risk of acquiring infections due to drug-resistant organisms include the following: nursing home patients; patients with frequent hospital admissions or prolonged hospital stays; patients with chronic illnesses requiring steroid therapy; patients with catheters, such as subclavians; and patients with incisions and other openings into the body.

How are MRSA and VRE transmitted?

MRSA

The main route of transmission of MRSA is by healthcare workers' hands that have become contaminated by contact with a patient who is either infected with or carries the organisms. People may carry the organism in their nose or on the skin. Some people are carriers, and others can become infected through boils, wound infections, pressure ulcers, etc. MRSA commonly infect wound, exit sites, and access sites. Environmental surfaces may also be contaminated with MRSA and act as a reservoir for the bacteria.

VRE

Enterococcus are normal flora of the gastrointestinal and female genital tracts. Because of this, most infections with these microorganisms have been attributed to sources within the patient. However, recent reports indicate that enterococci, including VRE, can spread by direct patient-to-patient contact or indirectly via transient carriage on hands of personnel or contaminated environmental surfaces and patient-care equipment.

Can a patient with MRSA and VRE safely dialyze in the outpatient facility?

Standard infection control or universal precautions recommended by CDC should provide sufficient protection against the transmission of MRSA in the dialysis unit.

The CDC standard precautions include:
- **Wash hands after touching blood, body fluids, excretions, and contaminated items, even when wearing gloves.** Also, wash hands after gloves are removed, between tasks, and between procedures on the same patient to prevent cross contamination of different body sites.
- **Wear gloves when touching blood, body fluids, excretions, and contaminated items.** Gloves should be put on before touching mucous membranes and nonintact skin, and they should be removed promptly after use.
- **Wear a mask and eye protection or face shield.** These will protect the mucous membranes of the eyes, nose, and mouth during procedures that are likely to cause splashing or spraying of body fluids.
- **Wear a gown for protection from skin contamination and soiling of clothing during procedures and patient-care activities.**
- **Handle patient-care equipment that is soiled with body fluids and excretions in a manner that prevents skin exposures and contamination of clothing.** Make sure reusable equipment is not used for the care of other patients until it has been sanitized.

In addition to these standard precautions, patients with VRE who have draining wounds not contained by dressings, who have diarrhea or are incontinent, who have poor hygiene or are confused and are handling their dressings, etc., should be dialyzed in a separate room or area. It is important to dedicate the use of noncritical items, such as stethoscope or sphygmomanometer, to a single patient or group of patients who are infected with or are carriers of VRE. If such devices are to be used on other patients, adequate cleaning and disinfect]ing must first take place.

How about sterilization and disinfection procedures in the dialysis unit?

All dialysis units must have written policies and procedures that deal with disinfection of the dialysis fluid pathway of the hemodialysis machine. These procedures are targeted to control bacterial contamination and have nothing to do with preventing bloodborne infections. The procedures generally consist of using sodium hypochlorite (bleach) on a regular basis (according to manufacturers' instructions) and a sterilant overnight at certain intervals (e.g., every 100 hours of use). Studies have shown that the HIV virus is inactivated rapidly after being exposed to commonly used chemical germicides at concentrations that are much lower than used in practice. The much hardier HBV virus is also known to be inactivated by common household bleach. Suggested concentrations of sodium hypochlorite prepared daily range from 500 ppm (1:100 dilution of household bleach) to 5000 ppm (1:10 dilution).

What about cleaning other surfaces?

Machine surfaces, patient chairs, and other surrounding furniture and equipment, such as an infusion pump, should be routinely wiped down with a 1:100–1:10 bleach solution following every patient treatment. Environmental surfaces such as walls, floors, and other surfaces should be routinely cleaned consistent with good housekeeping practices. Extraordinary attempts to disinfect or sterilize these surfaces are not necessary. Blood spills should be cleaned immediately. Linen soiled with blood or body fluids should be transported in leak-proof bags.

What about waste disposal?

There are two kinds of waste seen in the dialysis unit; regular trash and infectious waste. Regular trash, which is mostly paper and plastic, can be disposed of by the usual practice. Infectious waste, which is usually defined in a dialysis unit as "bloody," must be disposed of in specially labeled red bags. Various states have laws regarding the definition of infectious waste and its disposal.

Has peritoneal dialysis waste tested positive for HIV?

HIV antibody have been detected in the dialysate waste of AIDS patients. To date there are no national guidelines for the disposal of waste dialysate from AIDS patients.

Are there additional precautions that should be taken when caring for the patient on home peritoneal dialysis?

Universal precautions must be observed with all patients when there is possibility of contact with blood or body fluids. In addition, each renal unit devises its own criteria for safe disposal of waste fluids for the patient both at home and in the unit setting. Patients at home should be instructed to drain their bags into the toilet and then seal the empty bag in a plastic bag before disposal with household garbage. In the CAPD unit a toilet or sluice should be used whenever possible. Many units use a 1:10 bleach solution following the dialysate. Some units suggest adding 10 ml of bleach to the bag before disposal. If a sink is used for waste disposal, a bleach solution should follow the waste and preferably sit for 30 minutes.

Psychosocial Aspects of Dialysis Therapy

Mara Hersh-Rifkin and Martha H. Stoner

Dialysis, as a means of prolonging life for an indefinite period, took on new psychosocial implications on July 1, 1973, when the Medicare End-Stage Renal Disease Program (Public Law 92-603, Section 2991) became effective in the United States. The Medicare act made major financial coverage available to 90 percent of patients with renal failure, without regard for age or complicating disease processes.

Psychosocial issues were recognized by medical and mental health professionals as impediments to adjustment and satisfactory quality of life for ESRD patients long before Medicare entered the dialysis picture. This became even more apparent when federally supported dialysis treatment was determined to be the right of all persons with kidney failure. Some of the psychosocial factors include: changes in an individual's work and family situation, financial concerns, and the stress of living with a life-challenging illness.

Is it possible to predict how a patient will react to maintenance hemodialysis?

Little work has been done to help healthcare professionals predict how patients will react to the multiple changes and stresses associated with life on dialysis. Most studies have involved small numbers of patients and showed little agreement regarding predictive parameters. An individual's method of coping with past life stresses remains the best single indicator of his or her adaptability to daily life with dialysis. Frustration tolerance, aggression, denial of the sick role, and obsessive-compulsive characteristics are personality traits that can be evaluated and used to help predict a patient's potential adjustment to dialysis.

An evaluation of the patient's coping methods is conducted, in part, by a mental health professional (usually a clinical social worker) on the dialysis treatment team. An in-depth psychosocial evaluation that includes interviews with both the patient and his or her family is conducted by the social worker at the initiation of chronic dialysis treatment. Based on this evaluation, a treatment plan is formulated to include psychosocial counseling and community resource referrals that can enhance the patient's ability to cope. Often the social worker can provide support and reassurance to both patient and family as well as help alleviate pressing resource needs, such as assistance with financial and insurance problems.

What are the stages of adjustment to dialysis that a patient with ESRD may experience?

When the onset of ESRD is gradual, the patient has time to adjust to the idea of dialysis and to make well-informed treatment choices. The initial response to dialysis itself can be one of relief, especially if the patient has been feeling ill for a period of time. Unfortunately, some patients delay beginning dialysis until they are quite ill and then may require the initiation of dialysis on an emergency, hospitalized basis.

When the onset of ESRD is sudden, there can be an acute crisis phase of adjustment, often marked by feelings of shock, disbelief, desperation, and depression. In such cases, a crisis intervention approach by a trained mental health professional is indicated. Three stages of patient adjustment to dialysis have been identified:

- *The "honeymoon" period* is defined as a patient's initial response to dialysis, which can last from a few weeks to 6 months or more. Usually, this phase is one of physical and psychological improvement and is accompanied by renewed feelings of hope and confidence. During the "honeymoon" period, patients may respond to staff in a positive and grateful manner. This does not mean that patients do not also experience periods of anxiety and depression but rather that they may view dialysis in a more positive way overall because they feel better than they did before the initiation of dialysis.

- *The period of disenchantment and discouragement* is marked by reduced feelings of confidence and hope and can last from 3 to 12 months. This phase is usually triggered when an individual returns to some previous routine or employment and is forced to confront the limitations dialysis places on these activities. During this time, feelings of sadness and helplessness may arise.

- *The period of long-term adaptation* is characterized by the patient's arrival at some degree of acceptance of the limitations, shortcomings, and complications that dialysis brings into his or her life. Patients can experience long periods of contentment alternating with episodes of depression. Adaptation often can be facilitated by a return to some form of meaningful work or by settling down to doing little or no work at all. Incorporation of diet and activity restrictions and the dialysis procedure into the daily lifestyle is part of long-term adaptation.

These periods of adjustment are presented as general guidelines only. Not all researchers and practitioners agree about this sequence of phases. There is not always a linear progression from one stage to another, and for individual patients the various stages may be much briefer or much longer than indicated above. Further, patients may shift back and forth from stage to stage for a variety of reasons, including medical complications.

How can the quality of life of a patient on dialysis be evaluated?

Quality of life is a phrase that is sometimes used interchangeably with such terms as *life satisfaction*, *well-being*, and *morale*. Usually, quality of life is defined as encompassing major areas of functioning in the physical, psychological, and social realms. Further, feelings about this issue are relative perceptions for each individual, and any attempt to evaluate quality of life must take into account the significance of these highly subjective perceptions. What is an intolerable situation for one patient may not be for another.

Several instruments developed to measure quality of life for research purposes may be used for clinical assessment as well. In addition to using formal measures, dialysis personnel should provide patients with opportunities to talk about their own feelings and perceptions regarding their quality of life.

What can be done to enhance the quality of life for dialysis patients and their families?

Evaluation and planning for psychosocial intervention should begin before the patient actually needs dialysis. Patients and their families should be educated about dialysis and be encouraged to participate actively in deciding various aspects of the treatment program, including the type of dialysis. Evaluation of the type of dialysis to be used for a patient should include an assessment of the challenges he or she is facing, as well as personal, family, work, and social considerations. It is essential for staff to identify individuals who are at great risk for psychosocial dysfunction because early introduction of vocational and psychotherapeutic counseling (for the individual or family) can increase the patient's rehabilitation potential and improve his or her quality of life.

Once a patient has begun dialysis, the dialysis staff needs to institute interventions to maximize the positive and minimize the negative effects of dialysis on the patient's quality of life. Such interventions might include counseling by the dialysis social worker or other mental health professional who is familiar with the dynamics of ESRD and the dialysis process.

What are common sources of stress for dialysis patients?

Patients with ESRD are confronted with severe limitations and demands upon themselves and their families. They must contend with changes in family relationships, such as role reversal and deteriorating sexual responsiveness, and with accompanying feelings of guilt, depression, and loss. The threat of reduced job responsibility or unemployment can contribute to feelings of worthlessness and loss of self-esteem. Many patients experience conflict between the need to be dependent on a machine and on other people and the desire to remain independent. They may feel that they have relinquished control of their lives to the dialysis team. Underlying many of these feelings is the basic fear of dying. The patient's dependence on the dialysis machine can be a constant reminder that he or she has been rescued from death.

How can the dialysis team assist patients and families in coping when dialysis becomes necessary?

Dialysis patients and family members who regard renal failure and the need for dialysis as a loss may grieve over that loss. Dialysis personnel should be familiar with the issues of grief and the grieving process and be prepared to provide appropriate intervention or call upon a resource person, such as a psychiatric nurse, social worker, psychologist, or psychiatrist, as needed. If members of the dialysis team are able to recognize periods of exceptional stress and use appropriate crisis intervention approaches, they can help patients cope with such periods and prevent major adjustment problems.

Patients who are unable to accept the restrictions imposed upon them by dialysis may become depressed and unable or unwilling to adhere to their dialysis regimen. When this occurs, the diminished quality of life and increased potential for death should be addressed by prompt recognition and social work or psychotherapeutic intervention.

What are some psychologic reactions and common coping mechanisms of patients on maintenance dialysis?

Anxiety is the initial reaction for most patients and families faced with the prospect of life on dialysis. Such anxiety is entirely normal, and dialysis staff need to reassure patients that this is the case.

Depression may occur early on during the treatment process. Again, this is a rational reaction to the prospect of a limited and risky life that will require totally different objectives than would have been planned otherwise.

Hostility and anger are frequent reactions of patients on dialysis. Hostility toward dialysis personnel and the medical regimen is actually a reaction to the limitations imposed by the disease, but the anger is displaced to the treatment staff and procedure.

A difference of opinion exists as to the role that the *denial* mechanism plays in patients who have become stabilized on dialysis. To staff involved in the primary care of these patients, denial seems to be a common defense that allows the patient to cope with the realities of the situation while regarding them as not a part of his or her real self. Denial used in this way can be very useful for the patient because it shuts out negative aspects of the illness. However, denial can be carried to extremes, subverting medical management, and the result can be disastrous.

Do emotional factors affect the patient's long-term survival?

Successful life with a dialysis regimen requires a willingness and ability to adhere to dietary and fluid restrictions, medication regimens, and dialysis procedures. Most people adjust to these restrictions and show great responsibility.

In what ways does nonadherent behavior affect the patient's physical condition?

Nonadherent behavior can be manifested in a number of ways:
- Nonadherence to the prescribed diet is a manifestation of the denial mechanism gone astray. This can contribute to increased morbidity and even mortality.
- Ingestion of excess fluid represents denial of kidney failure with potentially harmful results.
- Inadequate care of vascular or peritoneal access is sometimes a problem. A clotted or infected vascular access may not be discovered until time for a dialysis treatment. With peritoneal dialysis, use of an improper technique may lead to infection.
- Manipulation of treatment time can be another manifestation of nonadherent behavior. Skipping treatments and shortening treatment times are examples of this behavior.

Such behaviors can contribute to malnutrition, neuropathy, bone disease, cardiac failure, and the like. If these behaviors persist, they result in physical deterioration and, in extreme cases, death—a form of passive suicide.

How can such adverse behaviors be countered?

Patients sometimes resent consultation with a psychiatrist. In such cases, the patient may be defensive and unwilling to admit that a problem exists or that problems may have an emotional basis. Even if the psychiatrist is recognized as a member of the treatment team, there is a tendency to avoid such counsel. Group sessions that involve patients as well as family members and are guided by a skilled and accepted social worker or psychiatric nurse (using the psychiatrist as a resource person) may be a more readily accepted form of help. Within such a group setting, ventilation, sharing of problems, and discussions with peers can help resolve many problems. The psychiatrist, psychiatric nurse, or social worker can also help medical and other personnel deal with a patient's resistant behaviors. These professionals can offer reassurance and suggest approaches to help other members of the dialysis team assist the patient in handling the challenges of dialysis.

What emotional problems are commonly seen in family members?

Anxiety is a common and normal response in family members, particularly when the patient first begins dialysis. With the passage of time, other stresses may bring added reactions. The continued drain on financial resources and the need for role changes within the family may create additional problems and resentment. Often, a patient on dialysis may become increasingly dependent, demanding and irascible. Resenting the loss of a positive self-image and self-esteem, either real or imagined, he or she may react in an antagonistic manner toward the rest of the family. Family members, in turn, may become hostile toward the patient and then feel guilty for having these feelings.

Nurses and other dialysis personnel can provide opportunities for family members to ventilate hostility and anxiety through the use of active listening techniques. Staff can offer reassurance that these are normal reactions. Furthermore, other team members may act as liaisons with the psychiatrist or social worker in developing a realistic plan to help the patient and family resolve problems that arise.

What are some of the physical problems that can adversely affect the psychosocial adjustment of dialysis patients?

Insomnia, chronic pruritus, neuropathy symptoms, muscle cramps, and bone and joint pain are some of the most commonly identified physical problems that contribute to a diminished quality of life for patients on dialysis. Ongoing assessment of the physiological response to ESRD and dialysis therapy is essential. In many cases, medical management can alleviate the physical problems, enhancing the patient's psychological adjustment and improving his or her quality of life. Some patients need to be encouraged to report physical symptoms, as they may otherwise assume that nothing can be done about them.

How does the dialysis procedure itself affect the psychosocial adjustment of dialysis patients?

The time commitment is probably the single aspect of the dialysis regimen that exercises the largest influence on a patient's adjustment to treatment. The time demand may interfere with the patient's ability to perform activities of daily living, resulting in loss of independence and, ultimately, lowered self-esteem and depression. Dialysis personnel need to work with the patient to design the least restrictive regimen possible. Encouraging the patient to perform self-care activities and to maintain some degree of independence will sustain a more positive psychosocial adjustment.

How does social support influence the psychosocial adjustment of patients on dialysis?

Social support, both in terms of quantity and quality, has been associated with better levels of psychological adjustment in persons living with any chronic illness. Family members are usually the greatest source of social support for a patient. However, to maintain their ability to be supportive of the patient, family members may need the assistance of dialysis personnel. In addition, patients and family members should be encouraged to continue to participate in social and leisure activities both within and beyond the family. The dialysis social worker can provide referrals to patient and family support groups and community resources for socialization. Caregiver groups, peer support, and senior-citizen centers can be included as appropriate.

What type of relationship should there be between the dialysis patient and the nurse or technician?

It is not uncommon for a dependence to develop between dialysis personnel and patients. This type of relationship may be very satisfying to the nurse or technician and may fulfill a desire to be needed. However, an excessively close relationship may cause the professional to exercise faulty judgment, which can be detrimental to the patient. Patients need to be encouraged to do things for themselves, whenever possible, to preserve and promote a sense of independence.

It is best if one staff person can be responsible for working with a given patient and his or her family. This helps prevent the problems that can be created by inconsistent responses to questions. In their anxiety, people tend to ask slightly different versions of their questions of everyone. The result can be ambiguity and chaos. Questions should be answered consistently, accurately, and honestly, and this is best accomplished if one team member serves as the primary information source for each patient and his or her family.

Do patients have unrealistic expectations of dialysis therapy?

It is not uncommon for patients to expect a greater degree of curative capability than dialysis can actually provide. Dialysis provides a lifesaving therapy, but it does not *cure* uremia. The patient and his or her family still must live and cope with a chronic illness.

How may these problems be countered?

Patients and their families need to be well informed and have a solid understanding of the disease process *and* the necessary treatment. A well-planned and well-executed patient education program is a vital aspect of the care of any person with ESRD.

Patient and family group meetings, held at regular intervals and guided by a qualified team member, can provide a great deal of support and problem-solving of a self-help nature. Patient care conferences involving all members of the dialysis team should be held regularly to keep all personnel current on patient problems and how they are being approached. Otherwise, with a large number of patients, the effort can become fragmented.

Is the sexual dysfunction experienced by many dialysis patients emotional in origin?

Sexual dysfunction in dialysis patients involves both emotional and organic factors. Organic elements that contribute to decreased sexual functioning are thought to include severe anemia, impaired testosterone and other hormonal levels, and increased PTH levels. These conditions can lead to reduced fertility and libido. Medications, particularly some antihypertensive agents, also may contribute. In addition to these organic causes, depression also seems to be an important element in the sexual dysfunction of dialysis patients. Even with correction of anemia with EPO, sexual dysfunction is still a major problem.

Both the patient and his or her partner need to be aware of the potential for sexual dysfunction and be provided with a framework for discussion about sexuality. In many cases, the nephrologist or mental health professional will need to initiate the discussion about sex, rather than expect patients to bring the topic up on their own. Together, the physician and social worker can provide a forum for discussion. Counseling may be helpful in some cases, and it should be possible for a couple to work out acceptable alternatives.

What degree of rehabilitation may be anticipated for dialysis patients?

Rehabilitation can be defined in both broad and narrow terms. Using a liberal definition, rehabilitation may be considered successful if an individual is able to fulfill family role responsibilities and occupy himself or herself with meaningful activities.

As defined in the narrow sense, meaning the return to a prior level of functioning, dialysis patients may have limited rehabilitation potential. Homemakers and students frequently are able to resume their customary activity schedules with minor limitations. The growing number of ESRD patients with concurrent illnesses and accompanying sensory and motor deficits has resulted in a decrease in the proportion of patients able to return fully to their previous level of functioning. With improved dialysis techniques and the correction of anemia, it is increasingly realistic for ESRD patients to consider returning to some type of work after commencing dialysis.

How can a dialysis patient's rehabilitation potential be enhanced?

In recent years there has been an increased focus on rehabilitation in the dialysis population. The dialysis social worker can refer patients to state vocational rehabilitation programs that can be helpful in assessing the patient's potential and identifying alternative sources of employment. These programs may include an educational component with referral to job training or educational programs within the community college system or at local universities. In some cases, financial assistance is available to low income patients.

What are Advance Directives (ADs)?

An AD is a written document that an individual completes that specifies in advance what kind of medical treatments he or she wants or does not want in the event of an incapacitating condition. In 1991, a federal law, The Patient Self-Determination Act (Danforth Bill: Public Law 101-508) went into effect. The Law applies to most healthcare organizations and providers. It requires that patients be given information concerning their legal rights to make decisions about the medical care and treatment they are about to receive. An AD can be a Durable Power of Attorney for Health Care or a Living Will. Requirements for what needs to be specified vary from state to state. This is a hard subject to discuss with anyone but can be particularly difficult to explore with someone who is confronting a life-threatening illness. Often it is the role of the social worker to provide information about AD to patients and their families, but all staff should be familiar with the law and issues surrounding Advance Directives.

What about patients who decide to discontinue dialysis?

In planning the treatment regimen, the staff should include a comprehensive and open discussion about the options available to patients. The right not to begin dialysis and the right to withdraw from dialysis are among these options. Such decisions are based on the specific needs and desires of the individual patient, with consideration of his or her medical condition. A decision to discontinue or not to initiate dialysis is usually made in conjunction with family members, the physician, and other members of the dialysis team, including the chaplain and the psychiatrist. In general, older persons who have complications because of underlying illnesses are more likely to discontinue dialysis than are younger individuals. When a patient has elected to discontinue dialysis, members of the professional team need to provide supportive care with an emphasis on physical and emotional comfort.

In what ways can the ESRD patient achieve more control over his or her own situation?

Patients who previously led very independent lives may be at increased risk for psychosocial difficulties with the onset of dialysis treatment. It is especially important that these individuals be given opportunities to participate in their treatment regimens as much as possible. Patients may feel a greater sense of control over their situation if they are encouraged to perform self-care dialysis on the hemodialysis unit or during home hemodialysis. PD can be a positive choice for patients with a need or desire for freedom from dialysis schedules.

Pediatric Hemodialysis

Helen Currier and Eileen D. Brewer

Treating children is complicated by the fact that they are still growing and developing, and chronic renal insufficiency and ESRD interfere with this normal growth and development. Thus, pediatric nephrology nurses must have a comprehensive knowledge of pediatric nursing and childhood growth and development.

What is family-centered care in a pediatric patient population?

The concept of family-centered care developed from an awareness that young patients' emotional and developmental needs are best be met by incorporating their families into the plan of care.

What are the staffing considerations for a pediatric hemodialysis population?

The hybrid of services that a pediatric dialysis facility provides necessitates a good method of matching resources to patient workload activity. The best choice is a time/motion study-based, statistically validated, patient-dependency classification system. A patient-dependency system takes into account factors such as developmental age versus chronological age and matches care requirements with the appropriate numbers of staff at each skill level. The patient-dependency system captures the care requirements of a patient who may be less ill, but is more dependent due to age, developmental level or cultural requirements, or who requires more frequent or different types of interventions than other patients with the same diagnosis. Because of the many pediatric patient-dependency categories, staffing requirements for pediatric care comprise a complex matrix that is most easily implemented with a staffing and scheduling system that targets staffing by skill level. As a patient's dependency level increases, increased caregiver skills are usually required. The system must also recognize the potential for day-to-day variation in an individual child's care requirements and in the staff required to provide that care. Determining staffing by matching caregiver-to-patient ratios with patient ages or sizes can be a disadvantage, since ratios presume that all patients with the same age or weight necessarily require the same level of care every day.

How can a pediatric facility maximize operations when it has a small patient base?

Many pediatric dialysis facilities maximize operations by cross training nursing staff in both acute and chronic renal replacement therapy. During orientation the pediatric dialysis nurse learns how to manage all of the therapies furnished by a particular facility. Commonly these include the pediatric modalities of hemodialysis, peritoneal dialysis and continuous renal replacement therapy. Some pediatric dialysis facilities offer additional extracorporeal therapies such as hemoperfusion and plasmapheresis. Orientation can take anywhere from six weeks to three months, depending on prior experience and learning opportunities. Simulated clinical experiences in a skills laboratory can supplement learning experiences. A broad orientation plan and a gradual progression to independence with a designated preceptor guiding the progress toward acquisition of knowledge and mastery of skills has worked best in our experience.

Is there a place for technical support in the care of children on hemodialysis?

Some programs employ technicians for well-defined tasks, such as preparing equipment for dialysis or assisting registered nurses with children who are not developmentally delayed and who weigh more than 35 kg. A well-defined orientation plan, competency list, and method of documenting progress are important. Some states have specific stipulations for technical support personnel; check with the state Department of Health for specific state guidelines.

What are the causes of acute renal failure in children?

Acute renal failure in children usually results from hypoperfusion of the kidneys due to septic shock, hypotension, severe dehydration from gastroenteritis or from acute blood loss from surgery or an accident. The pathology is that of acute tubular necrosis. Acute tubular necrosis can also occur after nephrotoxic drugs, especially aminoglycoside antibiotics and amphotericin B. The most common cause of primary acute renal failure in children in North America is the *hemolytic uremic syndrome*. Acute post-streptococcal glomerulonephritis, though common in children, rarely leads to acute renal failure severe enough to warrant dialysis.

What are the causes of ESRD in children?

The causes of ESRD are different for children than for adults. About two-thirds of the cases in children are caused by congenital urinary tract anomalies, such as posterior urethral valves, obstructive uropathy, reflux nephropathy, renal dysplasia and neurogenic bladder associated with spina bifida, or hereditary diseases, including cystinosis, hyperoxaluria and autosomal recessive polycystic kidney disease. The other one-third are caused by acquired kinds of glomerulonephropathy, like focal segmental glomerulosclerosis or membranoproliferative glomerulonephritis. Unlike ESRD in adults, diabetic nephropathy, chronic hypertension, autosomal dominant polycystic kidney disease, and membranous glomerulonephritis are rarely causes of ESRD in childhood and adolescence.

When is hemodialysis the right choice for pediatric ESRD patients?

The preferred modality of treatment for ESRD for most pediatric patients is renal transplantation. If a pediatric patient needs chronic dialysis, home peritoneal dialysis is the usual choice, but may not always be possible. Some family situations are unable to support chronic peritoneal dialysis. Some patients may have lost peritoneal function from previous abdominal surgery or peritonitis. Currently younger children, including infants and toddlers with ESRD, who have failed peritoneal dialysis and who are not yet eligible for transplantation or who are waiting on the cadaveric transplantation list, require chronic hemodialysis. Technical advances in equipment and vascular access catheters have made chronic hemodialysis possible even in small children. Some adolescents may choose hemodialysis because of concerns about body image or their ability to comply with the discipline of chronic peritoneal dialysis and the need for daily treatment.

What is the significance of body surface area to renal function in pediatrics?

Normal serum creatinine concentration increases with age and body mass. The normal serum creatinine level in a 2-year-old is 0.4 mg/dl, while in an adult it is about 1.0 mg/dl. If it were 1.0 mg/dl in a 2-year-old, that child would have renal failure with about a 60 percent reduction in renal function. In order to compare parameters of renal function in different sized pediatric patients from infancy to adolescence, creatinine clearance and other measures of glomerular filtration rate are usually normalized to the average adult body surface area of 1.73 m^2. The normal range for creatinine clearance in a pediatric patient older than 2 years of age is $100–120 \text{ ml/min}/1.73 \text{ m}^2$. When the creatinine clearance decreases below $10–15 \text{ ml/min}/1.73 \text{ m}^2$, the pediatric patient has ESRD.

Is there a preferred measure of weight for children?

The preferred measure of weight in children is metric, since most therapies are prescribed per weight in kilograms. Consistent use of the metric system to measure weight in children lessens calculation error. If a kilogram scale is not available, convert pounds to kilograms by dividing by a factor of 2.2.

Are there particular considerations when choosing a hemodialysis station location for the child dialyzing in an integrated pediatric and adult care facility?

Because of the higher dependency of the pediatric hemodialysis patient, especially those weighing less than 35 kg, the station for hemodialysis should be within easy access and centrally visible. In the event of an emergency in another patient, every effort should be made to protect the child from viewing the stressful event.

Do children ever require isolation?

Communicable diseases, such as varicella (chicken pox), are common in childhood. In addition to isolation for bloodborne pathogens, children may need to be isolated during periods when they are at risk of manifesting communicable diseases after recent exposure. Each facility should develop general recommendations for isolation for children exposed to communicable diseases, like varicella to avoid exposure of susceptible adult patients.

What is the safe limit for extracorporeal volume for a child?

The safe limit for extracorporeal volume in a child is 10 percent or less of the child's blood volume (Table 20-1). This blood is returned to the patient at the end of the treatment, unless it is needed for laboratory tests. In this case, no more than 3 percent to 5 percent of the child's blood volume should be removed on a given day. Many laboratories have microcontainers for blood sampling for small children or use minimal blood volumes for tests to help avoid excess blood loss in pediatric patients.

Table 20-1   Approximate Blood Volume by Age

Age	Total Blood Volume
Premature infants	90–105 ml/kg
Term newborns	78–86 ml/kg
>1 month–1 year	78 ml/kg
>1 year–adult	74–82 ml/kg
Adult	68–78 ml/kg

How does one calculate extracorporeal volume?

Extracorporeal volume is the total volume of the dialyzer plus the blood lines. Specific values are available from product manufacturers.

Can hemodialysis treatment be done when the extracorporeal volume exceeds the safe limits?

When extracorporeal volume is 10 percent to 12.5 percent of blood volume, the system must be primed with a volume expander such as 5 percent albuminized saline. When extracorporeal volume exceeds 12.5 percent of blood volume, reconstituted whole blood may be the safest for priming and is imperative when extracorporeal volume is 15 percent or more. There are specific dialysis products designed to minimize extracorporeal blood volume for small children, and these must be used to avoid the expense and risk of using blood products routinely. The pediatric nephrologist decides how much, *if any*, of the system prime is returned to the patient at the end of the treatment, based on the patient's specific albumin or hemoglobin deficit.

How is replacement blood transfusion volume calculated should a pediatric hemodialysis patient suffer an acute blood loss (i.e., clotted system)?

To replace acute blood loss associated with hemodynamic instability, transfuse packed red blood cells at 10 ml/kg body weight or more, depending on the estimated amount of blood lost and the child's hemoglobin prior to the loss.

What are the vascular access considerations in pediatrics?

The smaller the pediatric patient, the more difficult it will be to establish adequate access for hemodialysis. In patients weighing less than 10 kg, an indwelling catheter of appropriate diameter placed in a major vessel will be the only option. It is important for the catheter not to come close to or exceed the vessel size, which will lead to obstruction of normal venous flow. Dual and single-lumen cuffed catheters are now available for use even in very small children (5- to 10-kg body weight). In the hands of a skilled pediatric access surgeon, an arteriovenous loop graft in the thigh may be possible for patients >10 kg, and a primary arteriovenous fistula in the forearm, for patients >15 kg. In general, permanent access is extremely difficult when the patient is smaller than 20 kg and should be placed only by a surgeon or pediatric nephrologist skilled in these procedures.

Do children require special dialyzers?

In choosing the dialyzer for a pediatric hemodialysis patient, the dialyzer surface area (available from the product manufacturer) often approximates the child's body surface area. Dialyzers as small as 0.22 m^2 are available. The type of dialyzer chosen should be based on the blood volume of the dialyzer as well as the prescription for dialysis adequacy and the ultrafiltration coefficient. Hollow-fiber dialyzers are preferred because of their low compliance.

Are there special pediatric blood lines?

Many manufacturers offer neonatal or pediatric-size blood lines, which offer a substantial decrease in volume over adult lines. As these specialized blood lines tend to be shorter in length, caution should be taken to secure the lines so that there is no tension on the patient's access site.

Are there hemodialysis machines specifically for children?

Volumetric hemodialysis equipment that is used for adults can be safely used for children. Volumetric equipment decreases the margin of error for fluid removal. Note that *all* hemodialysis system manufacturers warn of the potential variance from target of 10 percent for fluid removal, which is especially important in the small patient, where 10 percent can be a substantial amount compared to the patient's total body water.

Can reprocessed dialyzers be safely used for children undergoing hemodialysis?

Only a few pediatric care facilities practice reuse. Reuse is more widely practiced in larger integrated pediatric and adult care facilities.

How is pain associated with hemodialysis managed in children?

For the discomfort of fistula needle insertion, pain management options include topical anesthetics (e.g., EMLA Creme) or subcutaneous 1% lidocaine at the needle insertion sites. Some children, often preschoolers, find topical anesthetics ineffective and subcutaneous 1% lidocaine "just another stick." For these patients a fistula needle insertion without anesthetic may be the best tolerated option. Additional pain management techniques include deep breathing, distraction (e.g., blowing bubbles or inverting a glitter wand), or visual imagery, such as focusing on a softly colored light. Remember that crying is a *normal* response to pain or to fear of a needle before there is pain. The key to pain management success includes a consistent approach and good communication with the patient/family. The team should take every opportunity to soothe anxieties, to offer an array of pain management options, and to positively reinforce desired behavior, such as holding still.

If a child must be immobilized for needle insertion, minimize the personnel involved and focus on immobilizing the child's joints to prevent movement that will interfere with successful needle placement. Children less than 10 kg are best swaddled. Only rarely should a child require restraints, and then only for a short time period. When restraint is deemed necessary, a medical order should be written and refreshed with each hemodialysis treatment for which restraint is used.

Is sequential ultrafiltration used in children?

Sequential ultrafiltration (UF) is only appropriate in older children and adolescents. Small infants requiring 5% albuminized saline or reconstituted whole blood prime should not have sequential UF. Prolonged UF in a small child can lead to hypothermia because the blood compartment will not be warmed by dialysis fluid.

How does one determine the target weight for a child on hemodialysis?

If the patient is growing, his or her weight should be gradually increasing. Target weight is the weight at which a patient with an adequate Kt/V is normotensive and euvolemic. Noninvasive inline monitoring devices, such as the CritLine, can help refine target weight determinations during a dialysis treatment. In growing children target weight should be reassessed at least monthly or more often when indicated by hypertension. Fluctuations in weight can occur frequently in children due to changes in dietary intake, compliance with fluid restrictions, or vomiting and diarrhea. Chronic fluid overload in children may masquerade as false weight gain and fool even the experienced dialysis nurse.

What is the optimal blood flow rate for a pediatric hemodialysis patient?

The optimal blood flow rate (Qb) is a function of what the access will allow as well as the desired Kt/V. A Qb of 200–350 ml/min/1.73m^2 has been optimal to achieve these goals in our pediatric unit.

How does intradialytic monitoring differ in children?

The advent of volumetric hemodialysis equipment has made the procedure much safer in children. Blood pressure monitoring intervals should match the individual patient's care requirements. Blood pressure should always be done immediately after initiating the hemodialysis and at least hourly thereafter. When a patient is perceived to be unstable, monitoring intervals should decrease. Resist the urge to take blood pressure measurements every 15 minutes or half hour just because the patient is a child. The child may just become agitated and uncooperative, creating technical difficulty obtaining reliable readings. Monitors designed to noninvasively and automatically measure systolic and diastolic pressure, mean arterial pressure, and pulse rate for neonatal or pediatric patients are effective and versatile. They continue to monitor during most clinical crises when other indirect measurement methods may fail. Acute hemodialysis treatments in unstable patients nearly always require continuous arterial pressure monitoring for safety.

In addition to blood pressure measurement in patients weighing less than 20 kg, continuous monitoring of heart rate (ECG) and oxygenation (pulse oximeter) is required to detect deterioration in patient condition, which is most often related to acute fluid removal. Continuous nursing assessment is also needed to pick up subtle changes of impending hypotension, like irritability or yawning or fidgety movements. Since these subtle signs vary from patient to patient, their inclusion in the individual patient's plan of care will facilitate communication of a particular patient's care to the entire team.

What is high blood pressure (HBP) in children?

Blood pressure differs by gender and increases with age and size, so parameters for hypertension will be different from adults as shown in Table 20-2 for boys. Girls and shorter children at a given age have slightly lower blood pressure than boys and taller children for age. Blood pressure must be taken with an appropriately sized cuff, the air-filled bladder of which should have a width equal to approximately 40 percent of the circumference of the arm, measured at a point midway between the olecranon and acromion, and a length sufficient to extend around the arm at least 80 percent of the circumference. Cuff size is not standardized by industry, so the name "infant," "child," or "small adult" on the cuff should be disregarded, and the above parameters should be followed for proper sizing. If a cuff is too small, the blood pressure measurement will be falsely high. An oversized adult cuff or large thigh cuff will be needed for obese adolescents.

Table 20-2   High Blood Pressure (>95 Percentile for Age)

| Age Group (Boys) | Significant BP* Based on height (Ht) percentile | | Severe HBP** |
	Ht 5%	Ht 95%	All
BP percentile	95%	95%	>99%
1 mon–1 year	98/55	106/59	>115/75
1–3 years	104/63	113/67	>118/82
4–6 years	109/72	117/76	>124/84
7–10 years	114/77	123/82	>130/86
11–13 years	121/79	130/84	>134/90
14–17 years	132/85	140/89	>144/92
>17 years	No data	No data	>150/100

*Adapted from Update on 1987 Task Force on HBP, 1996. Complete tables for each year of age (1–17 years) by height percentiles (5, 10, 25, 50, 75, 90 and 95%) and gender can be found in the tables of the National High Blood Pressure Education Program Working Group on Hypertension Control in Children and Adolescents.
**From Second Task Force on BP Control in Children, 1987.

What is the significance of latex in the pediatric hemodialysis setting?

Certain groups of children are at high risk for developing latex allergy. Children with spina bifida have a 10 percent to 60 percent risk of developing an allergy to latex. Other children who require clean intermittent urinary catheterization are also at high risk. Repeated exposure to latex products is purported to be a significant risk factor to trigger a reaction, which can begin as contact urticaria or can be as dramatic as an anaphylactic reaction. There are two basic exposure routes: direct mucosal contact and airborne latex particles. Treatment of latex allergy is best directed to preventing exposures from the numerous items, like gloves and catheters, which contain latex. In addition to identifying pediatric patients at risk, each facility should develop protocols for latex precautions.

Are there any differences in heparin requirements during a pediatric hemodialysis?

The adult guidelines for heparinization and activated clotting time (ACT) monitoring can be used for children. To achieve a target ACT of 1.5 times normal, begin with a loading dose of 25–50 U/kg and a continuous infusion of 10 U/kg/hr. Increase the loading dose by 10–25 U/kg and the continuous infusion by 5 U/kg/hr as needed to achieve the desired ACT. Once the usual heparin requirement is established for a given patient, one should resist the temptation to sample blood unnecessarily for ACTs. Heparin requirements may be different if a chronic patient receives new vascular access or has surgery or gastrointestinal bleeding. Neonates, especially premature infants, who require hemodialysis or continuous renal replacement therapy need tight heparinization as they are at high risk for cerebral hemorrhage.

How does anemia management differ in children?

Two multi-center trials have shown that pediatric patients <5 years old frequently require initial recombinant human erythropoietin in higher doses, approximately 300 U/kg/wk, than older pediatric patients and adults. Achieving target iron levels to support erythropoiesis requires the administration of supplemental iron, either orally or intravenously. When administering intravenous iron dextran, heed the differences in pediatric test doses, i.e. 10 mg for patients weighing <10 kg and 15 mg for those weighing 10–20 kg, and pediatric dosing by body weight. The Dialysis Outcomes Quality Initiative (DOQI) Clinical Practice Guidelines note the differences in anemia management in children and are a good guideline to follow for pediatric care. (See page 333 for additional information on NKF-DOQI.)

Why are children with ESRD short in stature?

Growth retardation is a significant consequence of ESRD in children. The age of onset of chronic renal insufficiency (CRI) is an important variable affecting growth—the younger the patient at the onset of CRI, the greater the potential for growth retardation. Many factors contribute to poor growth, including chronic metabolic acidosis, sodium wasting and chronic dehydration, chronic fluid overload, poorly controlled renal osteodystrophy, anorexia and malnutrition from poor caloric intake, steroid therapy for underlying renal disease control and disturbances of normal growth hormone regulation. To best achieve normal or catch-up growth, efforts should be made to correct as many of these abnormalities as possible before the patient needs chronic dialysis.

How can growth be maximized in a pediatric hemodialysis patient?

To maximize growth potential during chronic hemodialysis, efforts should continue to include correcting acidosis, minimizing fluid overload, controlling renal osteodystrophy, and promoting optimum nutrition, and should also include optimizing dialysis adequacy. Each patient's height and target weight should be monitored closely (at least every 3 months) until the bone growth plates close. Head circumference as well as length and target weight should be measured in children under age 3 years. Gender-specific growth charts should be maintained and plotted quarterly, or more frequently if the patient is falling off his/her percentile on the growth chart. When height falls below the fifth percentile for age in a child >1 to 2 years old, initiation of recombinant human growth hormone therapy should be considered. Children with CRI and ESRD are relatively resistant to normal levels of growth hormone, so supplementation can help normalize their growth and improve muscle mass.

What are the toileting concerns in the child with ESRD?

Facilitate toilet training when the child is developmentally ready. The child with ESRD may have no urine output or a small amount of urine daily. Some children, usually those with congenital renal disease, like dysplasia or obstructive uropathy, may have a large volume of urine output daily and little concentrating ability. Young children with large urine volumes often continue to have nighttime bed wetting, because of their obligatory urine loss during the night when they are too sleepy to feel the need to get up and urinate in the toilet.

Can children who are receiving hemodialysis treatments go to regular school?

Most school-aged children on hemodialysis are able to attend school regularly with their peers. Missing school is often related to hospitalizations or the hemodialysis treatment schedule. When scheduling hemodialysis, every attempt should be made to facilitate school attendance. School constitutes a framework for daily behavior that imposes discipline and regularities, skills which are essential to achieving adult independence and ultimately entering into the job market.

What are options for measuring functional status in children?

Denver II Developmental Screening Tests are easy to perform and recommended for the assessment of children less than 6 years of age. Developmental delays are not uncommon in this chronically ill population. Another functional status tool for older children is the Children's Health Questionnaire, which is the pediatric version of the SF 36.

How does emergency preparedness need to be adapted when caring for children?

Medical emergency. The facility *must* be equipped with the appropriate pediatric-sized airways, airmask bag units (AMBUs), and endotracheal tubes. As most pediatric drug doses are based upon weight, it is wise to have an emergency drug list with precalculated doses for each individual pediatric patient. There should always be a pediatric advanced life support (PALS) certified nurse and nephrologist readily available.

Fire. Fire drills must be adapted to each child's developmental understanding. Many child-friendly resources, such as coloring books and fact sheets, are available through the National Fire Protection Association (NFPA) or the Fire Divisions of the local Department of Public Safety.

Disasters. When local disasters such as floods, tornados, hurricanes, or earthquakes strike, pediatric hemodialysis treatment becomes a priority. If a disaster can be anticipated, some pediatric patients may benefit from preemptive hospitalization.

Does pediatric hemodialysis cost more than adult hemodialysis?

Pediatric hemodialysis costs are higher because of the increased cost of supply items and services. Pricing is not as competitive for disposables in this low volume specialized market. Staffing for the increased patient dependency in pediatrics demands increased caregiver skills or more nurses. Exception requests based on atypical service intensity are available through HCFA to enable pediatric centers to increase their center-specific Medicare reimbursement rate to compensate for more costly operating conditions.

When do children transition to adult care?

Optimally, early preparation should begin during the stage of late adolescence (ages 17–21 years), which is characterized by the teenager's having developed the ability to define future goals, make close and intimate friendships, and begin rapprochement with parents and other authoritative adults. During the stage of mid-adolescence (ages 14–17 years), a teenager is at the height of risk-taking behavior, peer conformity, poor future orientation and parental conflict, which is a very difficult time to implement the transition to adult responsibilities. Some patients who are developmentally delayed may not be ready at age 17 years. Transition preparation includes teaching self-care skills, such as taking responsibility for adhering to a medication schedule, arranging clinic visits, and arriving for treatments on time. Ideally, late preparation should also incorporate a visit accompanied by a trusted nurse and/or social worker to the adult dialysis center. Actual transfer to adult care should occur between 18 and 21 years of age, depending upon patient readiness, disease management and availability of service. Being in an integrated pediatric and adult care facility should not preclude having the adolescent participate in a defined transition preparation program to be sure the patient is ready for the demands of adult-oriented care.

ESRD in the Elderly

Susan K. Hansen

Since the early 1990s, at least 45 percent of new patients entering the ESRD program in the United States each year have been over 65 years old. This percentage is increasing; the figure for 1995 was 47.8 percent. The same trend appears in dialysis programs all over the world. Regardless of the treatment modality selected, some changes are required to adapt the therapy to the special needs of geriatric patients. As will become clear during the course of this chapter, besides presenting some limitations, elderly patients bring certain assets to their treatment regimen.

Are the causes of ESRD different in elderly patients?

Not really. The most common cause is nephrosclerosis secondary to either diabetes or hypertension. Causes such as chronic glomerulonephritis and pyelonephritis are as common in elderly patients as in younger, although there may be slightly more elderly patients with an "unknown" renal diagnosis (biopsies are rarely done in elderly patients with renal failure of undetermined cause).

How do elderly patients differ from younger ESRD patients?

Comorbid conditions are much more common in older patients and can complicate the treatment of ESRD. Examples of significant comorbidities include an impaired cardiovascular system, osteoporosis, non–insulin-dependent diabetes, delayed protein synthesis/reduced protein intake, impaired pulmonary function, impaired cognitive function, poor vision, poor mobility and/or poor coordination.

Although not physical factors, adverse psychosocial and socioeconomic factors also complicate treatment regimens for a larger proportion of the elderly than younger patients.

Can elderly patients benefit from renal replacement therapy?

Many, perhaps most, elderly people can benefit from renal replacement therapy, often returning to a level of physical functioning and quality of life that is either equivalent to that of people their age without ESRD or at least acceptable to the patient.

Some patients, usually but not necessarily elderly, may not benefit from treatment. Examples of such patients might include those with irreversible dementia, or extremely debilitating or imminently terminal comorbid conditions, such as cancer or advanced congestive heart failure. However, there are few firm medical or community standards with respect to withholding treatment and decisions regarding initiating therapy varies with individual physicians and/or family members.

What is trial dialysis?

The concept of trial dialysis is gaining favor in some areas. A patient in whom the value of therapy is questionable may be given treatment (usually hemodialysis) for a clearly defined period to see whether explicitly described clinical goals can be achieved. Examples of such patients might include those with unexplained dementia, potentially reversible acute renal failure, unexplained worsening of congestive heart failure, personality change, and adult failure-to-thrive syndrome. The duration of treatment, specific goals and subsequent actions (continue/discontinue) are agreed to in advance by the medical team and family and, in some cases, the patient. This allows the patient every opportunity to benefit from treatment, if that is possible, and if not, provides the family and patient time to adjust and the knowledge that every effort was made.

Are all ESRD treatment modalities available to elderly patients?

Yes, subject to the usual considerations, such as adequate vascular access or an intact peritoneal membrane. In the United States at the end of 1996, for example, 57 percent of ESRD patients were over the age of 60.

Can elderly patients be successfully transplanted?

Certainly. Although the proportion of elderly ESRD patients who qualify for transplantation is not as high as that of younger patients, graft survival in those who do receive transplants is about the same. Kidneys are becoming more available to elderly recipients, as some transplant surgeons believe that organs donated by an older person should go to an older person. Elderly patients often require less intensive immunosuppressive therapy, due to the fact that their immune systems may already be compromised by age.

While patient survival is not as good at that of younger patients, due to an increased number and severity of complications, data now exist to show satisfactory results for transplantation in elderly patients. By the same token, dialysis is also safer than ever for the elderly, so making a decision between modes of therapy is not simple.

What are the advantages for elderly patients in being on peritoneal dialysis (PD)?

PD, unlike hemodialysis at the present time, is a home dialysis therapy. Patients benefit from being at home in a number of ways. They are spared the considerable time, effort and expense of being transported to and from a dialysis center, for one. The transportation effort is, in itself, very debilitating for some elderly patients. Home dialysis patients are in full charge of administering their own therapy, for another. This not only fosters independence but preserves their usual lifestyle, allowing patients to perform exchanges at their convenience, within reason, rather than conform to a rigid in-center schedule.

Patients on PD do not need a vascular access, with its attendant problems (although they must have a peritoneal access catheter, with *its* attendant problems), and many elderly patients have inadequate peripheral vessels. Because PD is a continuous—or at least daily—therapy, blood chemistries and fluid status approach a steady state; thus PD patients do not suffer the effects of the rapid biochemical and fluid changes common in hemodialysis. This can be a significant advantage since elderly patients are more prone to adverse reactions to these changes. For example, PD patients with diminished cardiac reserve experience less orthostatic hypotension or other cardiac symptoms in response to fluid removal. Slow, continuous therapy allows better correction of brain electrophysiological and cognitive function abnormalities, which incurs less risk of destabilizing the fragile mental equilibrium of some elderly patients.

Another advantage of daily therapy is that dietary and fluid restrictions are less rigid, which can be important for those with diminished appetites or impatience with restrictions.

Can elderly patients learn to do peritoneal dialysis (PD)?

Yes, many can do very well by themselves, and others can do PD with assistance from family members. In addition, several assistive devices are available, which allow patients who are blind or have limited dexterity to perform their own fluid exchanges. Automated, overnight dialysis systems eliminate all but a single connection and disconnection procedure.

What are the disadvantages of PD for elderly patients?

The incidence of certain complications (dementia, hernias, s. epidermis peritonitis, abdominal and catheter leaks) is higher in elderly PD patients compared to younger PD patients and compared to elderly hemodialysis patients.

If the patient frequently requires significant ultrafiltration, the resulting increased dialysate glucose concentration can significantly suppress the appetite, resulting in substantial malnutrition. This can be difficult to diagnose, at least initially, since dry weight may be stable or even increase (dextrose provides many calories but little nutrition). This can be a special problem with elderly patients, who are already at higher risk for malnutrition.

Loss of the opportunity to socialize during in-center therapy may also be a drawback, as many elderly people are socially isolated.

What are the advantages of hemodialysis (HD) in treating elderly ESRD patients?

At the present time, most hemodialysis in the United States is provided as an in-center therapy. There may be psychosocial advantages for elderly patients in the human interactions of dialysis center treatment, as mentioned above.

Another advantage is frequent observation by trained personnel. Elderly patients are more prone to complications of both ESRD and dialysis. When they develop such complications, elderly patients often exhibit less obvious symptoms. Earlier recognition and intervention (with resulting reductions in patient discomfort and healthcare costs) is more likely in a dialysis center setting.

Modern hemodialysis equipment, with its sophisticated monitoring and UF control systems, is better able to provide controlled rates of biochemical and fluid removal and, thus, provide safe and comfortable treatments for a larger range of elderly patients than was possible in the past. Some patients prefer short, thrice weekly treatments rather than continuously being on dialysis, as with PD. Treatment "burnout" is less common in the HD population. Also, many elderly patients grew up in an era when physicians and nurses—not patients—were expected to provide healthcare. Self-treatment, whether in a dialysis center or at home, is not acceptable to every older person.

Is hemodialysis more complicated in elderly patients?

Some practitioners claim that elderly patients are easier to dialyze. They tend to have lower fluid gains, lower creatinines and lower urea generation rates; thus they do not necessarily require extremely aggressive treatment, with its higher risk of intradialytic complications. Also, older people are generally more compliant with all facets of the treatment regimen and express higher life satisfaction than younger patients.

With one exception, the nature and frequency of intradialytic complications is similar to that of younger HD patients. The exception is hemodynamic instability, which is more common in elderly people: thus, intradialytic cardiac arrhythmias and hypotensive episodes are likely in this group. In most cases, episodes of hemodynamic instability can be minimized, and often prevented, if staff members are properly trained in the methods to achieve this.

Measures to prevent hypotensive episodes include using an extracorporeal circuit with the smallest possible priming volume, equipment with a volumetric ultrafiltration control system, and a bicarbonate dialysate with sufficiently high sodium, calcium and dextrose levels to help maintain blood pressure during ultrafiltration. Ultrafiltration and/or sodium modeling can help, as can using cool dialysate (35.5–36.0° C) No patients, especially the elderly, should be allowed to eat during dialysis, as blood is diverted from the peripheral circulation (where it maintains BP) to the digestive organs immediately after a meal. As a result, hypotension is usually inevitable. There is now ample evidence that a brief episode of simple exercises, especially if performed during the last hour of dialysis, is an effective way to support blood pressure and minimize muscle cramping. Dietary sodium, protein and fluid intake and the antihypertensive medication regimen should be reevaluated on a regular basis.

Arrhythmias are common in elderly hemodialysis patients and may not be associated with any detectable symptoms. They arise in conjunction with anemia, hypokalemia, hyperkalemia, acidosis, hypoxia, hypotension, hypertension, digoxin, or cardiac abnormalities due, for example, to metastatic calcifications, amyloid deposition, or cardiac hypertrophy. Arrhythmias that are associated with symptoms such as weakness or hypoxia should be reported to the physician, who may elect to adjust the patient's diet, dialysate composition, or medication prescriptions. Nasal oxygen may provide symptomatic relief for hypoxia. Transfer to PD may be necessary, if feasible, for patients who do not respond to the aforementioned measures.

What are the disadvantages of hemodialysis (HD) in the elderly?

As mentioned above, patients with significant cardiovascular disease do not tolerate the rapid biochemical and hemodynamic changes that accompany hemodialysis procedures and are at higher risk of intradialytic complications. As also mentioned, debilitated elderly people undergo considerable physical and emotional stress in relation to the thrice-weekly transportation to and from the dialysis center. Patients in either group would probably do better with a daily home dialysis regimen, such as PD or daily home HD, if that is feasible. Elderly patients may also experience more vascular access problems.

It is important to realize that older patients whose comorbidities are no more severe than those seen in younger patients do as well.

What special precautions should be taken with respect to monitoring the nutrition of elderly patients?

All patients lose nutrients during dialysis, whether HD or PD. Compared to the general dialysis population, elderly patients are at higher risk of malnutrition, in addition to being less likely to replace the nutrients lost during treatment. For this reason, staff must be able to recognize, indeed regularly probe for, factors that signal poor nutrition.

In addition to the usual impediments to good nutrition, elderly people experience a number of losses that interfere with their ability to achieve good nutrition. There are physical losses, such as loss of teeth, loss of senses of taste and smell, which make eating difficult or uninteresting; or loss of mobility, making it difficult to get to the grocery store or prepare meals.

Mealtime, often an occasion of social interaction, can remind the elderly of their social losses, such as loss of spouse, companions or access to community support. Some patients have psychological conditions, such as dementia, depression or just mental inertia, which can impede their will to eat. Financial constraints can enter the picture, as many elderly live on fixed incomes and may have to make choices between paying for heat or for food, for example. Medical factors such as anorexia, constipation, and medication effects can interfere with eating. Even with adequate meals there can still be nutritional losses due to vomiting, diarrhea, or loss of protein through persistent exudates from wounds or sores. Some of the factors that impede good nutrition can be corrected if they are recognized.

Suspect malnutrition if the patient has an increase in episodes of intradialytic hypotension or symptomatic congestive heart failure, develops depression or dementia, reports episodes suggestive of hypoglycemia (when not on hypoglycemic agents), a steady decline in dry weight, or symptoms of adult failure-to-thrive syndrome.

A low predialysis BUN is always due to poor nutrition, not great dialysis. Resist the temptation to decrease dialysis; such patients usually need more dialysis, not less. By the same token, patients who are unstable during dialysis should not be taken off early. This leads to underdialysis, which decreases appetite, leading to lower plasma protein levels and, shortly, to even greater intradialytic instability.

The physician or dietitian should be contacted if any of the situations discussed in this section are identified.

What are the problems with medications in elderly ESRD patients?

Dialysis patients, especially elderly ones, are likely to take a great many drugs. Elderly patients are much more susceptible to drug reactions and interactions. Thus, the dose of each drug must be carefully calibrated by the physician, taking into consideration many factors such as the poor intestinal absorption, impaired hepatic clearance and alteration in distribution space common in the elderly. Various elements can alter the patient's response to the prescribed dosage or combination of drugs, therefore, any unexplained change in physical or mental condition should be reported to the physician.

However, the main issue for staff is to check with the patient on a regular basis to: (1) determine whether the patient is having problems taking all of the prescribed medications, and (2) be alert to the possibility of polypharmacy (the tendency of some elderly people to see several physicians and, unknown to each physician, acquire multiple prescriptions from each).

Does exercise play a role in the treatment of elderly ESRD patients?

It certainly does. Properly prescribed exercise can play a significant role in the rehabilitation and subsequent preservation of the ability to perform the normal activities of daily life. This not only provides a better quality of life for the patient but reduces the need for expensive hospitalizations and/or home health aides.

Of special importance to hemodialysis dialysis staff is the now ample evidence that a brief period (i.e., 10 minutes) of exercise, such as pedaling a stationary bicycle, especially during the last hour of hemodialysis, can reduce the incidence and severity of muscle cramps and hypotension. A special device can be constructed from a bicycle wheel and pedals which allows the patient to remain seated in his dialysis chair while exercising.

What are the outcomes of the various ESRD treatment modalities in elderly patients?

In terms of treatment selection, the most recent information available (*USRDS* 1997) offers these statistics at the end of 1995: 82.4 percent of US patients aged 65 or older were receiving in-center HD, 0.7 percent were on home HD, 9.8 percent were on PD, and 5.8 percent had a functioning transplant (1.3 percent were on an unspecified form of therapy).

One-year mortality was 31.3 percent for patients aged 65–74 years, and 45.5 percent for those over 75. This is an improvement over earlier years (in 1984, for example, the mortality figures were 38 percent and 53 percent, respectively) and may reflect not only an improvement in ESRD therapy over that period but also increasing experience with treating elderly ESRD patients. The mortality rate of elderly ESRD patients is noticeably greater than that seen in younger ESRD patient age groups (18.4 percent for 45- to 64-year-olds; 10.7 percent in 20- to 44-year-olds; and 5.3 percent in 0- to 19-year-olds), a trend noted in the non-ESRD population as well.

Management of Quality in Dialysis Care

Karen Schardin, Martha H. Stoner, Gail Wick

Like all of health care, dialysis programs are undergoing a revolution in accountability. The government, accrediting and regulatory agencies, payers, and patients are holding health care organizations accountable for the delivery of high-quality, low-cost health care. Health care providers are being asked to explain the rationale behind their decisions and plans of care. Increased competition in the managed care environment also demands that providers be responsive to quality and cost issues. Continuous Quality Improvement (CQI) is a method to address those concerns. CQI must be supported by a leadership style of Total Quality Management (TQM), in which all members of the organization are motivated to go beyond meeting minimum standards by complying with regulatory requirements as they continuously evaluate their performance with the goal of improving care and outcomes.

What is Continuous Quality Improvement?

CQI is the ongoing process of identifying opportunities to improve quality. CQI involves collecting data about the current situation, identifying ways to improve the performance, introducing new and better approaches and methods to achieve desired outcomes, and then evaluating the interventions. When CQI is operating as intended, important aspects of care in need of improvement are identified before problems occur. All personnel contribute to CQI by being vigilant in recognizing care practices in need of improvement. A patient-centered perspective and questioning (e.g., "What about my work interferes with my ability to do what needs to be done to have the best possible outcome for patients?") are effective ways to identify practices in need of improvement. The goal of CQI is to use data to make objective decisions without placing blame or finding fault.

What is the origin of CQI?

Quality management efforts began in manufacturing, where the focus was on inspection of products. Quality management experts, such as W. Edward Deming, recognized that it was not enough to just evaluate the end product. He introduced the principles of CQI to improve and manage the production processes to achieve a quality product.

What are the basic tenets of quality management?

Efforts to manage quality in health care continue to be influenced in particular by three sets of guides: Deming's 14 points; Donabedian's structure, process and outcomes framework; and JCAHO's 10 steps. Basic tenets of CQI/TQM are a focus on customers, broadly defined to include personnel and patients, and a commitment to gather and use data to identify opportunities to improve quality outcomes by modifying processes that result in higher quality care at less cost. Efforts to achieve quality are dynamic and continual and everyone in the organization is involved and responsible. Failures in quality are more often due to flaws in processes than the failure of people doing the work.

Why is CQI relevant for health care and for dialysis programs?

The health care industry is one of the largest and most costly industries in America. CQI was introduced to the health care industry in part as an effort to slow the ever-increasing percent of the gross domestic product devoted to health care. Care provided to people with ESRD, specifically dialysis, is costly. Dialysis is provided to about 217,000 Americans at an annual cost of $11.1 billion. The cost of dialysis care mandates efforts to decrease cost without sacrificing quality of care.

What is the connection between quality and cost?

Health care personnel are committed to providing high-quality care to patients. Consideration of the costs of that care has not always been attended to, and providers may not realize that poor care is costly. For example, if a satisfactory dialysis is not achieved for any number of process or system reasons, the patient may have outcomes that require hospitalization for emergency treatment and additional dialysis. The end result is increased cost and poor financial performance.

How is CQI different from Quality Assurance (QA)?

QA was an early effort to address quality care issues in health care. QA, initiated in response to requirements of accreditation organizations, tended to use retrospective data collection, in which audits of medical records identified problems. These audits evaluated documented, existing problems, but improved quality of care did not necessarily result. CQI is a more proactive method, focused on seeking every opportunity to improve processes and systems to achieve quality outcomes. Concurrent collection of data for analysis is a vital aspect of CQI. Rather than documentation of problems, the focus of CQI is evaluation of interventions to improve quality.

Does CQI meet a need in dialysis facilities?

As a high-volume, high-risk, problem-prone, and high-cost health care program, dialysis is a model for CQI. Dialysis facilities can use CQI techniques to identify processes in need of improvement, to implement interventions or corrective actions, and to evaluate cost and quality outcomes.

What are some CQI concepts and terms important to know?

A *process* is a series of interrelated activities to achieve a desired outcome or goal. Processes are those things dialysis personnel do to achieve well-dialyzed patients. Preparing the dialyzer, assessing the patient, and conducting the treatment with vigilant surveillance of both the patient and the machine are examples of processes that influence how well the patient is dialyzed. *Standards* define quality by specifying rules that apply to key processes and the results expected. They are written values communicated to all members of the organization. Professional organizations that establish standards for dialysis nurses include the ANNA Standards of Clinical Practice for Nephrology Nursing. Such standards specify a desired patient outcome (the patient will be free of vascular access complications), identify the nursing management aspects of care including assessment parameters (assess vascular access for patency and evidence of complications) and interventions (use aseptic technique in handling vascular access), and patient teaching.

Clinical indicators are valid and reliable measures used to evaluate important patient care services. They are events that are compared to some specified universe of events to encourage a focus on desired outcomes. Individual providers and dialysis facilities are encouraged to identify indicators relevant for specific settings. Organizations involved in specifying indicators are the JCAHO, NCQA, and the ESRD Networks. An indicator for a dialysis facility might be the number of times it is necessary for personnel to use more than one needle per venipuncture to initiate dialysis as compared to the total number of venipunctures done

A *benchmark* is a frame of reference for clinical practice. It is an objective way to compare a facility's processes and outcomes with its own past performance or with external standards. A benchmark can be gold standard or the industry's best practice. Benchmarking is a goal-setting process that recognizes that providers and the internal organization may not have the best answers for the problem being addressed. It is a process of comparing the care provided and its outcomes with what is considered the best. An example of a benchmark for a dialysis facility might be to compare the average Kt/V with what the industry has set as the standard.

An *outcome* is the result obtained from some action or intervention. The outcome must specify who will do what and by how much within a time period. For instance, a dialysis facility might identify an outcome, as personnel will reduce the number of second sticks required to initiate dialysis to 5 percent within 3 months following a skill refinement workshop.

What are some tools used in CQI?

Quality improvement efforts use the scientific method to search for the root cause of a problem, find it, and fix it. FOCUS is a CQI tool to help examine and analyze a specific process. The first step is to *Find* a process to improve by analyzing data. Statistical control is used to distinguish between common and special causes of variation in processes. Data are displayed in control charts to track performance. Variations outside of the control limits are special cause variances and require investigation. For more detailed instruction on the use of statistical control and other tools like flowcharts, Pareto charts, cause-and-effect (fishbone) diagrams, and run charts, refer to a CQI reference text.

The next step is to *Organize* a team to work together to improve the situation. To *Clarify* is the next step and involves collecting and analyzing data specific to the process being targeted for improvement. A cause-and-effect diagram might be useful in the clarifying phase.

In the *Understand* phase, health providers examine data for the causes of variation and the changes over time.

The final FOCUS step is to *Select* a method of improving outcomes and initiate the PDCA cycle of CQI.

What is the PDCA Cycle?

PDCA refers to Plan-Do-Check-Act, a framework for implementing the methods to improve outcomes selected during the FOCUS process.
Plan, the first step in instituting a change for improvement, requires an investment of time since a hastily determined solution may not produce the desired result. Using brainstorming techniques encourages all members of the team to contribute ideas to the plan. Reviewing relevant literature is a critical element of planning. One outcome of planning by the multidisciplinary team may be a decision to develop a clinical care pathway or to adopt a clinical practice guideline as a way to improve the quality and cost outcomes of an important aspect of care.

Once a plan is agreed upon, the second phase of PDCA, *Do*, is applied. Typically, *Do* means implementing an intervention and conducting a pilot study to see if the change is effective.

During the *Check* phase, results of the trial are checked against the objectives of the plan and modified as needed.

The final phase of the PDCA cycle is *Act*, in which the findings of the pilot study guide implementation of solutions in a more comprehensive, facility-wide initiative. Ongoing monitoring to make certain that improvement persists over time is necessary.

What role do the ESRD Networks play in quality management?

A collaborative effort involving ESRD Networks, HCFA and other organizations is designed to improve ESRD care by collecting and analyzing data about clinical characteristics of adult dialysis patients. Two of the initiatives are the ESRD Core Indicators project and the National ESRD Anemia Cooperative Project.

What are the foci of the ESRD Networks' key indicators?

The care indicators are adequacy of dialysis, desirable hematocrit value, optimal nutritional status, and control of blood pressure. Reports generated can be used by dialysis facilities to compare their unit's results with national findings, or benchmarks. These data can then lead to quality improvement projects designed to improve patient care within a facility.

Does the National Kidney Foundation (NKF) have a quality improvement initiative?

In March of 1995, the NKF established a Dialysis Outcome Quality Initiative (NKF-DOQI) to develop evidence-based clinical practice guidelines to improve the care of ESRD patients. The guidelines were completed in 1997 and are being translated into practice through professional education programs. Adoption of the guidelines will be evaluated for their impact on patient outcomes.

Does everyone agree with the quality management movement in health care?

Some health care providers resist quality improvement efforts because they believe the quality of their practice is ensured by their professionalism. Some people resent what they perceive to be external interference and controls. Still others believe that the time required for quality improvement is counterproductive. These negative impressions and resistance will, with time, diminish when they are countered successfully with a patient-centered perspective and acceptance of the goal of CQI to use data to improve quality and cost outcomes of care, as well as positive experiences with an effective TQI program.

How can I learn more about CQI/TQM in health care?

Books, journals, the Internet, and professional organizations, such as ANNA, are great resources for additional information about quality health care and the specific techniques of CQI/TQM.

Renal Care and Information Technology

Cedric Tuck-Sherman

Although information technology has been used to support renal billing and administration for many years, the use of clinical management systems in renal care has been limited.

What is driving the need for information technology in renal care?

Several factors are driving the need to capture better information in renal care. They include pressure to improve health outcomes, a trend towards managed care, and increased competition between renal providers.

Health Outcomes

Perhaps the most important reason to capture information is the need to better understand health outcomes. There is significant controversy and tremendous practice variation in the treatment of renal patients. For example, there is limited understanding as to why the United States experiences relatively poor morbidity and mortality rates. Is it due to short treatment times, dialyzer reuse, higher cormorbidity? Information systems must be used to collect and analyze comprehensive, robust information to better understand the cause and effect of different treatment regimens for different patient profiles.

Managed Care

Another factor driving the need for electronic information is the movement towards managed care. The way the renal market is evolving, certain renal organizations are creating renal specialty managed care groups. These organizations are subcontracting services to nephrology practices, dialysis centers, hospitals, and transplant centers for renal care. To manage in this new environment, these organizations and their subcontractors need to seamlessly exchange information throughout the continuum of care. Each provider in the treatment chain will have access to complete clinical information from which to base decisions. On the financial side, all costs will need to be closely monitored in order to measure profitability, decide subcontracting terms, and provide risk management information for future managed care bidding.

Competition

Most dialysis facilities belong to a group of centers ranging in size from a few to hundreds of centers. In order to leverage their competitive strength, renal provider organizations of all sizes must consolidate their clinical and financial information.

In a managed care environment, renal providers will need good clinical and economic information to remain competitive. They will not only need to manage their cost structure, but they will be expected to demonstrate the quality of delivered care and will be required to implement standardized clinical guidelines. Smaller organizations can leverage information technology to share data with other like providers and across the continuum of care in order to realize some of the advantages of the bigger players.

What value can information technology provide nurses and other dialysis personnel?

Process Management

One of the things that computers do well is manage processes. Call them care plans, protocols, assessments or algorithms, much of what renal care providers do is process oriented. Information technology provides the opportunity to automate these processes by providing guidance at the point of care. This fosters compliance with treatment guidelines and facilitates standardization to best-demonstrated practices.

Administration Management

Administrative activities play a big part in renal patient care. There are countless reports that must be completed to document care activities and collect payments: care plans, compliance reports, HCFA reports, management reports, claims, etc. Information technology can automatically create and print or submit all types of documentation, thus freeing up time for dialysis professions to spend on higher value activities such as direct patient care.

Health Outcomes Management

"Health outcomes" generally refers to the measurement of the clinical and financial results of delivered patient care. By tracking a full set of critical variables in the care delivery process (including demographics, medical history, and all treatment activities), information technology can statistically correlate variables to outcomes and help identify the optimal treatment pathway to maximize clinical results and reduce the overall cost of care. These "best demonstrated practices" can then be standardized and incorporated into standard protocols.

How can information technology support the caregiving process?

Accommodate Different Perspectives

Each type of dialysis professional uses the patient medical record in a different way. Nephrologists, nurses, technicians, social workers, dietitians, and administrators access and contribute information in the medical record that is specific to their role. A paper chart, however, remains the same regardless of who is using it. Information technology can recognize each type of dialysis personnel and present information in a format that best suits their needs. In this way a physician and an administrator can each access the patient database from a perspective that makes the most sense to their respective tasks at hand (i.e. clinical evaluation versus billing).

Provide Quick and Easy Access to Information

A key role of information systems is to present complete and up-to-date lab values, medications, procedures, and other pertinent information to renal care professionals at the point-of-care to support clinical interpretation and decision making. Information technology can call up and display information from the patient database in value-adding presentations that include data trending (e.g., labs), comparisons (e.g., labs to medications), and calculated algorithms (e.g., Kt/V). The information system's ability to support patient encounters at the point-of-care depends on how the system is set up in the dialysis facility. Such a system set-up is outlined in Fig. 23-1.

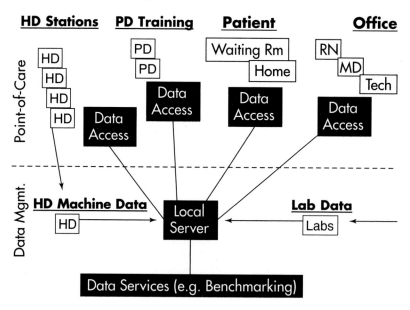

Fig. 23-1 Systems can be set up to provide access to the database throughout the dialysis facility with access to outside information, including labs and other sources of information.

Manage a Variety of Patient Encounters

By combining the ability to accommodate different perspectives and to manage processes, information technology can support a variety of patient encounters. Take, for example, a hemodialysis treatment. There are a number of complex activities that need to occur from the time the patient arrives at the center for treatment until the patient leaves to go home. Information technology can provide guidance throughout the dialysis treatment with the timely delivery of information and data collection templates. A good renal care system should support all aspects of a dialysis treatment including set-up of the dialysis machine, evaluation of the access site, recording of pre and post treatment parameters, managing the dialysis flow sheet, administrating intradialytic medications, and recording nurse and discharge notes. Other encounters from a physician's ward round to an administrator's billing review should likewise be supported by information technology.

Support Care Planning

Long-term and short-term care plans are an important part of renal care. Information systems can provide a dynamic environment in which to create and implement care plans. A well-designed system can, for example, maintain a library of task items that an individual provider or interdisciplinary care team can use to plan the management of patient problems. A scheduling module can then create reminders to providers when tasks are due.

Create Alerts

Clinical information systems can also provide "ticklers" that create alert messages or recommend actions based on newly received data. A complication or unusual lab value, for example, can trigger an alert or call-up a protocol based on pre-determined instructions. Let us say a dialysis unit considers an albumin level below 3.5 to warrant special attention. The lab module, within an information system, can be programmed to: recognize an abnormally low albumin value based on quality assurance parameters, trigger a malnutrition assessment for the dietitian to conduct, and send a message to all care team members.

Manage "To dos"

Managing "to dos" is also an important part of patient care. Electronic clinical systems can integrate task management and communication into the electronic patient records to allow providers to create reminders for themselves and others in the care team. At the appropriate time, these tasks and messages are presented to each respective provider.

What can be done with the data once it has been collected?

In addition to managing information at the point-of-care, reports can be generated to analyze clinical and economic data. There are several ways in which the database can be accessed and utilized to improve health care management.

Standard Reports

The type of reports available in any given information system depends on the type and quality of data collected. A comprehensive dialysis information system should be capable of providing value-added reports to support renal care providers, including adequacy of dialysis, nutritional status, anemia, vascular access, blood pressure control, and renal osteodystrophy. This is in addition to basic clinical reports such as demographic, laboratory, medication, diagnostic, and hospitalization information. On the administrative side, dialysis systems should generate renal billing, accounting, and regulatory reports such as HCFA's 2728.

Ad-hoc Reports

It is impossible to anticipate every report that might be needed from a database. Therefore information systems should be able to accommodate queries and generate ad-hoc reports. A typical means of querying a database is through a series of filters. Using filters, an investigator can "mine" the database based on specific criteria. For example, an investigator could look at diabetic patients, treated on protocol A and compare specific outcomes (i.e. adequacy, anemia, clotted access) with the same type of patients treated on protocol B. Once created, these ad-hoc reports can usually be added to the library of standard reports for future use.

Benchmarking and Other Data Services

The statistical value of data increases with the quality and volume of information collected. Good information systems provide the means for organizations to reach outside of their traditional boundaries to share data with other providers in the continuum of care, and to benchmark their performance against aggregated databases of like providers. These types of data services can help address the unanswered questions regarding renal health outcomes and provide an extension to the continuous quality improvement process.

How can the data be used to improve the caregiving process?

Support Research

The same tools that can be used to manage the process of care delivery and measure health outcomes can also be used to support clinical research. Information technology can be used to create protocols and manage the intervals, encounters and events that make up a clinical trial. If designed for research, information systems can ensure compliance to the protocols including management of inclusion/exclusion criteria for patient selection and run algorithms for randomization. For the information system, the only difference between day-to-day treatment and clinical research is the degree of control imposed on the processes of care. Controlling processes is something information technology does very well.

Process Improvement (CQI)

Information technology is a powerful tool for supporting the Continuous Quality Improvement (CQI) process. This is generally accomplished in a three-step continuous loop. First, patient records are maintained using the guidelines and assessments embedded in the system. Then reports (standard and ad-hoc), as well as benchmarking and other data services, are used to investigate outcomes and identify best-demonstrated practices. Finally, the guidelines and assessments that are embedded in the point-of-care management modules are improved based on the findings. The process starts over again to form a continuous quality improvement loop (see Fig. 23-2).

Is electronic medical data safe from loss and unwanted access?

The maintenance and exchange of patient information is relatively new and appropriate safeguards must be put in place to protect confidential information from loss and unwanted access. If information technology is properly utilized, electronic medical records can actually provide a safer and more secure medium for sensitive data than paper-based records. Procedures can be put in place to regularly back up databases and to control access to individual patient records by

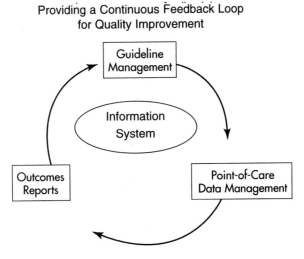

Fig. 23-2 Well-designed information systems provide an inherent process for continuous quality improvements (CQI).

provider type or even individual provider. The risk of loss of data and/or invasion of privacy comes from improper or insufficient safeguards. While the healthcare industry continues to develop standards for electronic data protection and access, it is up to systems vendors and provider organizations to ensure that the proper procedures are put into place.

Technology is constantly changing. How can an organization ensure that its information system doesn't become obsolete?

Even the most advanced information technology today will quickly become obsolete without continued maintenance and upgrades.

In selecting an information system, there are certain standards and platforms that are more adaptable to change. The technology platform and software design should be flexible in order to accommodate process changes in the organization as well as new treatment technologies. Selecting a vendor that is committed to continually improving the products and that provides a comprehensive maintenance and upgrade plan is essential.

One of the biggest difficulties in implementing an information system is ensuring seamless integration with existing databases. Few medical information systems function in isolation. Dialysis information systems should ideally be interfaced with the lab systems, with the hemodialysis machine, and with administration systems (such as billing). In addition, hospital-based dialysis units may also be interfaced to pharmacy, admission/discharge, radiology, pathology, and other systems. To facilitate the setup and maintenance of these interfaces, the dialysis system should be compliant with the healthcare industry's standard interface protocols (such as HL7). The database should also be ODBC compliant (Open DataBase Connectivity) to ensure easy access for interfacing and reporting. Finally, the system's database should be scalable to accommodate the growth of data collected over time.

How is the cost of purchasing a new generation renal information system justified?

Implementing a dialysis information system involves hardware, software, installation, training, maintenance and support costs. Although these costs are not insignificant, they can be justified economically.

Increased Revenues

By its very nature a clinical management system used at the point-of-care ensures complete capture and documentation of billable events. Information regarding billable activities including dialysis treatments, medications, procedures, examinations, etc., are recorded by the clinical management system and passed to billing. Because of this direct link from clinical to billing, the likelihood of missed charge opportunities is greatly reduced.

Improved Operating Efficiency

A key benefit of dialysis information systems is that the time it takes to collect data and generate clinical and administrative reports is dramatically reduced. Data parameters (e.g., patient name, lab test result, and dialysis machine readings) should only have to be entered once, whether manually or automatically from machine or systems interfaces. Once entered the data can be displayed for use in various clinical situations or accessed for clinical and administrative reporting.

Reduced Cost of Care

In supporting the management of processes, administration and health outcomes, information technology can help reduce the cost of care. Standardizing care around best-demonstrated practices not only improves the quality of care but can reduce the costs associated with practice variation. And health outcomes management can help identify opportunities to cut costs without cutting the quality of care.

Improved Marketability

Payers, Medicare and private insurers are demanding improved outcomes, more services and better data from renal care providers. Organizations will need to satisfy these demands in order to survive. Information technology can help collect and manage the information necessary to compete in the emerging marketplace.

In summary, renal care information technology has evolved beyond managing billing and administrative needs to addressing the clinical management of renal patients. For clinicians, information systems provide real-time access to medical records, while electronic clinical pathways enable them to make more informed clinical decisions. Administrators use the powerful analytical tools and comprehensive databases provided by good information systems to identify opportunities to increase revenues and safely reduce costs.

Dialysis information systems are rapidly becoming an integrated part of renal care management. In doing so, they are eliminating much of the administrative burden of collecting and reporting clinical and administrative data, freeing up time for dialysis personnel to focus on higher value-adding activities.

References and Recommended Readings

Association for Advancement of Medical Instrumentation: *AAMI standards and recommended practices, Dialysis, vol. 3*, Arlington, VA, 1996, AAMI.

Aronoff GR, Erbeck KM: Prescribing drugs for dialysis patients. In Henrich WL, editor: *Principles and practice of dialysis*, Baltimore, 1994, Williams and Wilkins.

Aweeka FT: Dosing of drugs in renal failure. In Young LY, Koda-Kimble MA, editors: *Applied therapeutics: the clinical use of drugs*, ed 6, Vancouver WA, 1995, Applied Therapeutics, Inc.

Bailie GR: Acute renal failure. In Young LY, Koda-Kimble MA, editors: *Applied therapeutics: the clinical use of drugs*, ed 6, Vancouver, WA, 1995, Applied Therapeutics, Inc.

Baillod RA: Home dialysis: lessons in patient education, *Patient Educ Couns* 26(1-3):17-24, 1995.

Bellamo R: Choosing a therapeutic modality: hemofiltration vs. hemodialysis vs. hemodiafiltration, *Sem in Dial* 9(2):88-92, 1996.

Bennett WM, et al.: *Drug prescribing in renal failure: dosing guidelines for adults*, ed 4, Philadelphia, 1999, American College of Physicians.

Berwick DM, Godfrey AB, Roessner J: *Curing health care: new strategies for quality improvement*, San Francisco, 1990, Jossey-Bass Publishers.

Blagg CR, Mailloux LU, Introduction: The case for home hemodialysis, *Adv Renal Replace Ther* 3(2):96-98, 1996.

Blagg CR: Home hemodialysis, *Semin Dial* 7:293-296, 1994.

Bloembergen WE, et al.: A comparison of cause of death between patients treated with hemodialysis and peritoneal dialysis, *J Am Soc Nephrol* 6(2):184-191, 1995.

Bloembergen WE, et al.: A comparison of mortality between patients treated with hemodialysis and peritoneal dialysis, *J Am Soc Nephrol* 6(2):177-183, 1995.

Brater DC: Dosing regimens in renal disease. In Jacobsen HR, Striker GE, Klahr S, editors: *The principles and practice of nephrology*, ed 2, St. Louis, 1995, CV Mosby.

Brown WW: Geriatric dialysis patients. In Henrich WL, editor: *Principles and practice of dialysis*, Baltimore, 1994, Williams & Wilkins.

Burrows-Hudson S: CQI and anemia management: maximizing positive outcomes, *ANNA Journal* 24(2), 254-261, 1997.

Burton B, Gross S, Vichek DL: A CQI approach to improved vascular access outcomes, *NNI*, January 1995, 33-36.

Centers for Disease Control. Fax Service—Document #231117. *Managment of Exposure HIV/HBV*, 1996.

Centers for Disease Control. Fax Service—Document #370105. *Hospital Infections Program: Methicillin-Resistant Staphylococcus Aureus*, 1996.

Centers for Disease Control and Prevention: TB/HIV: *The connection: what health care workers should know*, 1993.

Centers for Disease Control and Prevention: Guidelines for preventing the transmission of mycobacterium tuberculosis in health care facilities, *MMWR* 43(RR-13), 1994.

Centers for Disease Control and Prevention: Occupational exposure to HIV, *MMWR* 45(22), 1996.

Centers for Disease Control and Prevention: Recommendation for preventing the spread of vancomycin resistance, *Infection Control Hospital Epidemiology* 16(2), Feb. 1995.

Centers for Disease Control: Hepatitis B virus: a comprehensive strategy for eliminating transmission in the United States: Recommendations of the Immunization Practices Advisory Committee (ACIP), *MMWR* 40(RR-13), 1991.

Centers for Disease Control: Protection against viral hepatitis: recommendations of the Immunization Practices Advisory Committee (ACIP), *MMWR* 39(RR-2), 1990.

Chertow GM, Bullard A, Lazarus JM: Nutrition and the dialysis prescription, *Am J of Neph* 16(1):79-89, 1996.

Clinical practice guidelines for peritoneal dialysis adequacy: a report from the peritoneal dialysis adequacy work group of the National Kidney Foundation—Dialysis Outcomes Quality Initiative, Madison, WI, 1997, Medical Education Institute.

Coastal Video Communications Corp.: *Bloodborne pathogens training handbook*, Virginia Beach, VA, 1993.

Coastal Video Communications Corp.: *Drug-resistant organisms: a clinical approach*, Virginia Beach, VA, 1997.

Coastal Video Communications Corp.: *Tuberculosis: back from the past, training handbook*, Virginia Beach, VA, 1993.

Craddock PR, et al.: Hemodialysis leukopenia: pulmonary vascular leukostasis resulting from complement activation by dialyzer cellophane membranes, *J Clin Invest* 59:879-888, 1977.

Cronin RE: Mechanisms of nephrotoxic injury. In Jacobsen HR, Striker GE, Klahr S, editors: *The principles and practice of nephrology*, ed 2, St. Louis, 1995, CV Mosby.

Cutler RE, Forland SC, Hammond PGS: Pharmacokinetics of drugs and the effect of renal failure. In Massry SG, Glasscock RJ, editors: *Textbook of nephrology*, vol 2, ed 3, Baltimore, 1995, Williams & Wilkins.

Danforth Bill: Public Law 101-508, Omnibus Budget Reconciliation Act (OBRA) 1990.

Daugirdas J, Ing T: *Handbook of dialysis*, ed 2, New York, 1994, Little, Brown & Company.

Davidman M, Olson P, Kohen J: Iatrogenic renal disease, *Archives of Internal Medicine*, 151(9):1809-1812, 1991.

Deming WE: *Out of the crisis*, Cambridge, 1989, MIT, Center for Advanced Engineering Studies.

Dialysis Outcomes Quality Initiative: *Clinical practice guidelines for the treatment of anemia of chronic renal failure*, New York, 1997, National Kidney Foundation.

Dickens BM: Ethical and legal issues in geriatric nephrology, *Am J Kid Dis*, 16(4):375-377, 1990.

Donabedian A: Quality of care: how can it be assessed? *JAMA* 260, 1743-1748, 1988.

DuBose TD, Jr., et al.: Acute renal failure in the 21st century: recommendations for management and outcomes assessment, *Am J Kid Dis* 29(5):793-799, 1997.

Eknoyan G, et al.: What are the major changes in dialysis practice recommended by the dialysis outcomes quality initiative (DOQI)? *Sem in Dial* 10(3):151-157, 1997.

Elasy T, Anderson R: Changing demography of acute renal failure, *Sem in Dial* 9(6):438-443, 1996.

Evans RW, et al.: The quality of life of patients with end-stage renal disease, *N Engl J Med* 312(9):553-559, 1985.

Favero M, Bland L, Alter M: *Dialysis-associated infections and their control*, U.S. Department of Health and Human Services, Public Health Services, Centers for Disease Control and Prevention. Reprint from *Hospital infections*, ed 3, Boston, 1992, Little, Brown and Company.

Floege J, et al.: Clearance and synthesis rates of beta 2-microglobulin in patients undergoing hemodialysis and in normal subjects, *J Lab Clin Med* 118(2):153-165, 1991.

Forni L, Hilton P: Continuous hemofiltration in the treatment of acute renal failure, *Current Concepts* 336(18):1303-1309, 1997.

Friedman EA: A symposium on dialytic therapy for the diabetic ESRD patient, *Sem in Dial* 10(4):193, 1997.

Gokol R: CAPD—Clinical management and medical complications. In Briggs JD, et al., editors: *Renal dialysis*, London, 1994, Chapman & Hall.

Golper TA, Bennett WM: Use of drugs in renal failure. In Massry SG, Glasscock RJ, editors: *Textbook of nephrology*, vol 2, ed 3, Baltimore, 1995, Williams & Wilkins.

Gutierrez A, et al.: Effect of in vivo contact between blood and dialysis membranes on protein catabolism in humans, *Kidney Int* 38(3):487-494, 1990.

Habach G, et al.: Hospitalization among United States dialysis patients: hemodialysis versus peritoneal dialysis, *J Am Soc Nephrol* 5(11):1940-1948, 1995.

Haire-Joshu D: *Management of diabetes mellitus: perspectives of care across the life span*, ed 2, St. Louis, 1996, Mosby.

Hartigan M, Thomas-Hawkins C: Circulatory access for hemodialysis. In Lancaster L, editor: *Core curriculum for nephrology nursing*, ed 3, Pitman, NJ, 1995, ANNA.

Henrick WL, ed: *Principles and practice of dialysis*, Baltimore, 1994, Williams & Wilkins.

Hestin D, et al.: Renal transplantation in patients over sixty years of age, *Clin Nephrol* 42(4):232-236, 1994.

Himmelfarb J, Safirstein R: Introduction: Recent advances in acute renal failure, *ARRT* 4:1-2, 1977.

Hostetter TH, Nath K: Nutritional requirements of diabetics with nephropathy. In Klahr S and Mitch W, editors, *Nutrition and the kidney*, ed 2, Boston, 1993, Little, Brown and Company.

Ikizler TA, Hakim RM: Nutrition in ESRD, *Kid Int* 50(2):343-357, 1996.

Ikizler TA, Himmelfarb J: Nutrition in acute renal failure patients, *Advances in Renal Replacement Therapy* 4(2 Suppl 1):54-63, 1997.

Ishikawa K: *What is total quality control? The Japanese way*, Englewood Cliffs, NJ, 1985, Prentice Hall, Inc.

Jacobsen HR, Striker GE, Klahr S, eds.: *The principles and practice of nephrology*, ed 2, St. Louis, 1995, Mosby.

Jick H: Adverse drug effects in relation to renal function, *Am J Med* 62(4):514-517, 1977.

Johnson C, Simmons W: *Dialysis of drugs*, New York, 1996, The McMahon Group.

Johnson KB, editor. *The Harriet Lane Handbook*, ed 13, St. Louis, 1993, C.V. Mosby Company.

Jones MR: Preventing malnutrition in the long-term peritoneal dialysis patient, *Sem in Dial* 8(6):347, 1995.

Katz JM, Green E: Managing quality: A guide to system-wide performance management in health care, St. Louis, 1997, Mosby-Yearbook, Inc.

Keane WF, et al.: Peritoneal dialysis-related peritonitis treatment recommendations: 1996 update, *Peritoneal Dialysis International* 16(6):557–573, 1996.

Kopple JD: The nutrition management of the patient with acute renal failure, *J of Parenteral and Enteral Nutr* 20(1):3, 1996.

Kutner NG, Brogan DJ: Assisted survival, aging, and rehabilitation needs—comparison of older dialysis patients and age-matched peers, *Arch Phys Med Rehabil* 73(4):309-315, 1992.

Kutner NG, et al.: Fulfilling the promise—linking rehabilitation interventions with ESRD patient outcomes, *Dial & Transpl* 26(5):282-292, 1997.

Liponi DF, Winter ME, Tozen TN: Renal function and therapeutic concentrations of phenytoin, *Neurology* 34(3):395-397, 1984.

MacDonald J, et al.: Identifying a new reality: zero vascular access recirculation using ultrasound dilution, *ANNA Journal* 23(6):603-608, 635, 1996.

Mackay K, Moss A: Acute dialysis of patients with multiple organ dysfunction: should it be done? *Sem in Dial* 9(5):412-476, 1996.

Markell MS: Diabetes and dialysis. In Fine R, Gentile D, Nissenson A, editors: *Clinical dialysis*, Connecticut, 1995, Appleton & Lange.

Markell MS: Hemodialysis for end stage diabetic nephropathy. In Fine R, Nissenson A, editors: *Dialysis therapy*, Philadelphia, 1993, Hanley & Belfus.

Matzke GR, Frye RF: Drug therapy individualization for patients with renal insufficiency. In Dipiro JT: *Pharmacotherapy: A pathophysiological approach*, ed 3, Stamford CT, 1997, Appleton & Lange.

McCarthy JT, et al.: Improved preservation of residual renal function in chronic hemodialysis patients using polysulfone dialyzers, *Am J Kidney Dis* 29(4):576-583, 1997.

Mehta R, Martin R: Initiating and implementing a continuous renal replacement therapy program, *Sem in Dial* 9(2):80-87, 1996.

Mehta R: Modalities of dialysis for acute renal failure, *Sem in Dial* 9(6):469-475, 1996.

Mehta RL: Continuous renal replacement therapies in the acute renal failure setting: current concepts, *Advances in Renal Replacement Therapy* 4(2 Suppl 1): 81-92, 1997.

Mid-Atlantic Renal Coalition: Overview of CDC guidelines addressing tuberculosis: screening and management in healthcare facilities, Plymouth Meeting, PA, 1995.

Mid-Atlantic Renal Coalition: Reducing the spread of vancomycin-resistant enterococcus in the dialysis setting, Plymouth Meeting, PA, 1996.

Mooraki A, et al.: Selected outcome criteria and adequacy of dialysis in diabetic and elderly patients on CAPD therapy, *Adv in Perit Dial* 10:89-93, 1994.

Movilli E, et al.: Effect of age on protein catabolic rate, morbidity, and mortality in uremic patients with adequate dialysis, *Nephrol Dial Transplant* 8(8):735-739, 1993.

Moyer L, Alter M, Favero M: Hemodialysis-associated hepatitis B: revised recommendations for serologic screening, *Sem in Dial* 3(4), 201-204, 1990.

National Heart, Lung, and Blood Institute: Report of the second task force on blood pressure control in children, 1987, *Pediatrics* 79:1-25, January 1987.

National High Blood Pressure Education Program Working Group on Hypertension Control in Children and Adolescents: Update on the 1987 task force report on high blood pressure in children and adolescents, *Pediatrics* 98(4 Pt 1):649-658, October 1996.

National Kidney Foundation: *A guide for patients and their families*, New York, 1993, NKF.

National Kidney Foundation: *What you should know about infectious diseases: a guide for renal facilities*, New York, 1996, NKF.

Nephrology News & Issues: Issues in water treatment: a brief overview of the new FDA guidelines, *NNI*, October 1996, 9-10.

NIDDK: Kidney disease of diabetes (On-Line), 1997. Available: URL: http://www.niddk.nih.gov/

Niu PC, et al.: How can the care of elderly dialysis patients be improved? *Sem in Dial* 5:31-33, 1992.

Occupational Safety and Health Administration: Occupational exposure to bloodborne pathogens: final rule, *29CFR* 1901-1030; Federal Register, 1991.

Painter PL, et al.: Effects of exercise training during hemodialysis, *Nephron* 43(2):87-92, 1986.

Price C: Acute renal failure—a sequelae of sepsis, *Crit Care Clinics of No Am*, 6(2):149-154, 1994.

Price C: An update on continuous renal replacement therapies, *AACN Clin Issu in Crit Care Nsg*, 3(3):597-604, 1992.

Price C: Continuous renal replacement therapies (CRRT). In Lancaster, *Core curriculum for nephrology nursing*, Pitman, NJ, ed 3, 1995, Anthony J. Jannetti.

Price C: Continuous renal replacement therapy: the treatment of choice for acute renal failure, *ANNA J* 18(3):239-244, 1991.

Proceedings of the 3rd International Symposium on Daily Home Hemodialysis held in conjunction with the 18th Annual Conference on Peritoneal Dialysis, Denver, Colorado, February 1997, *Home Hemodialysis International* 1:1-48, Toronto, 1997, Multimed Inc.

Renal Physicians Association Working Committee on Clinical Practice Guidelines: Clinical practice guidelines on adequacy of hemodialysis, *Clinical Practice Guideline*, no. 1, Washington, DC, December 1993.

Report of the Expert Committee on the Diagnosis and Classification of Diabetes, *Diabetes Care* 20:1183, 1997.

Rodriguez D, Lewis S: Nutritional management of patients with acute renal failure, *ANNA J* 24(2):232-241, 1997.

Salusky IB: Nutritional management of pediatric patients on chronic dialysis. In Nissenson AR, Fine RE, Gentile DE, editors: *Clinical dialysis*, ed 3, Norwalk, Conn, 1995, Appleton & Lange.

Sepulveda S, Davis L, Schwab S: Blood transfusion during heparin-free hemodialysis, *Kidney Int* 51(6):2018-2021, 1997.

Sherman R, et al.: Recognition of the failing vascular access: a current perspective, *Sem in Dial* 10(1):1-4, 1997.

Sommadossi JP, et al.: Clinical pharmacokinetics of gancyclovir in patients with normal and impaired renal function, *Rev Infect Dis* 10(suppl 3):S507-S514, 1988.

St. Peter WL, et al.: Chronic renal failure and end stage renal disease. In Dipiro JT: *Pharmacotherapy: A pathophysiological approach*, ed 3, Stamford CT, 1997, Appleton & Lange.

Swan SK, Bennett WM: Use of drugs in patients with renal failure. In Schrier RW, Gottschalk CW, editors: *Diseases of the kidney*, vol 3, ed 6, Boston, 1997, Little, Brown, and Company.

Teehan BP, Hakim R: CAPD—Quo vadis? *J Am Soc Nephrol* 6(2):139-143, 1995.

Tzamaloukas AH: In Daugirdas JT, Ing TS, editors:*Handbook of dialysis*, ed 2, Boston, 1994, Little, Brown and Co.

United States Pharmacopeial Convention Drug Information (USPDI): *Drug information for the health care professional*, ed 18, Rockville, 1998, United States Pharmacopeial Convention, Inc.

United States Renal Data System, *USRDS 1998 annual data report*, Bethesda, MD, April 1998, National Institutes of Health, National Institute of Diabetes and Digestive and Kidney Diseases.

United States Renal Data System: *USRDS 1998 annual data report*, Washington, DC, 1998, US Department of Health and Human Services.

US Department of Health and Human Services: *A manual on water treatment for hemodialysis*, Rockville, MD, 1989, Public Health Service, FDA.

US Department of Health and Human Services: *Guidance for the content of premarket notifications for water purification components and systems for hemodialysis*, Rockville, MD, 1997, Public Health Service, FDA.

Vlchek DL, et al.: *Quality assurance guidelines for hemodialysis devices*, 1991, Conifer, CO, Dialysis Management Inc.

Vlchek DL, Seroka AM: Practical applications of continuous quality improvement in renal care, *Nephrology News & Issues* 36-44, April 1992.

Vogel SC: Access to the bloodstream. In Gutch CF, Stoner MH, Corea AL, editors: *Review of hemodialysis for nurses and dialysis personnel*, ed 5, St. Louis, 1993, Mosby–Year Book, Inc.

Winchester JF, Kriger FL: Hemodialysis and hemoperfusion in the management of poisoning. In Massry SG, Glasscock RJ, editors: *Textbook of nephrology*, vol 2, ed 3, Baltimore, 1995, Williams & Wilkins.

Woods JD, et al.: Comparison of mortality with home hemodialysis and center hemodialysis: a national study, *Kidney Int* 49(5):1464-1470, 1996.

Young DS: Implementation of SI units for clinical laboratory data, *Ann Intern Med* 106(1):114-129, 1987.

Zarama M, Abraham PA: Drug-induced renal disease. In Dipiro JT, editor: *Pharmacotherapy: A pathophysiologic approach*, ed 3, Stamford, CT, 1997, Appleton & Lange.

Nephrology Organizations and Resources

Lowanna S. Binkley, Kathy Bender, Nancy Gallagher, Martin V. Hudson, Kathy Law, Mary M. Macaluso, Georgina Randolph, Karen C. Robbins, and Philip M. Varughese

For healthcare providers who are practicing within a dialysis unit or nephrology program, it becomes important to know where to turn for specific information for patients or for staff. Several organizations can be good resources for the practitioner who is seeking information.

Knowing how to use these resources can be key to a successful practice. Most of us do not take full advantage of the educational and informational resources available to us from organizations and from the manufacturers of the products we use every day. These organizations are listed by category, followed by an alphabetical listing that gives a description of each organization.

Manufacturers of the products you are using will have the best available information about that specific product. It is in the best interests of the manufacturer to provide as much information as possible about its product(s), how to use the product(s), and other information that will maximize the product for the patient. Use these manufacturers as an important resource.

This Appendix provides information about voluntary and professional organizations of interest to health professionals caring for patients with ESRD.

Credentialing Organizations

Board of Nephrology Examiners, Inc., Nursing and Technology (BONENT)
PO Box 15945-282
Lenexa, KS 66285
(913) 541-9077
FAX: (913) 541-0156

National Nephrology Certification Organization (NNCO)
Inquiries to: Professional Testing Corporation (PTC)
1350 Broadway, 17th Floor
New York, New York 10018
(212) 356-0660
FAX: (212) 356-0678
e-mail: PTCNY@PTCNY.COM

Nephrology Nursing Certification Board (NNCB)
East Holly Avenue
Box 56
Pitman, NJ 08071
(609) 256-2321
FAX: (609) 589-7463
NNCB@mail.ajj.com

Patient Organizations

American Association of Kidney Patients (AAKP)
100 South Ashley Drive
Suite 280
Tampa, FL 33602
(813) 251-0725
e-mail: AAKPnat@aol.com
website: aakp.org

National Kidney Foundation (NKF)
30 East 33rd Street
11th Floor
New York, NY 10016
(212) 889-2210
800-622-9010
website: kidney.org

American Kidney Fund (AKF)
6110 Executive Blvd
Suite 1010
Rockville, MD 20852
(301) 881-3052
FAX: (301) 881-0898
e-mail:helpline@akfinc.org
website: akfinc.org

Professional Associations

American Nephrology Nurses' Association (ANNA)
East Holly Avenue
Box 56
Pitman, NJ 08071-0056
(609) 256-2320
e-mail:anna@mail.ajj.com
website: anna.inurse.com

National Association for Nephrology Technicians/Technologists (NANT)
PO Box 2307
Dayton, OH 45401-2307
(937) 586-3705
FAX: (937) 586-3699
e-mail: nant@nant.meinet.com and nefroworld.com

National Renal Administrators Association (NRAA)
11250 Roger Bacon Drive
Suite 8
Reston, VA 20190-5202
(703) 437-4377
FAX: (703) 435-4390
e-mail:nraa@nraa.org
website: nraa.org/renal/

Other Organizations

Association for the Advancement of Medical Instrumentation (AAMI) 3330
Washington Blvd
Suite 400
Arlington, VA 22201-4598
(703) 525-4890
FAX: (703) 276-0793
website: aami.org

United Network for Organ Sharing (UNOS)
PO Box 13770
1100 Boulders Parkway
Suite 500
Richmond, VA 23225
(804) 330-8500
FAX: (804) 330-8517 or (804) 330-8507
website: unos.org

What follows is an alphabetical listing of each organization, with a brief explanation about its function. Every effort has been made to provide the organizations' mission statements, or purpose.

American Association of Kidney Patients (AAKP) considers itself "the voice of all kidney patients" and was founded in 1969 *by* kidney patients *for* kidney patients. The purpose of this organization is to help patients and their families cope with the emotional, physical, and social impact of kidney disease. AAKP's purpose is to promote the welfare of kidney patients through education and advocacy. Self-help and patient education are key elements of local chapter activities. AAKP publishes *Renalife* on a quarterly basis and provides access to information on issues affecting the care and treatment of kidney patients through its informational clearinghouse.

American Kidney Fund (AKF) provides direct financial assistance to needy kidney patients. This organization publishes public and patient education brochures that are provided upon request, as well as a newsletter entitled *Clinical Strategies: the AKF Newsletter for Nephrology Professionals.*

American Nephrology Nurses' Association (ANNA) has as its stated purpose the obligation to set forth and update high standards of patient care, educate its practitioners, stimulate research, disseminate new ideas through the nephrology nursing field, promote interdisciplinary communication and cooperation, and address issues encompassing the practice of nephrology nursing. Association objectives center around the functional areas of education, clinical practice, representation and research. Any registered nurse licensed in the United States, Canada, or Mexico who is interested in the care of patients with renal disease is eligible for full membership. All others interested in the care of patients with renal disease are eligible for associate membership. Publications include *ANNA Journal* and the newsletter entitled *ANNA Update.* In addition to periodicals, ANNA publishes position papers and monographs devoted to nursing practice in nephrology, transplantation, and related therapies. For nurses interested in sitting for the NNCB examination, ANNA has developed a *Nephrology Nursing Certification Review Guide* and a model Certification Review Course to assist nurses in their preparation.

Association for the Advancement of Medical Instrumentation (AAMI) provides continuing information needed by healthcare professionals to keep up with changes in healthcare technology. They publish *Biomedical Instrumentation & Technology,* a bimonthly, peer-reviewed journal with solutions, news, and advice on aspects of medical technology; AAMI News is a newsletter that presents information on government policies and regulations, and national and international technology standards development; *Medical Device Research Report* aims to bridge the gap between academia and industry, facilitate technology transfer, and report on the public policy climate for medical device research.

Board of Nephrology Examiners, Nursing and Technology (BONENT) administers separate exams in the individual nephrology specialties of hemodialysis technology, hemodialysis nursing, and peritoneal dialysis nursing. Registered nurses, licensed practical nurses, and dialysis technicians who are actively working in ESRD and have a minimum of one year of experience are eligible to take the examination. To assist those interested in taking the exam, BONENT provides a study outline that includes a comprehensive bibliography. Successful completion of the examination entitles the applicant to use Certified Hemodialysis Technician (CHT), Certified Hemodialysis Nurse (CHN), or Certified Peritoneal Dialysis Nurse (CPDN) as a credential after his or her name.

National Association of Nephrology Technicians/Technologists (NANT) states that its mission is to promote the highest quality of care for end stage renal disease (ESRD) patients through education and professionalism. Its goals are to provide educational opportunities for the technical practitioner and other members of the integrated team; represent the technical professional in the regulatory and legislative arena; continue the development of technical professionals in leadership roles; achieve recognition for the role and significant contribution of the technical practitioner to the total care of the ESRD patient; and serve as a resource for the ESRD community to accomplish each of these goals. NANT provides manuals and study guides on dialyzer reprocessing, water treatment, dialysis technology, as well as selected reprints on technical aspects of dialysis. NANT also has audiotapes available from annual symposia, as well as multimedia packages of information on *Certification Issues*, *Re-Use*, *Access*, *Standards/Regulations*, *Water*, *Clinical Issues*, among others.

National Kidney Foundation (NKF) has a mission to prevent kidney and urinary tract diseases, improve the health and well-being of individuals affected by these diseases, and increase the availability of all organs for transplantation. NKF Goals include supporting research and research training, continuing education of health care professionals, expanding patient services and community resources, educating the public, shaping health policy and fund raising. Publications include: *American Journal of Kidney Diseases*, the official journal of the NKF, which includes peer-reviewed research papers as well as periodic position papers and proceedings from scientific symposia; *Advances in Renal Replacement Therapy*, a journal designed to meet the clinical needs of the multidisciplinary renal care team; *Journal of Renal Nutrition*, the official journal of the Council on Renal Nutrition; and the *Journal of Nephrology Social Work*, the official journal of the Council of Nephrology Social Workers. Other publications include newsletters for the various councils, pamphlets for the lay person to educate the public about various kidney diseases, and other general renal topics.

NKF-DOQI — The complete text of the NKF-DOQI Clinical Practice Guidelines is available in a variety of formats. A specially designed caddy houses a boxed set of five volumes (Hemodialysis Adequacy, Peritoneal Dialysis Adequacy, Vascular Access, Treatment of Anemia of Chronic Renal Failure, and Executive Summaries); each of these volumes is also available as a separate piece. In addition to the printed volumes, the full text of the NKF-DOQI guidelines is available on CD-ROM (PC and MAC compatible). For additional information and/or to order the NKF-DOQI Clinical Practice Guidelines, contact the National Kidney Foundation at (800) 622-9010.

National Nephrology Certification Organization describes itself as a fledgling certification organization with a unique mission: to create and administer subject-specific certification examinations for the dialysis technician/technologist. Currently there are two specialty examinations: (a) patient care technician and (b) biomedical (nephrology) technician. Upon successful completion of the examinations, the applicant can become a Certified Clinical Nephrology Technician (CCNT) or a Certified Biomedical Nephrology Technician (CBNT). As time and resources permit, other examinations will be developed.

National Renal Administrators Association (NRAA) is a voluntary organization representing professional managers of dialysis facilities and centers throughout the United States. Through education, networking, information, and governmental representation, NRAA aims to maintain competence and enhance professionalism throughout the renal community. Publications include *NRAA Journal*, published biannually, and the *President's Letter*, a monthly newsletter to keep members informed of key legislative decisions and regulations affecting renal professionals, along with regional news from across the country.

Nephrology Nursing Certification Board (NNCB) believes that certification serves as an added credential beyond nursing education and licensure, and therefore designs the examination to test the specific knowledge of the nephrology nurse. NNCB's purpose is to improve and maintain the quality of professional nephrology nursing care through the development, administration, and supervision of a certification program in the field of nephrology nursing. Those who successfully complete the certification process by meeting the eligibility criteria and passing a multiple-choice written exam are entitled to display the designated certification of Certified Nephrology Nurse (CNN).

United Network for Organ Sharing (UNOS) has a mission to advance organ availability and transplantation by uniting and supporting its communities for the benefit of patients through education, technology, and policy development.

By being aware of the resources that are available to the practitioner in the dialysis unit setting, the healthcare professional will be better prepared to assist his/her patients and family to cope with living a life with ESRD. Research has shown that the patient with a considerable support system lives longer than the patient with little or no support system. You play a key role in your patients' support system. Play this role wisely.

SI Units Conversion Factors for Clinical Chemistry Values Used in Hemodialysis

Component	Present Reference Range	Conversion Factor	SI Reference Range
Albumin (S)	4.0-6.0 g/dl	10	40-60 g/L
Alkaline p'tase (S)	30-120 U/L	0.01667	0.5-2.0 μkat/L
ALT (S)	0-35 U/L	0.01667	0-0.58 μkat/L
Aluminum (S)	0-15 μg/L	37.06	0-560 nmol/L
Ammonia (P)	10-80 μg/dl	0.5872	5-50 μmol/L
Amylase (S)	0-130 U/L	0.01667	0-2.17 μkat/L
Ascorbic acid (P)	0.6-2.0 mg/dl	56.78	30-110 μmol/L
AST (S)	0-35 U/L	0.01667	0-0.58 μkat/L
B$_{12}$ (S)	200-1000 pg/ml	0.7378	150-750 pmol/L
Bilirubin (S)	0.1-1.0 mg/dl	17.10	2-18 μmol/L
Calcium (S)	8.8-10.3 mg/dl	0.2495	2.20-2.58 mmol/L
Chloride (S)	95-105 mEq/L	1.00	95-105 mmol/L
Copper (S)	70-140 μg/dl	0.1574	11.0-22.0 μmol/L
CPK (S)	0-130 U/L	0.01667	0-2.16 μkat/L
Creatinine (S)	0.6-1.2 mg/dl	88.40	50-110 μmol/L
Digoxin (S) (toxic)	>2.5 ng/ml	1.281	>3.2 nmol/L
Ethanol (P)	100 mg/dl	0.2171	22 mmol/L
Ferritin (S)	18-300 ng/ml	1.00	18-300 μg/L
Fibrinogen (P)	200-400 mg/dl	0.01	2.0-4.0 g/L
Folate (S)	2-10 ng/ml	2.266	4-22 nmol/L
GGT (S)	0-30 U/L	0.01667	0-0.50 μkat/L
Glucose (P) (fasting)	70-110 mg/dl	0.05551	3.9-6.1 mmol/L
Hemoglobin (B)			
Men	14.0-18.0 g/dl	10.0	140-180 g/L
Women	11.5-15.5 g/dl	10.0	115-155 g/L

(continued)

Adapted from Young DS: Implementation of SI units for clinical laboratory data, *Ann Intern Med* 106(1):114-129, 1987.

B, Blood; *P*, plasma; *S*, serum.

Component	Present Reference Range	Conversion Factor	SI Reference Range
Iron (S)			
Men	80-180 µg/dl	0.1791	14-32 µmol/L
Women	60-90 µg/dl	0.1791	11-29 µmol/L
Binding capacity	250-460 µg/dl	0.1791	45-82 µmol/L
LDH (S)	50-150 U/L	0.01667	0.82-2.66 µkat/L
Magnesium (S)	1.8-3.0 mg/dl	0.4114	0.8-1.2 mmol/L
β_2-microglobulin (S)	0.8-2.4 mg/L	84.75	68-204 nmol/L
Osmolality (P)	280-300 mOsm/kg	1.00	280-300 mmol/L
Phosphorus (S)	2.5-5.0 mg/dl	0.3229	0.8-1.6 mmol/L
Potassium (S)	3.5-5.0 mEq/L	1.00	3.5-5.0 mmol/L
Protein (S)	6.0-8.0 g/dl	10.0	60-80 g/L
Sodium (S)	135-147 mEq/L	1.00	135-147 mmol/L
T_3 (S)	75-220 ng/dl	0.01536	1.2-3.4 nmol/L
Thyroxine (S)	4.0-11.0 µg/dl	12.87	51-142 nmol/L
Urea nitrogen (S)	8-18 mg/dl	0.3570	3.0-6.5 mmol/L
Uric acid (S)	2.0-7.0 mg/dl	59.48	120-420 µmol/L
Zinc (S)	75-120 µg/dl	0.1530	11.5-18.5 µmol/L

Conversion Table: Pounds to Kilograms of Body Weight

Kilo-grams	*Pounds* 0.0	0.1	0.2	0.3	0.4	0.5	0.6	0.7	0.8	0.9
40	88.00	88.22	88.44	88.66	88.88	89.10	89.32	89.54	89.76	89.98
41	90.20	90.42	90.64	90.86	91.08	91.30	91.52	91.74	91.96	92.18
42	92.40	92.62	92.84	93.06	93.28	93.50	93.72	93.94	94.16	94.38
43	94.60	94.82	95.04	95.26	95.48	95.70	95.92	96.14	96.36	96.58
44	96.80	97.02	97.24	97.46	97.68	97.90	98.12	98.34	98.56	98.78
45	99.00	99.22	99.44	99.66	99.88	100.10	100.32	100.54	100.76	100.98
46	101.20	101.42	101.64	101.86	102.08	102.30	102.52	102.74	102.96	103.18
47	103.40	103.62	103.84	104.06	104.28	104.50	104.72	104.94	105.16	105.38
48	105.60	105.82	106.04	106.26	106.48	106.70	106.92	107.14	107.36	107.58
49	107.80	108.02	108.24	108.46	108.68	108.90	109.12	109.34	109.56	109.78
50	110.00	110.22	110.44	110.66	110.88	111.10	111.32	111.54	111.76	111.98
51	112.20	112.42	112.64	112.86	113.08	113.30	113.52	113.74	113.96	114.18
52	114.40	114.62	114.84	115.06	115.28	115.50	115.72	115.94	116.16	116.38
53	116.60	116.82	117.04	117.26	117.48	117.70	117.92	118.14	118.36	118.58
54	118.80	119.02	119.24	119.46	119.68	119.90	120.12	120.34	120.56	120.78
55	121.00	121.22	121.44	121.66	121.88	122.10	122.32	122.54	122.76	122.98
56	123.20	123.42	123.64	123.86	124.08	124.30	124.52	124.74	124.96	125.18
57	125.40	125.62	125.84	126.06	126.08	126.50	126.72	126.94	127.16	127.38
58	127.60	127.82	128.04	128.26	128.48	128.70	128.92	129.14	129.36	129.58
59	129.80	130.02	130.24	130.46	130.68	130.90	131.12	131.34	131.56	131.78
60	132.00	132.22	132.44	132.66	132.88	133.10	133.32	133.54	133.76	133.98
61	134.20	134.42	134.64	134.86	135.08	135.30	135.52	135.74	135.96	136.18
62	136.40	136.62	136.84	137.06	137.28	137.50	137.72	137.94	138.16	138.38
63	138.60	138.82	139.04	139.26	139.48	139.70	139.92	140.14	140.36	140.58
64	140.80	141.02	141.24	141.46	141.68	141.90	142.12	142.34	142.56	142.78
65	143.00	143.22	143.44	143.66	143.88	144.10	144.32	144.54	144.76	144.98
66	145.20	145.42	145.64	145.86	146.08	146.30	146.52	146.74	146.96	147.18
67	147.40	147.62	147.84	148.06	148.28	148.50	148.72	148.94	149.16	149.38
68	149.60	149.82	150.04	150.26	150.48	150.70	150.92	151.14	151.36	151.58
69	151.80	152.02	152.24	152.46	152.68	152.90	153.12	153.34	153.56	153.78
70	154.00	154.22	154.44	154.66	154.88	155.10	155.32	155.54	155.76	155.98
71	156.20	156.42	156.64	156.86	157.08	157.30	157.52	157.74	157.96	158.18

Kilo-grams	Pounds									
	0.0	0.1	0.2	0.3	0.4	0.5	0.6	0.7	0.8	0.9
72	158.40	158.62	158.84	159.06	159.28	159.50	159.72	159.94	160.16	160.38
73	160.60	160.82	161.04	161.26	161.48	161.70	161.92	162.14	162.36	162.58
74	162.80	163.02	163.24	163.46	163.68	163.90	164.12	164.34	164.56	164.78
75	165.00	165.22	165.44	165.66	165.88	166.10	166.32	156.54	166.76	166.98
76	167.20	167.42	167.64	167.86	168.08	168.30	168.52	168.74	168.96	169.18
77	169.40	169.62	169.84	170.06	170.28	170.50	170.72	170.94	171.16	171.38
78	171.60	171.82	172.04	172.26	172.48	172.70	172.92	173.14	173.36	173.58
79	173.80	174.02	174.24	174.46	174.68	174.90	175.12	175.34	175.56	175.78
80	176.00	176.22	176.44	176.66	176.88	177.10	177.32	177.54	177.76	177.98
81	178.20	178.42	178.64	178.86	179.08	179.30	179.52	179.74	179.96	180.18

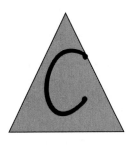

Sodium and Potassium Content of Selected Foods

Food	Amount	Grams	Sodium (mEq)	Potassium (mEq)
BREADS				
Biscuit	1 biscuit	35	9.5	1.0
Cornbread	1 piece	45	12.3	1.8
Cracked wheat	1 slice	23	5.3	0.8
Pumpernickel	1 slice	32	7.9	3.7
Rye	1 slice	23	5.6	0.8
Tortilla	6 in diameter	30	1.4	0.1
White	1 slice	23	5.1	0.6
Whole wheat	1 slice	23	5.3	1.6
CEREALS/GRAIN PRODUCTS				
All-bran	1 cup	56	24.7	13.3
Cornflakes	1 cup	22	9.4	0.7
Farina (instant)	1 cup	245	20.0	0.8
Farina (regular)	1 cup	245	—	0.8
Grits	1 cup	242	—	0.7
Macaroni (cooked)	1 cup	140	—	2.2
Noodles (cooked)	1 cup	160	0.1	1.8
Oatmeal	1 cup	236	—	3.3
Puffed rice	1 cup	14	—	0.4
Puffed wheat	1 cup	14	—	1.2
Raisin bran	1 cup	50	12.7	6.2
Rice (cooked)	1 cup	150	24.4	1.1
Shredded wheat (spoon sized)	1 cup	45	0.2	4.5
CHEESE				
Cheddar, processed	1 oz	28	13.8	0.6
Cheddar, unprocessed	1 oz	28	8.6	0.6
Cottage, creamed	3 ½ oz	100	10.0	2.2
Cream	2 tbsp	28	3.7	0.9
Swiss	1 oz	28	8.7	0.7

Food	Amount	Grams	Sodium (mEq)	Potassium (mEq)
EGGS				
Egg, whole	1 (medium)	48	2.6	1.6
Egg substitute	¼ cup	604	4.7	3.3
FATS				
Butter	1 tbsp	15	5.4	0.1
Margarine	1 tbsp	15	6.4	—
Oil	1 tbsp	14	—	—
FISH AND SEAFOOD				
Clams, soft, meat	4 large or 9 small	100	1.6	6.0
Cod, broiled	4 oz before cooked	95	4.6	9.9
Crab (canned or cooked)	½ cup	85	37.0	2.4
Oysters, raw	5–8 (medium)	100	3.2	3.1
Salmon, pink (canned)	⅖ cup	100	16.8	9.3
Sardines (canned in oil)	8 (medium)	100	22.2	14.4
Shrimp, raw	3 ½ oz	100	6.1	5.6
Tuna (canned)	¾ cup	100	34.8	7.7
FRUIT JUICES				
Apple juice, canned	1 cup	240	0.1	6.2
Apricot nectar	1 cup	240	—	9.3
Cranberry juice cocktail	1 cup	240	0.1	0.6
Grape juice, bottled	1 cup	240	0.2	7.1
Grapefruit juice, canned	1 cup	240	0.4	8.9
Orange juice, canned or fresh	1 cup	240	0.1	12.3
Orange juice, frozen (diluted)	1 cup	240	0.1	11.4
Pineapple juice, canned	1 cup	240	0.1	9.2
Prune juice, canned	1 cup	240	0.2	14.5
Tomato juice, canned	1 cup	240	20.9	14.0
FRUITS				
Apple, raw	1 medium (2 ½ in)	150	—	4.2
Applesauce, canned (sweet)	½ cup	150	0.1	2.5
Apricots, canned (sweet)	3 halves (medium)	100	—	6.0
Apricots, raw	2–3 (medium)	100	—	7.2
Avocado, raw	half (3 ¼ X 4 in)	100	0.2	15.5
Banana, raw	1 (medium)	150	0.1	14.1
Blueberries, raw	½ cup	70	—	1.5
Cantaloupe, raw	quarter (5-in diameter)	100	0.5	6.4
Cherries, raw (sweet)	15 large or 25 small	100	0.1	4.9
Cranberry sauce, canned	5 tbsp	100	—	0.8

Food	Amount	Grams	Sodium (mEq)	Potassium (mEq)
Dates, dried	10 (medium)	100	—	16.6
Figs, dried	5 (medium)	100	1.5	16.4
Fruit cocktail, canned (sweet)	½ cup	100	0.2	4.1
Grapefruit, raw	half (medium)	100	—	3.5
Grapes, domestic, raw	22 (medium)	100	0.1	4.1
Orange, raw	1 (medium)	206	—	7.0
Peaches, canned (sweet)	2 halves (medium)	100	0.1	3.3
Peach, raw	1 (medium)	100	—	5.2
Pears, canned (sweet)	2 halves (small)	100	—	2.2
Pear, raw	half (3 X 2 ½ in)	100	0.1	3.3
Pineapple, canned	1 slice (large)	100	—	3.8
Pineapple, raw, diced	¾ cup	100	—	3.7
Plums, prune type, raw	3 (medium)	100	—	4.4
Plums, purple, canned (sweet)	3 (medium)	100	—	3.6
Prunes, dried	10 (large)	100	0.4	17.8
Raisins, seedless, dried	⅝ cup	100	1.2	19.6
Strawberries, raw	10 (large)	100	—	4.2
Watermelon, balls or cubes	½ cup	100	—	2.6

MEATS

Food	Amount	Grams	Sodium (mEq)	Potassium (mEq)
Bacon, fried crisp	3 strips	23	10.9	1.4
Beef, lean (cooked)	1 slice	86	1.7	11.2
Ham, cured, lean	1 slice	60	22.5	6.1
Hamburger, lean (cooked)	1 patty	86	1.8	12.3
Liver, calf, fried	3 ½ oz	100	5.1	11.6
Pork, lean chop (cooked)	1 chop	68	1.8	9.9
Sausage, pork (cooked)	1 link	20	8.3	1.4

MILK/DAIRY PRODUCTS

Food	Amount	Grams	Sodium (mEq)	Potassium (mEq)
Buttermilk (from skim)	1 cup	245	13.8	8.8
Chocolate (2% fat)	1 cup	250	6.5	10.8
Half and half	1 cup	240	4.2	7.8
Lowfat (2% fat)	1 cup	244	5.3	9.6
Skim	1 cup	246	5.6	10.5
Whipping cream, heavy	1 cup	240	4.2	4.5
Whole (3.5% fat)	1 cup	244	5.3	9.0
Yogurt, low fat	1 cup	227	6.9	13.6

MISCELLANEOUS

Food	Amount	Grams	Sodium (mEq)	Potassium (mEq)
Nuts, mixed, unsalted	8–12 nuts	15	0.1	2.2
Peanut butter	2 tbsp	30	1.6	6.3
Sunflower seed kernels	3 ½ oz	100	1.3	23.6

Food	Amount	Grams	Sodium (mEq)	Potassium (mEq)
POULTRY				
Chicken, roasted	3 ½ oz	100	3.3	9.4
Turkey, roasted	3 ½ oz	100	5.7	9.4
SWEETS				
Honey	1 tbsp	20	—	0.3
Jelly	1 tbsp	20	0.1	0.4
Molasses, light	1 tbsp	20	0.7	7.7
Sugar, brown (dark)	1 tbsp	14	0.1	0.8
Sugar, white	1 tbsp	14	—	—
VEGETABLES				
Asparagus, canned	6 spears	115	11.8	4.9
Asparagus, fresh	5–6 spears	100	0.1	7.1
Beans, green, canned	½ cup	110	11.7	2.7
Beans, green, fresh (cooked)	1 cup	125	0.2	4.8
Beans, pinto (frijoles)	½ cup	193	47.9	17.8
Beans, white (cooked)	½ cup	100	0.3	10.7
Beets, canned	½ cup	83	8.5	3.5
Broccoli, frozen (cooked)	3 ½ oz	100	0.7	5.4
Broccoli, raw	1 stalk (5 ½ in)	100	0.7	9.8
Brussels sprouts, frozen (cooked)	3 ½ oz	100	0.6	7.6
Cabbage, raw, shredded	1 cup	100	0.9	6.0
Carrots, canned	⅔ cup	100	10.3	3.1
Carrots, raw	1 large or 2 small	100	2.0	8.7
Celery, raw	1 large or 3 small	50	2.7	4.4
Collards (cooked)	½ cup	100	1.1	6.0
Corn, canned	⅖ cup	100	10.3	2.5
Cucumber, raw	½ (medium)	50	0.1	2.0
Kale, frozen (cooked)	3 ½ oz	100	0.9	4.9
Lettuce	3 ½ oz	100	0.4	6.8
Lima beans, canned	½ cup	115	11.8	6.5
Lima beans, frozen (cooked)	⅝ cup	100	4.4	10.9
Mushrooms, canned (with liquid)	½ cup	100	17.4	5.0
Mushrooms, fresh	4 large or 10 small	100	0.7	10.6
Mustard greens (cooked)	½ cup	100	0.8	5.6
Okra, cooked	8–9 pods	100	0.1	4.5
Peas, canned	¾ cup	100	10.3	2.5
Peas, frozen	3 ½ oz	100	5.0	3.5
Potato, baked	2 ½ in diameter	100	0.2	12.9
Potato, mashed	½ cup	100	14.4	6.4
Spinach, canned	½ cup	90	9.2	5.8

Food	Amount	Grams	Sodium (mEq)	Potassium (mEq)
Spinach, fresh (cooked)	½ cup	90	2.0	7.5
Squash, summer (cooked)	½ cup	100	—	3.6
Squash, winter, baked	½ cup	100	—	11.8
Sweet potato, baked in skin	1 (small)	100	0.5	7.7
Tomato, raw	1 (medium)	150	0.2	9.4
Tomatoes, canned	½ cup	100	5.7	5.6

Glossary

AAMI Association for the Advancement of Medical Instrumentation. This organization set the standards and recommended practices for dialysis machines, reuse of dialyzers, electrical safety, monitoring and culturing of machines and water systems, cleaning of machines, quality of water used for dialysis, and methodology for bacteriology and culturing samples.

ACT Activated clotting time. ACT is a test to measure the clotting time of the blood.

acute Adjective used in two ways: to indicate that something is of short duration or sudden onset and to indicate a high degree of severity.

adsorb To cause particles or molecules in solution to stick to the surface of a solid material.

air embolus Air bubble carried by the bloodstream to a vessel small enough to be blocked by the bubble.

albumin A protein found in many body tissues. It disperses in water as a colloid and is an important fraction of blood plasma. Molecular weight is approximately 68,000 d.

allograft A graft, such as a kidney, taken from another person (Greek *allo*, other). The donor may be a blood relative or unrelated.

amino acids Building blocks of protein. Amino indicates that one or more hydrogen ions of an acid have been replaced by the radical (NH_2). Amino acids also contain carbon, oxygen, and frequently sulfur.

amyloid Abnormal protein material occurring in certain disorders as deposits in various body tissues. In ESRD patients, it results from long-time accumulation of beta-2 microglobulin.

analog A structure whose function is similar to that of another organ or structure of a different kind and origin.

anaphylaxis A particularly severe type of systemic reaction to a foreign protein or other substance. It results from previous sensitization to the particular substance and can be fatal.

aneroid Pressure gauge (positive or negative) that contains no fluid.

aneurysm A blood-filled sac formed by stretching and dilation of the wall of an artery.

angiogram X-ray film of a blood vessel obtained by injecting a liquid contrast material into the vessel.

anion   Ion carrying a negative (–) electric charge. Unlike electric charges attract one another; hence the negatively charged particle is attracted to the positive pole (the anode).

anterior   In front or toward the front position.

antibody   A protein produced in response to stimulation by antigen that can combine specifically with that antigen.

anticoagulant   Medication or chemical to prevent clotting.

antigen   A molecule capable of combining specifically with antibody, resulting in either an immune response or a specific tolerant state.

antiseptic   Chemical that stops the growth and reproduction of bacteria or germs; it does not necessarily destroy them.

anuria   Complete cessation of urine flow.

APTT/PTT   Activated partial thromboplastin time.

ARF   Acute renal failure.

arrhythmia   Any variation from the normal, rhythmic heartbeat.

arterial   Anything that has to do with an artery or arteries.

arteriovenous   Involving both artery and vein.

artery   Blood vessel carrying blood under pressure from the heart to the various parts of the body.

ascitic fluid   Ascites. An accumulation of fluid in the abdominal cavity. Usually contains protein to a varying degree.

aseptic   Free of bacterial or infectious organisms; sterile.

aspirate   Remove something by suction or negative pressure.

atherosclerosis   A type of arteriosclerosis (hardening of the arteries) caused by degeneration and fatty changes in the walls of the arteries.

ATN   Acute tubular necrosis.

atony   Lack of normal tone or strength.

autoclave   Device for sterilization of materials, using saturated steam under pressure.

autogenous   Produced within the organism itself.

azotemia   Retention of nitrogenous wastes (urea, creatinine) in blood and body fluid.

bacteremia   Presence of bacteria in the bloodstream.

bacteria   Small one-celled plantlike organisms; widely prevalent everywhere. Many kinds are harmless or beneficial; certain ones cause infections and may be dangerous.

biocompatible   Not causing change or reaction in living tissue. A biocompatible membrane would not damage blood cells, cause clotting, or release pyrogenic matter.

blood cells   Cellular elements of blood. Red blood cells are vital for transport of oxygen from lungs to tissues; white blood cells act to combat infection and destroy bacteria.

B₂M Beta₂-microglobulins.

bradycardia Slow pulse rate or heart rate.

bruit An abnormal sound or murmur heard by listening over a blood vessel with a stethoscope. Expected sound heard over a vascular access, shunt, or fistula, of a dialysis patient.

BUN Blood urea nitrogen. A chemical determination of the amount of nitrogen, derived from urea, present in the blood. Actual urea is 2.2 times the BUN value. Normal BUN is 9 to 15 mg/dl (3.0 to 6.5 mmol/L).

BUN-creatinine ratio Normal ratio is 10:1.

cachexia General ill health and malnutrition. Wasting.

calcium-phosphorus product Calcium (in mg/dl) multiplied by phosphorus; product should be less than 70.

calibrate Adjust or accurately set a measuring device by comparison with a known standard.

cannula Tube that is inserted into a body opening.

CAPD Continuous ambulatory peritoneal dialysis.

carbohydrate One of the three main categories of basic footstuffs; composed of carbon, hydrogen, and oxygen and readily used by the body for energy. Starches and sugars are carbohydrates.

cardiomyopathy Any weakness or dysfunction of the heart muscle. Usually there is dilation and enlargement of the heart.

catabolism Breakdown of body tissue at a rate faster than its restoration.

catheter A hollow tube for withdrawing or introducing fluid into a cavity or passage of the body.

cation Ion carrying a positive (+) charge, which is attracted to the oppositely charged electric pole, the cathode.

caudad Toward the tail or the tail bone.

CAVH Continuous arteriovenous hemofiltration.

CAVHD Continuous arteriovenous hemodialysis.

CAVU Continuous arteriovenous ultrafiltration.

CCPD Continuous cycling peritoneal dialysis.

CVVH Continuous venovenous hemofiltration.

CVVHD Continuous venovenous hemodiafiltration.

CDC Centers for Disease Control.

cellulose A complex carbohydrate polymer of form $(C_6H_{10}O_5)_N$. It is the fibrous support structure of plants. Treatment with heat and chemicals produces a semipermeable membrane.

cephalad Toward the head.

CHF Congestive heart failure; also HF for heart failure.

chloramine Chemical compound containing chlorine attached to nitrogen, forming NC1 groups.

CHT Certified Hemodialysis Technician.

clearance   Mathematic expression of the rate at which a given substance is removed from a solution, for example, the clearance of urea from blood by the natural or an artificial kidney. It is defined as the number of milliliters of solutions that would be completely cleared of a given solute in 1 minute.

CLIA   Clinical Laboratory Improvement Act

CNN   Certified Nephrology Nurse.

coagulation   Formation of a blood clot.

colloid   A very finely divided substance, larger than a molecule, which spreads throughout a liquid as tiny particles. A colloid does not actually dissolve in the liquid nor does it cross a semipermeable membrane. It does exert an osmotic effect proportionate to its concentration. Serum albumin is a colloid.

comorbid   A coexisting illness or disease process not directly related to the primary disorder. It may make the overall course more complicated or adversely affect the outcome.

compliance   Capacity to yield or stretch. Also, the adherence to a plan of care such as dietary and fluid restrictions.

compound   A distinctive substance formed by the chemical union of two or more elements in definite proportion by weight.

concurrent   As applied to a dialyzer, dialysis fluid and blood flow are in the same direction.

conductivity   Ease with which an electric current is carried or conducted through something. The conductivity of dialysate solution is proportional to its electrolyte content.

contaminate   Make dirty, impure, or unsterile.

convection   Movement of solute across a membrane caused by bulk flow of solution.

countercurrent   In a dialyzer the direction of flow of dialysis fluid and of blood are 180 degrees opposite one another.

CQI   Continuous quality improvement.

creatinine   One of the nitrogenous waste products of normal muscle metabolism. It is produced at a fairly constant rate in the body.

Crit-Line monitor   An arterial in-line medical instrument that provides continuous measurement of absolute hematocrit, percent blood volume change, and oxygen saturation in real time. It measures blood volume change based on the hematocrit since these two values have an inverse relationship. As fluid is removed from the intravascular space, the blood density increases. This is displayed in percent of blood volume change on a grid-like graph on the instrument's screen. With this device, it is possible to maximize ultrafiltration safely and prevent hypotension, cramping and other intradialytic complications associated with volume depletion. A disposable blood chamber is attached to the arterial side of the dialyzer and a photo-metric technology is utilized. This device will also measure access recirculation.

CRF Chronic renal failure.

CTS Carpal tunnel syndrome.

cyclosporine A An immunosuppressive medication, technically an undecapeptide. It is highly effective in controlling transplant rejection. However, it adversely affects kidney function.

cytomegalovirus (CMV) A group of species-specific herpetoviruses that infect humans and other animals. Often asymptomatic, but tends to exacerbate in immunosuppressed individuals, causing illness with cellular enlargement, cytoplasmic inclusions, and damage to various organs.

dalton One atomic mass unit. Named for John Dalton, a developer of the atomic concept.

debris An accumulation of fragments of miscellaneous material; rubbish or junk material.

degassing Process of importance in proportioning-delivery systems; removing the gases (largely air) normally dissolved in tap water.

deionize Remove the various solute ions from a solution. Usually it refers to a water treatment process that removes all the electrolytes from the water.

delta The Greek letter D (Δ), used in mathematics to indicate a differential or change between two points.

dextrose A simple sugar, readily used by body cells for metabolism.

dialysance Expression for the capability of a dialyzer to clear a given solute. It represents the net rate of exchange of a substance between blood and bath per minute per unit of blood-bath concentration gradient.

dialysate Dialyzing fluid that has been used; it contains solutes not originally present. Often applied loosely to any dialyzing fluid.

dialysis-quality water Water that by LAL testing is less than 1 ng/ml (negative) for mycobacteria and meets AAMI chemical analysis standards for water used for dialysis.

diastole Period of relaxation of the heart; its filling phase.

diffusion Spreading out or scattering of different kinds of particles among each other.

dilate Expand or make wider.

dilute Thin out or weaken. A solution is diluted (made less concentrated) by the addition of more solvent.

disinfectant Chemical that destroys bacterial-organisms.

distal In a direction away from the center of the body or from the point of attachment.

diuresis Increased output of urine.

diverticulum A pocket or pouch off the side of a tube or hollow vessel.

DOQI National Kidney Foundation's Guidelines, Dialysis Outcomes Quality Initiative.

dyspnea Shortness of breath.

dyspraxia Partial loss of ability to perform coordinated movements.

ecchymosis   An extravasation or oozing of blood into the skin, as with a bruise.

edema   Collection of fluid in body tissue; swelling, often soft and compressible.

effluent   The outflow from something (usually liquid).

electrolyte   Substance that separates into ions after going into solution.

embolus   Clot, or portion of a clot, carried by the blood flow from a distant vessel and forced into a small vessel and blocking it.

encephalopathy   Any gross dysfunction of the brain, temporary or permanent, that may result from anatomic damage, metabolic imbalance, or toxic agents.

endocarditis   Inflammation of the endocardium, or interior lining of the heart. A serious condition that can be fatal.

endogenous   Originating within the body. Metabolism of the nitrogenous constituents of cells and tissues.

endotoxin   A toxic substance produced and held with the cells of bacteria until they die or are destroyed, whereupon it may be released.

EPO   Recombinant erythropoietin.

equilibrium   State of balance between opposing forces.

erythrocyte   Red blood cell.

erythropoiesis   Process of making red blood cells by the bone marrow.

erythropoietin   A hormone, normally produced by the kidneys, that causes the bone marrow to produce red blood cells (erythrocytes). A synthetic form of the hormone, recombinant human erythropoietin, is used to treat anemia.

ESRD   End-stage renal disease.

ethylene oxide   A gas that may be used for sterilization of objects that might be damaged by heat. Articles must be dry and must be "aired" after sterilization.

euglycemia   Normal blood glucose value.

euvolemia   Normal intravascular volume.

exogenous   Originating outside the organism. Due to external causes.

extracorporeal   Outside the body.

febrile   Feeling feverish; having an elevated temperature.

fecal   Relating to a bowel movement or excretion from the bowel.

fibrin   Protein product formed during the clotting of blood, usually threadlike strands.

fibrinolysin   A substance that lyses, or breaks up, fibrin.

fistula   Unnatural opening or passage. As related to dialysis, a surgical opening between an artery and vein to fill the vein with arterialized blood for blood access.

flowmeter   Device for indicating rate of flow of a liquid past a given point.

flux   The rate of flow or change across or through a surface.

formalin   Disinfectant consisting of 40% formaldehyde gas in water.

gamma irradiation Gamma rays are a form of high-frequency, high-energy radiation emitted from radioactive atomic nuclei. They are very penetrating for a short distance and kill all bacteria, spores, and viruses that they strike.

globulin A class of proteins found in serum and tissue and of much larger molecular size than albumin. Certain serum globulins are involved in the immune response of the body and are called *immunoglobulins*. IgA, IgG, IgM, and so on.

glucose Same as **dextrose**.

gradient Rate of increase or decrease between two variables.

hematocrit The cellular proportion of blood expressed as a percentage when blood is separated into its liquid and cellular elements by spinning in a centrifuge.

hematoma Accumulation of blood that has escaped from a blood vessel into surrounding tissue.

hemofiltration Removal of water from the blood by ultrafiltration without dialysis. A volume of water with its solute load is removed by convective transfer. No osmolar gradient between body fluid compartments, which might cause symptoms, is generated.

hemoglobin Red, protein portion of the red blood cells that has the capacity to bind oxygen temporarily while it is carried throughout the body.

hemolysis Breakup of red blood cells so that the hemoglobin is released into the surrounding fluid. Hemolysis may result from mechanical, chemical, or osmotic injury.

hemolytic-uremic syndrome An acute illness, most common in children and usually brought on by toxic bacterial diarrhea. Involves breakup of red cells (hemolysis) with release of hemoglobin, thrombocyte destruction, vascular endothelial injury and acute kidney damage with azotemia and uremic symptoms and findings.

hemoperfusion Removal of noxious substances by passing blood over a column of charcoal or special resin that has high binding capacity. No dialysis or ultrafiltration is involved.

heparin Chemical that slows the natural clotting of blood.

hepatitis Inflammation of the liver, often caused by a viral infection but which can result from toxic agents or medication.

HFAK Hollow-fiber artificial kidneys.

Hg Mercury (Latin, *hydrargyrum*).

high-efficiency dialysis Nonconventional dialysis performed with a special dialyzer that uses a membrane of very large surface area, which allows middle molecular weight (up to 5000 d) solutes to be diffused across the membrane in significant amounts.

high-flux dialysis Nonconventional dialysis performed with a special dialyzer that uses a highly permeable synthetic membrane that allows low and high molecular weight solutes (up to 12,000 d) to be convected across the membrane.

hydrolysate A substance produced from the breakdown of another substance by the addition of the elements of water.

hydrophilic Water-loving; a substance that blends or combines well with water.

hyper- Prefix to indicate higher than or greater than some standard.

hyperglycemia A blood sugar level higher than normal.

hypertension Blood pressure that is higher than normal.

hypo- Prefix to indicate lower or less than the normal.

hypobaric Less than normal atmospheric pressure.

hypocalcemia Serum calcium value less than normal (normal: 9 to 11 mg/dl).

hypokalemia Serum potassium (Latin, *kalium*) less than normal (3 to 5 mEq/L).

hyponatremia Serum sodium (Latin, *natrium*) less than normal (135 to 145 mEq/L).

hypotension Blood pressure that is abnormally low.

hypovolemia Low volume within the vascular system.

iatrogenic A condition resulting from therapy or medical treatment.

icterus Jaundice.

idiogenic Something separate or independent, originating with an organ or cells.

IDPN Intradialytic parenteral nutrition.

in vitro A test done not in a living organism but in a synthetic environment for the particular test.

in vivo A test done in a patient or in a living experimental animal.

infarction An area of tissue destruction resulting from obstruction of the local circulation usually from embolism or thrombosis.

infuse Introduce a fluid into something.

intima (tunica intima) The inner lining of blood vessels.

intravenous Within a vein (abbreviated IV).

ion Atom, or group of atoms, that has an electric charge.

IPD Intermittent peritoneal dialysis.

ischemia A temporary deficiency of blood supply.

isotonic Having the same concentration or the same osmotic pressure (Greek *iso*, same or equal).

jaundice Deposition of bile pigments in the skin, producing a yellowish color, caused by liver disorder or disease.

K Potassium (Latin, *kalium*).

kinetic Having to do with motion or movement.

kinetic modeling Sometimes called *urea kinetic modeling* (UKM). A mathematical tool used to prescribe and monitor dialysis therapy and to assess protein intake.

Kt/V A calculation result derived from UKM. The Kt/V goal for adequacy of hemodialysis is not less than 1.2 for three times weekly and 1.9 for twice weekly. The goal for peritoneal dialysis is greater than 1.5.

k_{UF} The ultrafiltration coefficient, which ranges from 0.5 to 80 ml/hr/mm Hg, depending on the membrane.

labile Unstable or easily changeable.

LAL Limulus amebocyte lysate. An assay for endotoxin that uses a protein extract from the horseshoe crab *(Limulus)*. Values are given in nanograms or in endotoxin units (1 ng/ml = 5 EU/ml).

lateral To one side or the other.

lesion Any injury or wound or local area of degeneration.

leukocyte A white blood cell.

lipid A group of substances including fats and esters, a fatty or organic oily substance.

lot In manufacturing terminology a group of units manufactured at the same time, from the exact same material, or to the same specifications.

lumen The open space within a tube or container.

lyse To destroy or break up cells.

macerate To soften or break up by immersion in water.

malrotate To rotate or turn incorrectly or inappropriately.

manometer Instrument or gauge to indicate pressure.

medial Toward the middle or midline.

metabolism Chemical and physical processes by which living organisms produce and maintain their own substance and develop energy for their use.

metastatic Disease or disorder that is transferred from one organ or tissue to another area not directly related to the primary site.

methemoglobin Hemoglobin in which the iron is in the ferric form rather than the ferrous form of normal hemoglobin. In this ferric form, it cannot combine with oxygen to transport it in the normal way.

microalbuminuria Screening tests for the presence of albumin, or other protein in the urine, such as the widely-used "dipstick," generally do not detect protein in amounts less than 200 mg/dl. Sensitive analytical testing methodology measures much smaller or "micro" amounts.

microglobulin Beta$_2$-microglobulin is a protein (MW-11,800 d) produced by normal turnover of nucleated cells in the body. It is catabolized by normal kidney tubules. In ESRD, beta$_2$-microglobulin accumulates, leading to deposits of an abnormal protein—amyloid—in bone, joints, tendons, and elsewhere.

modeling Mathematical simulation using probability analysis to predict outcome from changes in the known variables of a particular process. Usually done by computer.

module Self-contained unit that may be combined with others of the same type to form a larger unit.

mole One molecular weight of any given substance expressed in grams.

molal Solution containing 1 mole of solute in 1 kg of solvent.

monitor To supervise or check on something; a mechanical or electronic device that checks or supervises some operation.

mono- Prefix indicating one.

mycotic A disease or disorder caused by a fungus rather than by a bacterial organism.

NCDS National Cooperative Dialysis Study. The study was a multicenter study to correlate patient outcome with amount of dialysis delivered.

necrosis Death of tissue.

nephrologist Physician who specializes in kidney diseases and their treatment.

nephron Basic functioning unit of the normal kidney.

nephropathy Abnormal functioning of kidney. It may result from trauma, inflammation, toxic agents, or metabolic disorder.

neuropathy Damage to or disease of nerves.

NPD Nocturnal peritoneal dialysis.

obtund Dull, stupid; poorly responsive.

obturator Metal rod or stylus that fits inside the tube of a trocar. It carries a sharp point and can be withdrawn from the trocar after insertion.

occlude Close off or shut off.

oliguria Daily urine output less than 400 ml, which is the minimum amount of *normal* urine that can carry away the daily load of metabolic waste products.

omentum Fold of peritoneum that hangs like an apron between the stomach and the anterior abdominal wall.

oncotic Osmotic pressure resulting from the presence of nonionic solutes and suspended materials such as plasma proteins.

OSHA Occupational Safety and Health Administration, a federal agency that edicts safety and health issues.

osmolality Osmotic effect of a solute based on the molal concentration of the solution.

osmometer Instrument for determining the osmolality of a solution. It operates by determining the precise depression of the freezing point of a solution, which is directly related to the concentration of particles of solute per unit amount of solvent.

osmosis Passage of solvent through a semipermeable membrane that separates solutions of differing concentrations.

osteitis fibrosa cystica Bone rarefaction with fibrous degeneration and cyst formation; a result of parathyroid overactivity.

osteoblast A cell that lays down new bone structure.

osteoclast A cell that resolves and removes bone structure.

osteodystrophy General term for defective bone formation; it includes osteomalacia, osteoporosis, and so forth.

osteomalacia Softening of bone caused by lack of calcium deposition.

osteoporosis Bone rarefaction or thinning caused by inadequate new bone formation.

palpitation Irregular jumping or pounding of the heart.

PAN A dialyzer made of polyacrilonitrile (synthetic) membrane.

parameter Quantity to which arbitrary values may be assigned, as distinguished from a mathematic variable, which can assume only values determined by the form of the mathematic function. Parameters measured in dialysis work are blood pressure, flow rates, conductivity, temperature, and so on.

parathyroid glands Four small glands, located on the posterior surface of the thyroid gland (*para*, beside, adjacent to). The parathyroid hormone is concerned with regulation of calcium in body fluid.

patent Open.

pathogenic Causing a disease or abnormal process.

peptide A compound of two or more amino acids in which the carboxyl group of one is linked to the amino group of the other. A *polypeptide* is a chain of such peptides connected in special sequence.

percutaneous Through the skin.

pericarditis Inflammation of the pericardium, the sac surrounding the heart.

peritoneal equilibration testing (PET) Measures the characteristic of the peritoneum in terms of solute transport and ultrafiltration.

peritoneum The smooth, serous (and permeable) membrane that lines the abdominal cavity and covers the loops of intestine, the liver, and other organs.

petechia A small spot or freckle formed by blood leaking into skin; usually occurs in crops (petechiae).

phlebitis Inflammation involving the walls of a vein.

phlebotomy Release of blood from a vein.

photocell Electronic device sensitive to light. An electronic circuit may be closed or opened by its response to light.

physiology Life processes and functioning of living organisms.

plasma Fluid portion of blood (without cellular elements) before clotting occurs.

plasmapheresis *Pheresis* denotes "taking something away," derived from Greek. Special filter units, usually hollow fibers, permit removal from serum of elements such as antibodies and immunoglobulins.

platelet   A small circulating white blood cell, about 25% as large as a red blood cell, primarily concerned with instituting clot formation on contact with any abnormal surface of the circulatory system or a defect in the integrity of the system.

PMMA   A dialyzer made of polymethylmethacrylate (synthetic) membrane.

polymer   A compound of the same elements in the same proportion as another but of differing molecular weight: $(CNOH)$, $C_2N_2O_2H_2$, $C_3N_3O_3H_3$, and so on. Many plastics are polymers of simple compounds.

pore   A very small opening or hole.

posterior   Behind or toward the back of something.

premorbid   Before an illness.

protamine   Substance that neutralizes the anticoagulant action of heparin by combining with it.

protein   An essential constituent of all living cells that is formed from complex combinations of amino acids.

protein catabolic rate (PCR)   Refers to a given patient's protein metabolism expressed in grams of protein per kilogram.

proteinaceous   Proteinlike, or material derived from protein.

proximal   Near to a point or near to the central area.

pruritus   Intense itching.

pseudoaneurysm (false aneurysm)   Sac or outpocketing on the wall of a vein.

Pseudomonas   Genus of bacteria found in soil, water, sewage, and air. They are often highly pathogenic and resistant to many antibiotics.

pulsatile   Rhythmic throbbing; a rhythmic forward thrust.

pyrogen   Any substance or agent that causes a fever.

Q_B   Indication of blood flow rate.

Q_D   Indication of dialyzing fluid flow rate.

qualitative   Identifying a substance as to kind.

quantitative   Identifying a substance by amount present.

radial   Located on the side of the forearm near the radius, the forearm bone that ends at the wrist near the base of the thumb.

red blood cells   See **blood cells**.

renal   Pertaining to the kidneys (Latin *ren*, kidney).

renin   A hormone produced in the kidney with important effects on sodium and potassium balance and on blood pressure.

resin   Substance capable of binding, chemically or physically, some other substance and rendering it inactive.

retrograde   In a backward manner, or opposite to the usual direction.

reverse filtration   During high-flux dialysis a gradient from dialysate to blood may occur, a reversal of the usual blood-to-dialysate gradient. This reversal of flow may carry bacterial or pyrogenic material into blood.

reverse osmosis (RO) The process of removing almost all solute from a solution by applying high pressure on it against a membrane permeable only to the solvent; used to purify water.

rhabdomyolysis Breakdown of muscle tissue with release of myoglobin into the circulation that may result from trauma or toxic substances. Myoglobin is toxic to the kidney and a cause of acute renal failure.

sclerosis An unusual hardening.

septicemia Bacteremia with growth and multiplication of organisms in the blood. It is usually severe and may be life threatening.

serum Fluid portion of blood remaining after a clot has formed.

shunt Short circuit or bypass; in dialysis usage, the system of tubing that connects the flow of blood from the arterial cannula to the venous cannula when they are not needed for actual dialysis.

SI units An extension of the metric system used by clinical laboratories. The amount of substance is reported as moles/L rather than g/L or mg/dl.

sodium modeling/variation Technique of raising the sodium concentration in the dialysis bath for part of the treatment to minimize hypotension during fluid removal.

solute A dissolved substance.

solvent A liquid capable of dissolving a substance.

sorbent An agent that acts by its adsorption effect.

sphygmomanometer Device for measuring the blood pressure by means of an inflatable cuff placed around an extremity.

spores Certain bacteria, in an inactive or resting stage, that are highly resistant to antiseptic effect.

Staphylococcus Genus of bacteria, some of which normally inhabit skin or other body surfaces. Some are pathogenic and may cause serious infection.

sterile Completely free of any living microorganisms.

subcutaneous Underneath the skin.

sump Depression, or low point, for collecting fluid.

syndrome A complex or set or symptoms occurring together.

synthetic Manmade; not occurring naturally.

systemic Affecting the entire body as a whole.

systole Contraction of the heart; its emptying phase.

tachycardia Excessively rapid heartbeat.

tamponade Compression or pressure on. Pericardial tamponade compresses the heart by pressure of fluid in the pericardial sac.

thermistor Small sensitive metal device that changes its electric characteristics with temperature change. These changes are sensed by electronic circuitry and displayed on an indicator or recorder.

thermocouple Measuring device using a pair of coupled dissimilar metal conductors that bend when a temperature difference exists.

thrombosis Clot formation.

thrombus   Clot formed in a blood vessel or a blood passage.

tight heparinization   Monitoring ACT to maintain a clotting of 90 to 120 seconds. This is used in managing the patient at risk for bleeding during the hemodialysis treatment.

tortuous   Full of twists or turns; winding.

TPD   Tidal peritoneal dialysis.

transducer   Device that transmits power from one system to another system. For example, a pressure transducer converts the pressure (power) at its sensing surface to an electronic force that can be shown on an indicator or recorder.

trauma   Injury or wound.

Trendelenburg position   A body position in which the head is placed at a 45-degree incline down on a table with the legs elevated.

trocar   Tube with a sharp point for making puncture wounds.

turbulent   Characterized by agitated or irregular mixing action.

ulnar   Toward the ulna, the forearm bone on the inner side when the arm is held in the classic anatomic position.

ultrafiltration   Filtration by a pressure gradient between two sides of a porous (filtering) material.

urea   One of the chief nitrogenous waste products formed by metabolism or breakdown of protein in the body.

urea reduction ratio (URR)   Another method to calculate adequacy of dialysis. The formula is percentage of urea reduction = $100 \times (1 - C_t / C_o)$.

uric acid   Breakdown product of certain proteins, known as *nucleotides*. Excessive amounts in blood may cause acute inflammation of joints known as gout.

urticaria   An allergic skin reaction; hives.

vascular   Having to do with the blood vessels.

veins   Blood vessels that return blood from various parts of the body to the heart. Usually they are under lower pressure and have thinner walls than arteries.

venospasm   Involuntary contraction or narrowing of a vein.

venous   Anything related to the veins.

vestibular   Having to do with the vestibule of the inner ear, which is concerned with maintaining balance.

virus   Submicroscopic, infectious, living agents that are causative factors of many illnesses. They are completely dependent on the cells of the host that they infect. They are not sensitive to antibacterial medications.

white blood cells   See **blood cells**.

xenograft   A graft of tissue or an organ taken from a different animal species.

Index